INFANT PSYCHIATRY

A New Synthesis

Monographs of the Journal of the American Academy of Child Psychiatry
No. 2

INFANT PSYCHIATRY

A New Synthesis

edited by
Eveoleen N. Rexford,
Louis W. Sander, and Theodore Shapiro

NEW HAVEN AND LONDON
YALE UNIVERSITY PRESS
1976

Library of Congress catalog card number: 75-2774
International standard book number: 0-300-01890-8
Designed by Sally Sullivan
and set in Baskerville type,
Printed in the United States of America by
The Colonial Press Inc., Clinton, Mass.

Published in Great Britain, Europe, and Africa by
Yale University Press, Ltd., London.
Distributed in Latin America by Kaiman & Polon,
Inc., New York City; in Australasia by Book & Film
Services, Artarmon, N.S.W., Australia; in Japan by
John Weatherhill, Inc., Tokyo.

Chapters 1, 2, 14, 17, and 18 are published in this
monograph for the first time. All other chapters are
reprinted from *The Journal of the American Academy of
Child Psychiatry*. Volumes 1–9 were published by International Universities Press, Inc., New York; Volumes 10–12 were published by Quadrangle, The
New York Times Book Co., New York; starting with
Volume 13, the *Journal* is being published by Yale
University Press, New Haven.

CONTENTS

III. THE DEVELOPMENTAL COURSE AND SOME
OF ITS VARIATIONS

IV. CLINICAL CONSIDERATIONS AND THE CHALLENGE
OF INTERVENTION

FOREWORD

Eveoleen N. Rexford, M.D.

The title of this Reader, *Infant Psychiatry: A New Synthesis,* may prove to be the most challenging and controversial aspect of the book. One may fairly ask: what is infant psychiatry or what might it be? What does it have to do with child psychiatry or the *Journal of the American Academy of Child Psychiatry?* And finally, what is being synthesized and by whom?

The Reader itself grew out of a confluence between my interest and a pragmatic count of requests for reprinting papers. When, within a few months, more than one compiler of anthologies asked for permission to reprint several *Journal* papers on infant and early childhood research, and a dozen persons, within the same period, asked for reprints of specific infant papers, I began to discuss with my colleagues on the Editorial Board the possibility of preparing an anthology in this area from papers selected from the *Journal of the American Academy of Child Psychiatry.*

Louis Sander of Boston University is a child psychiatrist and a psychoanalyst who has worked since 1954 as an investigator of infant-mother interactions. His own contributions were among the most frequently requested *Journal* articles. Theodore Shapiro is a child psychiatrist and child analyst, Director of the Children's Services at Bellevue Hospital, and a student of the language of schizophrenic children. Together, Sander and Shapiro have selected the papers to be included in the Reader. In the course of our discussions, something other than a compilation of published and soon-to-be published papers began to emerge. We all recognized the progress in infant research over the past decade. We knew that certain of the *Journal* papers were considered classics by those involved in infant work, that others brought corroborative data or presented new propositions, and still others addressed the issue of applying research findings from systematic observations to interventive efforts on behalf of babies at high risk. We began to see the opportunity to achieve more with the anthology than make available in one volume the *Journal* papers on infant research and services accumulating over a decade—namely, to involve child psychiatrists more actively in the problems of infancy.

Editor, Journal of the American Academy of Child Psychiatry, 1965–1975.

From the publication of the 1960 Boston University Symposium on Child Development in the first volume, we at the *Journal of the American Academy of Child Psychiatry* have looked for and welcomed papers on research in infancy and early childhood. Both Irene Josselyn and I believed that the broad range of appropriate child psychiatry concerns stretched far enough to include original and informative reports on studies of the development of babies and young children. Through the 14 years of publication, we have presented a number of such provocative papers—provocative in the sense of turning the clinical thinking of some of us to the challenges and opportunities in creating early intervention programs for infants and young children at risk, if we only knew or could learn enough to venture into such a field.

The background of our considerations regarding this book partook of two further factors: a particular aspect of the historical development of child psychiatry and the issue of the scope and magnitude of the child mental health problems in this country.

The stake of child psychiatrists in work with infants and young children has an honorable history in our field. For instance, Douglas A. Thom, author of *Everyday Problems of Everyday Children,* the Dr. Spock of the 1930s, founded his Habit Clinic for Child Guidance in 1921 in Boston in direct association with well-baby clinics operated by the Baby Hygiene Association of that city. During the 1930s, child psychiatrists and psychoanalysts met regularly with pediatricians in the historic Cornellian Corner group to exchange ideas and findings about infant care, mother-child interactions, and at-risk babies. Yale University School of Medicine, with the hearty support of Grover Powers, Professor of Pediatrics, pioneered in the collaboration of pediatricians, obstetricians, psychoanalysts, and child psychiatrists in developing such patterns of baby care as rooming-in and self-demand feeding. During the 1950s, John Rose from the Philadelphia Child Guidance Clinic established a service at St. Christopher's Hospital for problem newborns and young children who were not progressing well.

The Report of the Joint Commission on Mental Health of Children (1969) offered estimates of the magnitude and scope of child emotional and mental disorders in the United States: "It is estimated that about 0.6 percent are psychotic and that another 2 to 3 percent are severely disturbed. It is further estimated that an additional 8 to 10 percent of our young people are afflicted with emotional problems (neuroses and the like) and are in need of specialized services" (p. 253f.). The child psychiatrist daily encounters evidence of the number of children in his city and in his area who need his kind of help and will not receive it. He knows, too, how often the disturbances of the children he is seeing can readily be traced back into the child's early days. There are no carefully controlled studies which demonstrate that early intervention in infancy and early childhood will decrease the extent of emotional problems in the population at a later age. Nevertheless, it seems to us sensible that if at-risk mothers and babies can be helped to negotiate the early basic issues between them and the infant so helped to move along the developmental lines of growing capacity for relationship, self-differentiation, and tolerance of frustration, the likelihood is considerably greater that the child will progress reasonably well than if neither receives any special help. Until we have set up a number of well-planned and staffed intervention projects to study, we will continue having to reply, "We have no proof" when asked how we know early intervention will prevent or greatly ameliorate later emotional and mental illness, and others will use this reality to discourage any headway in developing the projects because "there is no proof."

In the early months of the Joint Commission, when concepts of child mental health care based upon the developmental model were prepared by the Committee on Studies, attention was focused upon the great potential for prevention and early intervention in collaborative work dealing with pregnant women and their deliveries and the care of their offspring in well-baby and problem-infant clinics. The Clinical Services Committee of the Joint Committee later revived the earlier interest, and child psychiatrists discussed enthusiastically their involvement in interventive work with high-risk babies and their parents.

Repeatedly, as with similar considerations in the past, many enthusiastic child psychiatrists lost interest when they decided that they knew little or nothing about the assessment of babies or about interventive techniques. Others who had access to research people in the infant field thought these specialists could teach the child psychiatrists through demonstration and discussion.

This book is intended to pick up these earlier experiences and suggestions about work with babies. It is intended as a stimulus and a challenge to child psychiatrists who have the opportunity to extend their activities into the earliest years if they can acquire the knowledge and skill to offer themselves as clinicians for infants who are not developing well or are unlikely to do so, and for their families.

It is clear to the empiricist that no great benefit can possibly accrue to the slow baby left alone for hours in his crib every day or the failure-to-thrive baby whose profoundly depressed mother can offer him only physical care and then be frantic as the child deteriorates. We do know of the increasing number of impaired babies who today survive the birth process and of many others who are saved from infectious deaths by antibiotics. The magnitude and seriousness of the problem of child abuse are more evident daily, as is the fact that intervention can often save these children and stabilize a home for them. We know something of the many children evidencing later retardation who had received only a minimal opportunity for human interchange during their early months. Blind babies, as Selma Fraiberg found, can often be rescued by systematic, planned programs from the helpless, isolated lives for which they had seemed fated. A large number of infants and young children in our population are at high risk of distorted or delayed development, personality disorganization, retardation, and mental illness. If preventive and early interventive measures offer some possibilities of promoting the progress of a number of these children, there seem humane and pragmatic reasons to institute well-planned and monitored projects in the near future.

Even though a reader may accept the reasoning offered to this point, he may still ask: why should child psychiatrists be encouraged to play a major role in programs of early intervention for high-risk infants? Let me here outline our ideas, which will be elaborated in the text of the book. In the first place, the child psychiatrist comes from a medical background. The principal caretakers of such babies have always been physicians. Even those child psychiatrists who have isolated themselves from medical settings or left off the effort to keep up with medical research and practice retain a framework of basic knowledge of the human body and the residue of ways of approaching physical diagnosis and treatment planning. The child psychiatrist can function in hospitals and clinics and approach other medical people with the preparation of shared background and experience. And for many child psychiatrists working in university and hospital settings for some years, the gap has been steadily narrowed, despite the frankly different orientation with which these specialists approach their work with children. The statistics of the American Association of Psychiatric Services for Children which show the shifting patterns of child psychiatric services from independent community clinics to hospital and medical school centers mean that a larger proportion of today's child psychiatrists are working in closer collaboration with their medical colleagues than was true a generation ago. We make no attempt to gloss over the differences in focus and philosophy between the child psychiatrist and the pediatrician or cardiologist, nor do we underestimate the tremendous advances in physical medicine during this same period of which the child psychiatrist cannot become master. Yet the child psychiatrist is a physician and an increasing number are assuming leadership in bringing current concepts and findings in neurology, endocrinology, and other special areas into their evaluations of children within their purview. The medical aspect of the medical specialist rubric has a reality of growing importance in the field of child mental health.

In the second place, the child psychiatrist has a crucial role to play in early intervention programs for high-risk babies because he is a clinician. This means many things: a skill, a point of view, a body of experience. It subsumes many of the attributes people discuss under the rubric of the art of medicine. "It isn't what he does, it is the way he does it." First in relation to the practice of physical medicine and then of psychological medicine, the child psychiatric clinician wants to learn what he needs to know to determine what, if anything, is awry and so base his recommendations upon his findings, but the diagnostic process takes place in a setting, an interaction between two or more people. The clinician's sensitivity to the spoken and unspoken communications from his patients and their families, their responses to him, the nuances of their mode of giving information, the hints they drop of their anxieties and defenses against them provides cues for him in which he embeds the factual data he elicits. So he knows more and can plan more skillfully for the person who is his patient and who has, or about whom others have, complaints or problems. Mothers and, indeed, fathers, too, are alert to every nuance of meaning of what the doctor says; what will be revealed of fact or worry can be determined by their perception of the physician's reaction, point of view, or finding. A doctor-parent relationship which adds psychological expertise to the basic clinician's skills can be a valuable asset for parents and babies needing help.

Thirdly, child psychiatrists in large numbers are involved in planning and trying to give service to large segments of our child population never served, or served ineffectively, before. In community mental health center programs over the country they are learning in a practical fashion where the children are who need or may need special developmental help, how they can be reached, what networks of resources are or might be made available. Their sophistication in what we have called for years "the psychosocial aspects of child care" has of necessity grown in large increments over the past decade.

Finally, child psychiatrists bring not only knowledge of personality development but their convictions of the great importance of the emotional, the psychological, the feeling and being portions of human life. Infancy and early childhood are the periods of the child's greatest and most definitive growth, not only physically, but in the unfolding of the basic modes of building a self and of adapting to his society. The physical, the endocrinological, the cognitive aspects of the growing baby can subsume a host of facts, research findings, and medical manipulations. All of these affect, often decisively, the being of the small child which is developing and so must be part of the considerations the child psychiatrist puts together in trying to understand the whole little being. Other specialists can, however, pursue their lines of interest without seeking the significance of their findings for the child and his parents. The child psychiatrist must synthesize: the better he can bring together and relate to one another the different areas of concern and data, the more effectively he can help promote the child's progression and mitigate the deleterious effects of developmental regressions.

Of course, not every child psychiatrist would be interested in infant work, nor should we seek to induce him to turn from older children to the babies. While every training program ideally should include experience on newborn services, problem-infant clinics, and well-baby services, many trainees will prefer to move on to practice in other areas. But for a substantial group, we believe, Infant Psychiatry would seem an attractive and sensible area of specialization.

It is to the latter that this book is primarily addressed. The infant psychiatrist requires skills, practice in examining babies and talking to their parents; he needs to polish up his capacities to relate to other professional people and to work collaboratively with pediatricians, nurses, surgeons, and neurologists. But he needs more: he needs an armamentarium of early interventive skills based on a knowledge of infants and their varied modes of development. Those in infant research and those pioneering in early intervention keep telling us they do not know enough. We are certain this is true, but we are sufficiently concerned about the import of the growing number of babies at high risk in our population that we are mounting this challenge: let us use what we do know.

Here is an anthology of some good papers on infant research and early intervention. Can these provide a beginning for some infant programs? Will this Reader stimulate the research people and the innovators in early intervention to write up more of their findings and ideas so that infant psychiatrists could have even more to work with? Can the Reader encourage at least a few child psychiatrists to seek out opportunities to participate in baby programs, bringing their skills, their interests, and the help the research people can give to their task? And can we so bridge the gap between pure research and its application to pressing human needs?

These are our hopes for this Reader. If, in 5 or 10 years, the *Journal* can publish another monograph which relegates many of the ideas of these papers and of ours into the historical attic, well and good. We would then have served the basic purpose of the *Journal of the American Academy of Child Psychiatry*.

INTRODUCTION

For the present and probably for some time to come, the psychiatric clinician stands on a no-man's land between biology and psychology. This is especially so for one interested in infancy. In attempting to bring coherence to this inherent complexity, the individual clinician is left to himself to order his data and to resolve in his practice the many dilemmas with which the data confront him.

It is our hope that this collection of papers on infant research and early intervention programs will provide child psychiatric clinicians with suggestions and facts to help them work with babies and their mothers, as well as excite their interest in this challenging field. The papers in this Reader come from two sources: issues of the *Journal* published largely during its first decade and a 1971 symposium on primary prevention and early intervention.[1]

The reprinted papers were selected for three principal reasons: (1) the paper is regarded as a classic often quoted elsewhere and worthy of being assembled with others in one volume; (2) the paper represents a pioneering effort, which although perhaps somewhat dated in 1975 provides important background, giving depth and perspective to more current formulations; (3) it presents case material, experiences, or points of view not readily found elsewhere which contribute in their own right to the subject matter of an Infant Psychiatry.

Those papers chosen from the 1971 symposium relate directly to work reported or ideas offered in the *Journal* papers. In some instances, they extend the suggestions in the earlier publications; in others, they offer a group of new data which bear upon the pioneering work; and in some instances, the symposium papers report upon the application of infant research findings to specific intervention programs.

This volume is intended to be a first consolidation: it is not intended to be a definitive, comprehensive, fully up-dated presentation of Infant Psychiatry. It is obvious that certain other papers from the *Journal* could have been included in a reader on Infant Psychiatry. The Emde and Koenig paper on "Neonatal Smiling, Frowning and Rapid Eye Movement States," Marion Blank's paper on "Maternal Influences" or the report of Fineman and her co-workers on "Spasmus Nutans," for

1. The symposium was entitled "Infant Observation and Longitudinal Study: Implications for Mental Health and Primary Prevention of Mental Disorders in High-Risk Situations." It was sponsored by the Committee on Prevention, Saul I. Harrison, M.D., chairman. It took place at the 18th Annual Meeting of the American Academy of Child Psychiatry in Boston, October 1971.

instance, contribute to one or another theme in the sections of the Reader. However, due to sharp limitations in space, we were forced to leave out papers which did not seem to us to contribute so centrally to our thesis. Similarly, symposium papers (which will be published in the *Journal* in the near future) such as Barbara Fish's study of "Infants at Risk for Schizophrenia" or Galenson's report on "The Choice of Symbols" were not included for the same reasons.

The field of infant research is expanding rapidly in many directions. Our focus upon presentations which came into the ambience of the *Journal* reflects the clinical preoccupations of most of our readers and our own wish to engage the child psychiatrist in an interest in clinical programs of Infant Psychiatry. In view of the space limitations which rising costs have imposed upon us, we could not, for instance, include papers on neurophysiology, sleep, or perception by research workers such as Graham, Cohen, Lewis, and Bower. It is our hope that the clinician who becomes intrigued with the infant studies included in this volume will seek out the research reports of such authors which both complement and support the points of view we espouse.

The plan of the papers in this volume offers one framework by which the variety of contributions relevant to the task of the clinician can be brought together, namely, that of the systems point of view. Among the most significant influences of the current infant research work is the new appreciation for the way in which principles common to all living systems characterize the human organism as well. The biologist, Paul Weiss, comments upon "the supreme role of harmony as a prerequisite for continued survival." Careful observers of the newborn and young infant sense their urgent need for harmony and coherence which appears to power many processes seemingly set into motion before birth. Following delivery, the baby's behavior is rapidly organized to achieve that coherence amid different circumstances and constantly changing demands and possibilities. This fluid state of adaptation emerges from the continuing adaptations of the various systems involved in organizing the infant's behavior.

We found therefore the systems approach useful in selecting and arranging the papers for this Reader. This viewpoint places the infant always in a context and in an ongoing continuity of exchange within that context. From this standpoint, organization of behavior at any one place in time, and the changes in organization of behavior during a child's development, are not considered to be issues belonging at the level of the individual but rather are viewed as issues properly belonging at the level of the system, that is, the baby in interaction with the caretaking environment. The infant and the caretaking milieu are the constituents of an open, interactive, regulative system, each component member participating in exchanges which mutually influence and regulate the behavior of the other.

Since we wished to emphasize the importance of these concepts, we did not arrange the papers by the familiar developmental stages, but chose instead to provide sections in which the focus would be placed upon the components of the system and their interactions. If one is to assess an infant at risk and determine what interventions may be feasible and useful, it is not sufficient to identify the infant factors which define the high-risk infant. One needs also to determine the effects of these factors in the particular parenting environment of that infant, and in turn the effects of the specific parenting environment on that infant's particular potentials and vulnerabilities. It is no longer enough to speak of an "average expectable environment": to understand the genesis of behavior, we need to fill in, for each infant-milieu pair, the categories of exchange which constitute the specific content of their regulative encounters at different age levels.

Within such an adaptive, interactive schema, the baby and his caretaking environment are viewed as subcomponents of the system, each having its own idiosyncratic characteristics and each having its own range of variations which must come to some kind of enduring coordination within the system. When an adapted state is achieved, the two become linked in an around-the-clock, usually episodic cycle of exchanges, required day after day for the proper regulation of the functions of each. Changes introduced into the interaction by the growth of the infant and the consequent appearance of new capabilities produce perturbations in the previously regulated system. These perturbations demand further mutual adjustments, leading to new specificity in interaction and to further idiosyncrasy in the content and configuration of exchanges in the system. Abnormalities in the infant, the caretaking milieu, or both, will result in particular characteristics of interaction necessary to achieve stable coordinations in the face of the deviation. Major gaps obviously still exist in our understanding of the more detailed mechanisms and dynamic factors by which the requirement for regulation of functions generates behavior and leads to mutual modification.

But the most elusive task in comprehending the various aspects of personality development lies in accounting for the way the whole, that is, the person, achieves and maintains a coherence comprising a myriad of parts, their varying levels of complexity, and their relations to one another. This essential coherence must be conserved and maintained, while at the same time the individual remains capable of a certain degree of modification and change.

It is precisely at this most important frontier that the infant psychiatrist can make a special contribution, based upon his particular training and clinical experience which range across the life span from infancy to adulthood. The infant psychiatrist must make his own new synthesis based upon his observations of baby and the caretaking milieu, upon his varied clinical experiences, his grasp of the variety of conceptualizations of developmental processes, and his assimilation of the ongoing flow of research findings from new empirical data.

In seeking to understand the whole person in the baby, the clinician has had to apply wisdom drawn from the observation of behavior later in life to order the empirical data he observed in the infant and young child. In the past, he has lacked systematic empirical data extending from the earlier to the later points of development as well as adequate concepts to permit him to select the most salient variables and assess their interactions in the necessary longitudinal perspective. The infant research of the past quarter century provides him with both data and concepts to which he can join his clinical experience in moving toward the comprehension of the whole person and of the development of personality organization from the early days on.

While Sections I and II deal with studies of the two systems of the baby and his caretaker, Sections III and IV present reports on clinical efforts to intervene with infants at high risk. The major gaps in data and conceptualization will become more evident to research worker and to clinician alike as the infant psychiatrist searches for an understanding which will permit him to modify or even prevent the slide toward deviant development in the baby at risk. The contributions of the clinician to the research field in identifying problems to be solved, questions to be asked, and concepts to be derived from both experimental and naturalistic investigation are highly significant to the task of understanding infant, and indeed, all of human development. Somewhat as the infant and his mother depend upon one another for gratification and for different types of support, so the research worker and the clinician may benefit mutually from the interactions of the clinic and the research laboratory. Much is said these days of the drawbacks of the medical-clinical experience in identifying and working with psychopathology. It is a historical fact, however, that experiences in clinical neurology and the related fields of neurohistology, anatomy, and pathology underlie much of what is understood of the functioning of the human central nervous system today. Good clinical observations from infant psychiatry can point the direction to and speak to the need for good research in areas not familiar to or hithertofore not considered by the research worker.

We assume therefore that we are speaking to a partnership between the clinic and the laboratory which promises mutual profit, albeit at this point we are directing our readers to the contributions of infant research to infant clinical programs, and to an expanded child psychiatry. We do so with a word of caution which the authors of the papers in this Reader have implicitly offered, namely, the developmental processes are highly complex. While all levels of infant behavior may presuppose a minimal substrate of intact brain function, they may also be studied independently or by means of systems according to the methods appropriate to each organizational level. How the detailed data derived from one level cohere with those of the next organizational level remains a crucial difficulty for any student of development. Changing hierarchic structures which emerge epigenetically from stage to stage require observational variations which make the sense of continuity we seek difficult to maintain. Recent research has indicated that what is observed at 1 month through a test appropriate to that period is not likely to correspond well with functional results observed at 6 months or 3 years by the use of other measures.

So, while we enthusiastically seek to engage the interest of clinicians in this field of Infant Psychiatry opening up before us, we urge our readers to accord the young persons the respect and disciplined approach which their complexity and our current state of partial knowledge warrant. Those in infant research are telling us what a marvelously complicated organism a newborn baby is and how finely attuned his interactions with his caretakers are. They challenge us to use their findings in a fashion respecting the intricacy and many variations in the developmental processes whereby the baby becomes a young child, then an older child, and finally an adult.

THE EDITORS

ACKNOWLEDGMENTS

We are grateful to the authors who have participated in the preparation of this Reader. They have assented graciously to several rearrangements of plans, to delays in publication as the *Journal* changed publishers, and to many deletions in their texts. All have shared our wish to bring this material before a wider audience and to encourage clinicians and research workers in the field of infancy to study and to collaborate together.

The Yale University Press found the manuscript and the topic congenial to their interests and we appreciate the celerity with which Mrs. Jane Isay and her staff have worked to make early publication possible. We have had in this endeavor, as with each issue of the *Journal,* the expert advice and the skillful collaboration of Mrs. Lottie M. Newman, and we are as always appreciative of them.

Mrs. Sheila King, editorial assistant to the Editor of the *Journal* for the last five years, helped in bringing these materials together, in working with authors, and in scrutinizing each latest suggestion of the Editors of the Reader. Her proofreading of the manuscript is her final contribution to an anthology in which she shares our investment. We thank Mrs. Alice Begish for compiling and checking the Bibliography. Mrs. Susan Bush deserves our warm thanks for patient typing and retyping and for keeping our confusion about a series of deletions to a minimum.

E.N.R.
L.W.S.
T.S.

PART I

Perspectives

1

A PSYCHIATRIST FOR INFANTS?

Theodore Shapiro, M.D.

William James declared that a difference, in order to *be* a difference, has to *make* a difference. In the light of this guidance does the suggestive title of this volume justifiably designate yet a new specialized concern for physicians? Pediatricians, developmental psychologists, child psychiatrists, and educators, among others, do overlap in their interest in children, while each has a vantage point distinguishable from those of the others. However, does the intersection of each discipline constitute the special vantage provided in the concept of infant psychiatry, or is the whole more than the sum of its parts?

Clearly, the pediatrician is concerned with the growth and development of the neonate as well as the detection of pathological deviation at biochemical and other levels. The developmental psychologist using naturalistic and experimental methods subject to statistical analysis has helped define the sequences and norms of stage- and phase-related behaviors. Recent ingenious experiments have been designed to tease out early cognitive structures and rescue the child investigator from his veterinarian's plight observing a nonverbal subject.

The educator has pushed his concerns farther and farther back in a child's life so that educational techniques and materials are now available for crib babies as well as for toddlers and nursery school children. As Piaget has noted, "The American Question" he hears so often when lecturing in the United States is: "Can we do it earlier?"

Child psychiatrists have more and more been asked to consult and intervene in the period of infancy as they have used their experience in advising parents and absorbed some of the data and expertise of the other disciplines concerned with early detection of deviance. This interest in early childhood began within adult psychiatry as retrospective reconstruction utilizing the developmental point of view. It continued in the child guidance clinics in cooperation with pediatricians concerning problems such as rumination, marasmus, and early deprivation.

This paper was specially prepared for this monograph.

More recently, child psychiatrists have carried out prospective studies
in the early detection of deviance, and they have studied systematically
temperamental and constitutional precursors to personality.

In his work the psychiatrist borrows the prestige and social impact of
the doctor-patient relationship from the rest of medicine. Parents, as
auxiliaries of infants' needs, come to physicians because of their anxiety, and their wish for help. At this point in our social history, the
physician, specialist or not, retains the image of a "natural" source of
pain relief. It is clear that he bears no innate qualities to so recommend
him, but the image has become firmly embedded in the public mind.
We believe his skills could in many instances be readily adapted to the
requirements of the discipline to be described. Psychiatrists, trained
both in the methods of clinical medicine and in psychological principles, represent source material for the new area of Infant Psychiatry.
The training of the child psychiatrist could readily be augmented to
include the experience necessary to do the work well, and in a few
centers such early interventive experiences are open to the trainee. The
following is a catalogue of the skills, work habits, and general competence which recommend psychiatric training as an apt starting point for
our new departure.

The psychiatric vantage point forces an appreciation of the impact of
early interpersonal relationships on the developmental course. Parents
are looked at as interacting participants in the developmental process
which does not permit a dichotomization of nature and nurture. Encounter with parents is viewed not only as a means of recovering children's histories and anamnesis. The psychiatrist integrates a general
awareness of the dynamic interplay of parental behaviors at each stage
of maturation and of the child's personality growth into a holistic long
view of personality development. From such a point of view, when the
child psychiatrist studies a child brought for some behavior or developmental problem, he does not conclude that "he'll grow out of it" or that
a parent is "neuroto- or schizophrenogenic." Rather, he asks, how does
this infant "thrive, fail, or survive" this or that influence, given his
genetic potential and maturational stage? The psychiatrist's training
emphasizes the synthesis of current influences among a bevy of concur-
rent events as well as the capacity to identify a hierarchy of emergent
psychic organizations as behavior changes with chronological age and
development.

These behavioral observations are complemented by a respect for the
conservative forces in personality development, not only of the infant
but of the parents. Psychiatrists' belief in therapeutic change is tempered by experience with the slow progress of human modifiability. Patience and toleration of passivity have become significant admixtures of
our enthusiasm. There is a distrust of simply instructing, because we

recognize that the unconscious needs of parents which so often con-
found and influence development adversely are not easily amenable to
education. How many times can a practitioner attest to his having instructed a parent in one or another technique of care, only to find that
comprehension or implementation has not been effective? Instead, the
psychiatrist utilizes the relationship with a parent through his awareness of transference and of identifications. The availability of these latter modalities to foster change provides a set of new possibilities for
"instruction" in child rearing which represent a more rational base than
those provided by "instinctive maternalism," imitation of ambivalently
regarded grandparents, or the use of the infant as narcissistic extensions of personal needs. And these are but a few of the possible distortions to which child rearing is subject and to which a clinician might be
alerted if he hopes to modify what seems to be the inevitable march of
personal growth toward neuroticism, character disorder, delinquency,
or even a generalized incapacity for work or experience of pleasure.

This catalogue should by no means suggest that the answers are at
hand or that our knowledge of the factors that influence behavior is
complete. This is far from the fact, but a group of child specialists who
are especially interested in an unintrusive, thoughtful investigative approach to infancy—one that is at the same time clinical in orientation—might well be expected to influence positively a child's growth in
a most crucial period of his life.

While all the disciplines mentioned focus on the child, the members
of no one discipline as yet embody the vantage point which emerges
from the sum of the papers presented in this volume. I invoke the sum
because if we look at each contribution in isolation, the orientation, the
tools, and the problem-solving techniques do not seem new, i.e., one
may be statistical, another experimental, another cross-sectional naturalistic, and yet a fourth an anecdotal individual case report. When the
whole scene is scanned, however, James's pragmatic measure of difference is justified. There emerges a discipline whose concern is a hu-
manistic, holistic view of the child growing up amid the reciprocal influence of his biological equipment and social experiences and of his
taking form as a unique individual who represents a new identity in an
ever emerging biosocial pool. It is here in the exploration and management of a growing personality, of rate of development and of possible
deviance that a new variety of clinician interested in infancy may
emerge. The contents of this volume will perhaps especially attract
those who have flirted with such an idea as well as challenge those for
whom it suggests a new departure.

Those acquainted with the history of pediatrics and psychiatry may
believe that what is presented has already appeared under older ru-
brics. No one familiar with the work of Milton Senn or the Bakwins

could suggest that holistic mergers have not been in the air before. In that sense, this volume does not claim priority, but to the extent that it focuses on the infant, his differentiation, and personality development as clinical concerns, it does coordinate a significant body of literature. If it is an example of historic recurrence, it is offered in a new climate of investigative competence.

2

INFANT OBSERVATION AND LONGITUDINAL STUDY

Implications for Mental Health and Primary Prevention of Mental Disorders in High-Risk Situations

Justin D. Call, M.D.

Current developments in the field of Infant Psychiatry mark the emergence of this field of inquiry from an infant mythology which has served both to inspire and to discourage serious scientific work in this area. The current resurgence of scientific interest in the early development of human infants is not the first such thrust we have known. Various steps along the path have been made since Darwin's study (1877) of his first male child in 1842.

The concept of primary prevention received renewed emphasis in the Report of the Joint Commission on Mental Health of Children (1969), but despite considerable advocacy of its merits, it has remained more of an ideal than an actuality. Primary prevention provides a clear guide to practice so long as the lines of "practice" are drawn broadly and idealistically, but it seems difficult to use and to test in specific cases and circumstances. Our task is to redefine and then use the concept appropriately in dealing with the problems of infant psychiatry and the development of human potential.

Primary prevention may be approached from either of two polar sets. The first polarity refers to interventions which are addressed either to the weakness or to the strength of the child, family, or social system being studied. A great deal has been said about the weakness: that is, how properly to label deficits in mental functioning and what to do about them in their incipient stages. Very little has been written or said about how to identify potentialities for psychological strength and

Presented at the 1971 symposium in Boston.

capacities for creativity in coping, let alone how best to insure that children, families, and social systems obtain social and psychological nutrients for optimal growth. Our tendency to look for weaknesses instead of strengths is due, I believe, to the cognitive comfort gained in being able to circumscribe deficits in function with a label. It is much more difficult to describe the endless varieties of normal human functioning.

The second polarity, often not acknowledged but still very important, refers to the alerting vs. the nonalerting characteristic of the problem, the loudness or the quietness of deficit functioning or symptoms in the person, family, or social unit. Crisis refers to the loudness of a problem, which in turn refers to how upset someone is about a problem. School phobia or dropout was a favorite crisis of the '50s. Drug abuse is the crisis of the early '70s. In our society the squeaky wheel gets the grease. The current use of crisis intervention as a method of treatment is very different from the utilization of crisis in approaching problems of primary prevention, originally described by Gerald Caplan (1959). Caplan made it clear that a crisis in a person, family, or community was most importantly a means of providing access to the psychosocial system involved: the mental health worker could thereby influence the system in the service of primary prevention.

Crisis intervention has become a dominant mode of approach to problems of mental health; mental health may currently be defined as the absence of crisis! Crisis has become an attractive target of administrators and the "here and now" practitioners of our time, and is an approach to mental health problems reflecting the social sanction of our media-oriented culture. The mass media have the capacity to focus the attention of society on a given issue, and hence to politicize automatically scientific as well as social issues. This kind of issue-making has, I believe, blinded many, including professional people, who are interested in the problems of mental health to the opposite position in this second polarity: namely, to low-amplitude, persistent phenomena which extend over time. Such low-amplitude problems slip through critical periods of psychological growth unnoticed by others because no one else is upset by them. Such problems may create long-lasting and devastating effects upon the person, recognized only at some later stage. When the difficulties are finally recognized, they are apt to be misinterpreted as due to some short-term recent circumstance. Examples of such low-amplitude, nonalerting phenomena are process schizophrenia, schizoaffective disorders, environmental retardation, child neglect (as opposed to battering), sadomasochistic character formation and life style, "as if" personality, learning impotence, lifelong social inhibitions, and problems in sexual identification. These phenomena often do have a beginning in the early years of life and may be associated with physical and emotional deprivation, or some other traumatic environmental influence operating upon a vulnerable organism. The effects of such influences are not revealed immediately in any easily identifiable, highly pathognomonic, specific, or alarming symptom, but are slowly incorporated in the fabric of the mind itself, influencing all aspects of mental life. Such phenomena can be recognized only by a long, sensitive look at subtleties in behavior and overall functioning. Once identified, such problems stand out sharply and dramatically, and the alarm for intervention can be sounded. Thoughtful longitudinal case studies and long-term follow-up studies can be of great value in identifying the significance of low-amplitude phenomena.

If we are to move steadily from the stage of mythology to a slightly more advanced stage of small- and large-scale theory of primary prevention, a theory which can organize our practice in such a way that it will be possible for us to attend to the obvious crises as well as the low-amplitude chronic deprivations, to the areas of weakness *and* strength in human potentiality and development, we shall have to recognize the very broad base of growing knowledge of human development. It is well to remind ourselves that members of many disciplines are at work, often investigating the same phenomena, while utilizing different theories and terminologies. I shall briefly mention the work of a few of our colleagues, using some illustrations from the literature.

Freud, whose roots were anchored in nineteenth-century biology and developmental neurology (Jones, 1953), maintained that man's instinctual drives, as well as variations in ego functioning, spring from a common ego-id matrix (Freud, 1937) which is of a physical-biochemical origin and under genetic control. He stated that some day man's mental disturbances might be successfully treated with chemicals. These speculations by Freud have, during the past 20 years, gained substantial support.

The major breakthroughs of the last few years in understanding how genes are constructed, how they replicate themselves, how they regulate enzymes, which in turn regulate protein synthesis, and how they transmit information to new generations of cells, all took place through the study of the lowly bacteria with the identical amino acids and double helix structure characteristic of the higher organisms, including man. This new knowledge coming from the study of bacteria effectively reduces the built-in prejudice of researchers against accepting or making use of findings from nonhuman species in understanding normal development and disease processes in man. Application of the principles derived from such studies has implications for all living organisms and for life itself. This breakthrough at the genetic level, like earlier embryological and evolutionary studies, makes it increasingly more difficult for any scientist to view man separately from other forms of life. All forms of life are joined together by chains of amino acids! What man learns of other life forms has increasingly become part of his own self-understanding. Thus, Jane van Lawick-Goodall's (1971) longitudinal, multigenerational studies of chimpanzee families in the natural environment, showing the lifelong significance of early attachments and the powerful bond between three generations of female chimpanzees, provides biological roots for our understanding of human attachment and for sex differences in attachment behavior. The Harlows' earlier work (1962) showed the importance of contact comfort and opportunities for clinging in the young rhesus monkey and the serious distortions in later development of rhesus monkeys deprived of maternal and peer contact, such as extended autoerotic behavior and lack of capacities of males to mate and females to conceive at adolescence; it thus provided additional proof of the importance of early object relations in organizing mammalian social sexual behavior. The studies of Kaufman and Rosenblum (1967) on the effect of early separation (4–6 months) on two closely related, but different species of monkeys, the Pigtail and the Bonnet, have shown that Pigtail infants react to separation from the mother first with agitation, followed by depression-withdrawal, followed by recovery, while Bonnets immediately increase ventral contact with other adults and become adopted by them. Kaufman's studies caution us against oversimplistic use of biological findings in understanding human behavior. Ivan Tors is currently making a worldwide film survey of the social life of mammals from "A" to "Z." His film (1971) on the social life of the African elephant, demonstrating the importance of the elephant's trunk as a highly evolved sensorimotor organ of adaptation, equivalent to the human hand in infant care and in social relations with other elephants, illustrates the deep biological roots of the snout area for these functions in man, as suggested in the studies of Rangell (1954), Hoffer (1949), and Call (1964). Thus, we have learned much and can expect to learn much more about our own needs and vulnerabilities from the study of other mammals.

Certainly we can no longer afford the narcissistic view that study of the rat tells us nothing about man. Even the description of fellow scientists as "rat psychologists" must now be looked upon as a special case of human chauvinism. Calhoun's (1962) findings of perverse sexual and social life in rats under conditions of overpopulation and his interesting data showing that "inferior," noncompetitive members of the species are more likely to initiate new forms of adaptation in the species (food storage in the rat) than are the healthy, aggressive, competitive members of the species give us some new questions to ask about ourselves as humans. Bennett et al. (1964) have now produced an impressive volume of work with the rat, showing that insufficient amounts of protein and sensory stimulation are clearly associated as interdependent variables in the formation of neurons in the young organism. Levitsky and Barnes (1972) demonstrated that the increased emotionalism associated with malnutrition in rats can be significantly reduced by increased handling of the young malnourished rat. Sheibel's (1962) neurophysiological studies of developing cortex in young kittens reared under conditions of sensory deprivation and under conditions of enriched sensory stimuli with the mother indicate early structural change in the number of dendritic processes within cortical neurons in that group reared under conditions of deprivation. Globus et al. (1973) have confirmed this finding, tracing the development of individual neurons under conditions of poor versus abundant sensory stimulation. They lend substance to what many have proposed, including Richmond and Lipton (1959), who suggested that the period of rapid growth of the brain in the human infant should be of specific concern with regard to later mental functioning. This view is one shared by Rene Dubos (1968) in a paper called "Environmental Freudianism," and by Benjamin Bloom (1964) in his important book on stability and change. The field of developmental biochemistry, as explored by Eiduson et al. (1964) and others, may provide us sufficiently detailed clues to the developmental aspects of enzyme systems and intermediary protein metabolism of the central nervous system to enable us either to protect certain vulnerable infants from central nervous system deficits, or to develop means of increasing the potential for development of the central nervous system itself.

Findings such as these regarding the rat and kitten, combined with some interesting cases of early psychopathological development in human infants, have convinced many of us that we should be looking much more carefully at the earliest phases of infant development if we are to detect variations in instinctual development or in apparatuses of ego autonomy. One fact which must be emphasized in evaluating the significance of either positive or negative environmental influences on the human infant is the relative dominance of biologically derived developmental patterns with which the human infant is endowed. Such underlying processes constantly influence the ways in which the infant responds to stimulation, trauma, or deprivation in the environment and insure his survival. Until such maturational patterns are more thoroughly understood, outcome prediction will continue to be difficult to make.

Part of our job also is to define more clearly what is meant by the average expectable environment (Hartmann, 1939), that environment which will allow opportunities for normal growth. A new challenge before us, and one which can be easily misinterpreted, is to define what environment is optimal for man's early development. Wolff and Feinbloom's (1969) recent review casts considerable doubt upon the possibility of increasing man's cognitive capacities simply by "enriching" the sensory field, notwithstanding the fact that deficits in function and structure result from sensory deprivation in the young.

The fields of genetics, population control, and what seems to be emerging as quality control for human impregnation and birth, are doors now only beginning to be opened. The immediate effects of applications of these studies should be fewer defective infants at birth, but it has yet to be demonstrated that such "quality control" could yield human infants with greater potential for mental development. David Rosenthal's (1971) careful probing of the interaction between genetic and environmental variables in schizophrenia has provided a model for such studies in other areas, and has laid to rest once more a recent flare-up of the nature-nurture controversy, an old battle sapping much strength and often leading nowhere.

A whole army of workers is now looking at the problem of high-risk in infancy, defined either in terms of genetic loading, physiological vulnerability, nutritional deficiency, birth trauma including drug effects, effects of drugs and radiation on the fetus, or of socioeconomic factors contributing to prematurity and low birth weight (which in itself is often associated with a high incidence of anomalies, including those of the central nervous system). A study by Halverson and Waldrop (1971) indicates that by a simple count of minor forms of first trimester congenital anomalies visible on the surface of the body, it is possible to predict some 70 percent of infants who will later show "the hyperactivity syndrome." They noted that great stress is placed upon the parents of such children: thus the possibilities for primary prevention are considerable here if we become more attentive to the specific needs of such a vulnerable child and his parent.

A new speciality called neonatology has grown up within pediatrics. Infant mortality has taken another downward trend in centers using fluid support and correction of acid base imbalance in infants showing difficulty at birth. Many infants are now surviving who would earlier have died, but these infants are at risk for neurological damage and for mental disturbance resulting from the interaction of the vulnerable infant with his family. Recent studies on Down's syndrome and other forms of organically caused mental retardation illustrate that efforts at environmental enrichment within the context of enduring family contact indeed prevents some of the deficits usually seen in such children. Fraiberg and Freedman (1964), working with blind infants who show no organic deficit, have demonstrated that the so-called blindisms, autistic behavior, and severe developmental retardation in speech and motoric behavior in these children, together with the greater degree of separation anxiety and much delayed capacity in achieving object constancy (in the psychological sense), can be prevented when adequately trained child workers provide the parents of blind infants with sensitive and empathic models of parenting behavior.

It is now quite clear that when specific defects of infants are diagnosed early, and when positive programs are developed for these babies, they have significantly increased probability for greater developmental potential and significantly less social dependence than do those infants whose deficits are diagnosed late and for whom no positive program is available.

Another rapidly growing field with much to offer is that of linguistics, including aspects of paralanguage, kinesics, and parakinesics. The developmental aspects of linguistics are increasingly useful for assessing mental functioning since the new linguistic theories of Chomsky (1965) have liberated linguistics from a purely structural view. One may now begin to concern oneself with the evolution of meaning as well as the evolution of sound.

A few models from the past continue to shine forth with renewed importance for infant researchers interested in primary prevention: studies by Fries (1937), Levy (1958), Mahler (1968), Spitz (1959), Benjamin (1959), Bayley (1943), Ernst Kris (1950b, 1951), and Pavenstedt (1961). The latter's abiding interest in problems of primary prevention and the way in which these problems dovetail with issues in early child development posed by psychoanalytic theory coincide with the work of many of us today. Piaget's (1936) work in cognitive development is receiving renewed attention in the climate of concern for the educational problems of children from all groups, and new questions are being formulated in terms of his theoretical structure.

As scientific knowledge gradually replaces mythology, certain themes appear and reappear: (1) the need for more operational low-level theories; (2) the relationship between theory and observation and between theory and practice; (3) the relationship between small-scale interventions with highly select samples and large-scale interventions to larger, less select populations by new workers; (4) the continued problem of defining the stages and particular stresses in the psychology of parenthood; and (5) the reminder that fathers are parents, too.

Many exciting approaches are open to those interested in primary prevention, and older strategies still present us with issues to explore. For instance, long-term case studies which synthesize data from many sources are still needed. New strategies for change, ranging from case management to better organization and integration of systems of medical and mental health care must be explored. The significance of the longitudinal study and of follow-up studies remains as telling today as it was 20 years ago when my teachers outlined some of the same points I am making in this paper.

I believe the papers chosen for this Reader broaden our understanding of child development in general and help us comprehend how complex the issue of primary prevention actually is. To that extent, they liberate us from the mythology of infancy, but leave us with a greater complexity of issues and interrelationships. But such has always been the outcome when man has peered into the mysteries.

PART II

A Context for the Consideration of Early Human Development

3

METHODOLOGICAL ISSUES IN
PSYCHIATRIC EVALUATION OF INFANTS

Leon Cytryn, M.D.

Some recent developments in child psychiatry point to the need for a comprehensive, standardized method for the psychiatric evaluation of infants.

The current trend is to integrate departments of child psychiatry into the general pediatric hospital setting and activity. Seeing children of all ages, including infants with developmental deviations and various disturbances of psychosomatic, behavioral, and affective nature becomes part of the psychiatrist's daily activities. Clinical work with hospitalized infants plays an important role in the teaching program for fellows in child psychiatry and for pediatric residents who rotate through such services. Efforts to impress these trainees with the crucial importance of the period of infancy in the development of the human personality have been hampered by the lack of a satisfactory clinical method of highlighting normal and abnormal personality traits in infancy. In planning research involving infants, one also becomes acutely aware of the lack of a uniformly adopted standardized method for the psychiatric evaluation of infants, which could serve as a basis for later comparisons.

The general public is becoming more aware and accepting of the existence of psychiatric difficulties and personality abnormalities in infancy. The number of requests for psychiatric evaluation of infants by pediatricians, family physicians, public agencies, and courts has been increasing. In these cases (which are bound to become more numerous) our having a standard method of investigation would help to improve the quality of services rendered. This in turn would facilitate public acceptance of the psychiatrist's role in the appraisal and treatment of infants.

Reprinted from the *Journal*, 7 : 510–521, 1968.

Such recent works as Anna Freud's Diagnostic Profile (1965) or the comprehensive methods used by Murphy (1968), Provence and Lipton (1962), Thomas et al. (1963), and others may well serve as a basis for a clinical diagnostic instrument applicable to infants. The construction of such an instrument presents several problems.

GENERAL CHARACTERISTICS

The principles of psychiatric evaluation of infants do not differ basically from those guiding the diagnostic process in older children. Like the latter, it is a dynamic process aiming at the evaluation of all growth-promoting and growth-retarding factors in the child and his environment (G.A.P., 1957). While the basic principles of psychiatric diagnosis may be applied to infants, certain characteristics of infancy require their modification. These characteristics include among others the problems of state (see chap. 5), the degree of dependence upon the mother, and the importance of the mother-child unit (Yarrow and Goodwin, 1965)

The patterns of behavior in infants are usually unstable, and the psychophysiological homeostasis is easily upset. In addition, the process of growth in all areas proceeds, especially in the first year of life, at an extremely rapid pace. The changes in infant behavior do not occur abruptly, but rather one pattern merges almost imperceptibly into the next one, with frequent oscillations between regressive and progressive trends. All this would seem to necessitate spacing the psychiatric evaluation of an infant over several weeks, rather than limiting it to a single examination. As the infant grows older, toward the end of the first year and in the second year of life, his neurophysiological apparatus acquires more stability. This permits more diagnostic certainty with each examination, increasing in direct proportion to the age of the child.

The assessment of the patient's customary performance under real-life circumstances is basic to the psychiatric approach. The limited adaptability of infants suggests that the examination preferably be conducted in the child's home and include samples of significant daily events such as feeding, sleeping, diapering, waking. If home visits are not feasible, care should be taken to provide, in the office, an atmosphere in which infant and mother can feel comfortable. A crib, bassinette, playpen, and other nursery equipment are essential.

The psychiatrist will of course have an opportunity to observe the mother-infant interaction during his examination, which should *always* include the mother or the mother substitute. Under unusual circumstances, such as in a hospital or institution, one is frequently compelled to examine the infant without his mother, but more caution in interpretation of the findings is then indicated. It is very helpful in such cases to have at least the infant's favorite nurse, child care worker, or aide present during the examination.

The evolution of a personality occurs in a context of an interpersonal relationship, and the mother-child interaction is a paradigm of such a relationship. Thus the mother's personality, her way of responding to the infant's changing needs in accord with her own conscious and unconscious wishes, motives, and beliefs have to be studied extensively. This, in addition to the evaluation of the rest of the family, would permit the psychiatrist to get a picture of the milieu in which the infant is destined to grow and to live. The complementary and contradictory traits in the infant and his family, their mutual "fit" and adaptation, can be ascertained only in this fashion.

HISTORY

The parents are the main suppliers of the developmental data. Their concerns may include such symptoms as feeding difficulties, sleep problems, failure to thrive or to relate, breath-holding spells, psychosomatic illness, and many others. While the parents' recall of details of the child's past tends to be distorted (Wenar, 1963), we know that this tendency is less pronounced in recalling recent events (Birch et al., 1962). Therefore, in infancy, with a relatively short lapse of time, we may get valuable information about the various phases of physical development, the child's mode of behavior since birth, about pregnancy and delivery, illness, hospitalization, feeding, sleeping and elimination patterns, response to people and inanimate objects, and a host of other details.

As is customary in child psychiatry, the parents can be interviewed either by the psychiatrist or by a psychiatric social worker. What matters is the competence of the interviewer, which should include a thorough knowledge of normal and abnormal infant development, and the progressive stages of infant-mother interaction.

COMPONENTS OF THE PSYCHIATRIC EVALUATION OF INFANTS

The psychiatric evaluation of an infant is, like that of older children, a composite of pediatric, neurological, psychological, and psychiatric examinations. In the first six months, all these examinations will converge, since the infant's repertoire of responses is relatively meager. As the infant grows older, one is more justified in breaking down the psychiatric evaluation into its traditional components.

The *physical examination* concerns itself with the general state of health of the infant, with his rate of body growth, the size of his skull, state of nutrition, and the presence of any acute or chronic illness, in-flammatory or congenital in origin. The obvious importance of these factors to the infant's total functioning requires no elaboration.

The *neurological,* or rather the *neurophysiological examination* concerns itself with the infant's neuromuscular equipment, the state of the sensory apparatus, and the infant's reactivity and activity patterns. It has to include the evaluation and time sequence of postural and other automatisms of infancy (Paine and Oppé, 1966). The functioning of the automatic nervous system also belongs in the scope of this examination, since it may influence the character of the child's response to stress, its speed, strength, and appropriateness (Richmond et al., 1962; Bridger, 1962). The hyper- or hyposensitivities of the sensory systems (Bergman and Escalona, 1949) should be explored in this context, as well as preferred sensory modalities, the state of awareness, arousal, excitability, and inhibition. The neurophysiological functioning of the infant is a dynamic process, subject to rapid changes and maturation and often capable of remarkable improvement.

The *psychological examination* may be performed by the psychiatrist if he is skilled enough in this rather specialized area, or else by a developmental psychologist. There are several good infant tests available which can be used (Gesell and Amatruda, 1941; Bayley, 1961; Cattell, 1940; Griffiths, 1954). In addition to the evaluation of the cognitive and motor functioning and integration, the psychological examination should ideally represent a broad framework, capable of incorporating the results of highly specialized research, as they become available, such as the development of smiling (Spitz and Wolf, 1946; Ahrens, 1954), crying (Karelitz et al., 1960), following (Bowlby, 1958a), and the object concept (Piaget, 1937). The evaluation of speech development will properly belong here. In essence, the psychological examination gives us a picture of the child's general equipment needed to meet life's contingencies and his use of this equipment under specified standardized conditions. There is a significant overlap between the neurophysiological and the psychological examination, especially in the very young infant.

THE ROLE OF THE PSYCHIATRIST

All the previously mentioned examinations, the physical, the neurophysiological, and the psychological, give us a picture of the child's potential, his strengths, weaknesses, vulnerabilities, and proclivities toward certain reaction patterns, which may be the foundation of his personality. How the infant really behaves under *his peculiar circumstances* and how he reacts to his particular life situation must also be determined. This kind of appraisal of the patient's intrapsychic balance and his life style in an interpersonal context has been traditionally the domain of the psychiatrist. The psychiatric examination of an infant, or better yet, the psychiatric examination of the infant-environment complex, need not stray in principle from the traditional pattern.

The intrapsychic balance of an infant, as compared with that of an adult, is probably more directly determined by his constitutional makeup. This would include among others the state of the sensorimotor apparatus, characteristics of autonomic functioning, drive patterns, and proclivity for particular defense mechanisms. By drive endowment we refer to "physiologically determined pressures such as are involved in metabolism and in as yet incompletely understood organic and tissue pressures that build up and call for relief in order to maintain homeostasis within the organism" (Lourie, 1966). The concept of congenital activity type refers to the amount of activity a newborn shows in response to certain stimuli (Fries and Woolf, 1953). Although such a general concept may be useful, more recent research (Bell, 1960) suggests the advisability of attempting to break this down into finer categories. For example, an infant might be rated as highly active with regard to eye movements, at the same time as he is found to be relatively inactive in gross motor movements. Another aspect of activity that may be useful to study is the infant's sleep pattern, since norms are now available for the first six months of life (Kleitman and Engelmann, 1953; Anders and Hoffman, 1973; Parmelee, 1973; Anders et al., 1971). In the area of drive endowment (Alpert et al., 1956) a breakdown of specific drives is also useful. The sucking drive should be considered under nutritive and nonnutritive aspects. The amount of biting would be another index of specific drive endowment.

The defense proclivities or patterns of dealing with anxiety may be manifested very early, and could be roughly divided into active or passive forms of behavior. For example, some babies react to frustration with prolonged massive motor discharge and others tend to withdraw into sleep. Using the reaction to unwanted food as another example, turning the head away would be a passive avoidance, whereas spitting the food out or firmly closing the lips would be an active rejection (Heider, 1966). These defense proclivities will be influenced very early by the environment. Yet it is likely that infancy affords the best opportunity to make the most accurate estimate of constitutional traits since they are relatively unobscured by the experimental overlay of later childhood (Wolff, 1966). However, immediately upon birth the environment and persons in it influence and effect reactions in the infant (Brazelton, 1962).

The infant's prevalent affect, especially the quality and degree of depressive mood or anxiety, must be carefully noted. An assessment also has to be made of capacity to delay gratification, frustration tolerance as well as control over motor, oral and aggressive drives. The degree and quality of response to anxiety-producing situations will reflect the child's reaction patterns and the stability of his emotional balance (Spitz, 1950). Frustration tolerance is characteristically low in general in this early period, and yet variations within the general pattern can be discerned. Sublimation potential on a very simple level may be reflected in an infant's ability to accept substitutes (e.g., a thumb in place of food, for a time). Regarding anxiety tolerance, one may differentiate an infant who cannot eat for two hours after a disturbing experience from one who takes fifteen minutes to recover.

In approaching the interpersonal facets of the infant's personality, one considers how he relates to mother, other family members, mother substitutes and strangers (Schaffer and Emerson, 1964b). The child's reaction to separation from his mother, his response to prohibition, and his drive for independence are noted; his state of tension or relaxation, trust or distrust, and basic warmth or remoteness can be estimated by the examiner.

The examiner should be equally observant of the mother's response to the child. Her feeling tone when she feeds him, diapers him, puts him to sleep or scolds him, gives us important clues as to how she relates to *this* particular infant (Brody, 1956). Also noted are her enjoyment of the child, or her annoyance and irritability, her anxiety over his state of health or his performance, and her fear of real or imaginary dangers. Of special importance is the evaluation of the perceptiveness and flexibility of the mother regarding the specific needs of the child, as well as her willingness and ability to act on her perceptions (Levy, 1958). A mother may correctly perceive her child's needs and yet be unable to fulfill them because of overwhelming dependent needs of her own. Another maternal characteristic to be studied is the ability to differentiate the infant from herself (Winnicott, 1960). Flexibility includes the ability to respond appropriately to a rapidly changeable and changing organism (Yarrow and Goodwin, 1965). To a compulsive mother the ever-changing patterns of early infancy can be particularly trying.

In addition to the central figure of the mother, there are many other factors in the environment which merit consideration. The role of the father, his direct involvement with the infant as well as his support given to the mother are often inadequately studied despite their crucial importance. Other factors to be considered are the presence of siblings or other household members and the stimulus potential of the physical aspects of the environment. Several home visits would provide a more accurate appraisal in view of the daily variations in the environment as well as in the child.

The cultural, religious, social, and ethnic characteristics, child-rearing practices, values, and attitudes of the child's community have to be explored. This is of particular importance in our country where we still see a number of cultural groups or subgroups living next to each other.

THE PSYCHIATRIC DIAGNOSTIC FORMULATION

The previously mentioned components of an infant's psychiatric evaluation are illustrative of the child's emotional, physical, and intellectual makeup, his assets and vulnerabilities, and the environment in which he grows. It remains the task of the psychiatrist to fit all the pieces into a meaningful, whole structure. It is debatable whether he has to perform all these examinations himself, and it may often be impractical in other than research or teaching settings. However, in addition to the usual psychiatric knowledge about normal and abnormal human behavior, he needs to be familiar with pediatric principles, neurological examination, and modern dynamic neurophysiological theories and should be acquainted with the psychological examination methods of his choice and their interpretations. Finally, he must be cognizant of cultural and social factors which may be decisive in the infant's fate. All this is a large order, but the task is too complex to be squeezed into a short-cut formula. For psychiatric screening purposes, or for use by pediatricians, less comprehensive methods will have to be devised, but this holds true of psychiatric examination of older children as well.

The psychiatrist has to weigh carefully evidence of strength and weakness; he must distinguish between permanent damage and a developmental lag. Above all he must be alert to the dynamic interplay between the infant and his environment; where do the child's needs and the needs of his environment coincide and where do they clash to the detriment of both? In other words, the psychiatrist has to appraise *the reality of the infant's life situation;* and using that as a background, he evaluates the infant's actual performance, his life style and its usefulness to his present and future satisfactory growth and adjustment.

The infant psychiatrist also has to be cognizant of the age-appropriate changes in the mother-infant interaction (chap. 11), and of the critical periods in the life of an infant when basic changes occur which cut across the specialty lines and involve neurophysiological, cognitive, and emotional maturation as well as physical growth (Caldwell, 1962; Greenacre, 1960). He has to be aware of the role of regressive behavior in the normal process of infant development (A. Freud, 1965). Only by taking all these factors into consideration can he make a sensible evaluation of the infant's personality, leading to useful recommendations.

THE PROGNOSTIC VALUE OF A PSYCHIATRIC EVALUATION
OF AN INFANT

Several factors limit the prognostic value of any infant evaluative method in our present state of knowledge. To begin with, the biological building blocks, i.e., the neurophysiological, neuroendocrinological, and biochemical states of the infant and young child, are responsive to both positive and negative environmental influences. Pediatric neurologists are extremely cautious in prognosticating in infancy, even in the presence of serious neuropathology. Sometimes even infants who are spastic at birth or have abnormal reflexes may recover or greatly improve when seen several months or a year later (Peiper, 1963). We do not yet know the exact nature of this recovery process. Perhaps it depends on the maturation and myelinization of the central nervous system or on its plasticity which permits certain functions to be assigned to alternative components when the customary ones fail.

The psychologists are equally cautious in making predictions on the basis of their examinations in early life, especially in infancy (Bayley, 1958). The experience of Skeels (1966), who saw the IQ of some infants increase from a severely retarded to normal or above-normal range with appropriate stimulation, is just one case in point. Gesell (1954) marveled at the great "hidden reserve" within the human organism which comes into play when needed and when the situation allows it.

Pediatricians, on their part, are constantly faced with many changes, often very drastic ones, which occur within the lifetime of a young child and affect vital areas such as his general vigor, activity patterns, and responsiveness.

As for the environment, especially the mother and the entire family unit, it is equally difficult to make valid long-range predictions. We cannot foresee the many life events which may contribute to the shaping of a child's mind. Sickness, death in the family, the arrival or death of a sibling, divorce or separation, operations, financial disaster, father's success or failure in his professional life, handicap or brilliance of a sibling, presence or absence of a mother substitute, maid or grandmother—these are only a few of the myriad possibilities or combinations of possibilities which may be decisive and yet impossible to predict.

The "complementary" or "contradictory" elements in the mother-infant interaction are also a very elusive subject for investigation. Certain elements in both mother and child may be complementary in early infancy and contradictory in later life or vice versa. Since we are dealing with two dependent variables, the number of possible combinations is very great and cannot be easily squeezed into a framework of a few characteristics of the infant and his environment, no matter how cleverly selected.

We may make, however, short-term predictions especially about the vulnerable, high-risk infants with various handicaps (Murphy, 1968) and point out the most likely possibilities which help us in making appropriate recommendations. This traditional role of the psychiatric evaluation is very useful despite our incomplete knowledge. But we should not expect from such an examination of an infant—a highly flexible organism with his entire life ahead of him—what we do not expect even from the psychiatric examination of an adult, whose physical and emotional makeup is relatively stable.

Summary

The need for a uniform, standardized psychiatric appraisal of infants is presented. The breakdown of such an appraisal into several components and its general characteristics and setting are discussed in detail. The role of the child psychiatrist is seen as a coordinator of the diagnostic team. Finally, the long-range prognostic limitations of an infant psychiatric evaluation are acknowledged.

4

THE CONTRIBUTION OF DEVELOPMENTAL NEUROLOGY TO CHILD PSYCHIATRY

Richmond S. Paine, M.D.

Evaluation of the disorders of the function of the nervous system in preschool children depends to a very large extent on knowledge of the evolution of the sensorimotor responses, of the acuity of sensory function, and of the postural patterns and automatisms during the years of infancy. Distortion in evolution in these sequences is one of the greatest sources of diagnostic information available to the neurologist or to the pediatrician.

Muscle Tone

The distribution of muscle tone in the newborn is quite different from that in the older child or adult and in the full-term newborn it is quite different from that in the premature. We have only to think of the usual posture assumed by the full-term newborn baby as being one of relative hypertonus in flexion: the upper extremities are flexed at the elbows, and the lower extremities are flexed at the hips and knees and are drawn up on the trunk. The premature is quite different, with predominant extension of the limbs. The differences in reflexes and automatisms which we see in comparing newborns with older babies or in comparing full-terms with prematures depend, I suggest, to a very large extent on the background of muscle tone on which they are executed.

Muscle tone in the newborn can be appraised as tone to palpation (that is, the "feel" of the muscle) or as resistance to movement (in this, there is a distinction between rapid and slow, passive manipulation of the limbs). Either of these would correspond to the French school's (Thomas and Sainte-Anne Dargassies, 1952) phrase *passivité*, and the degree of possible range of motion to *extensibilité*. The rebound after

Reprinted from the *Journal*, 4 : 353–386, 1965.

release is a characteristic of muscle tone which is almost peculiar to newborn infants. This is not the rebound of cerebellar disease but rather the phenomenon in which the newborn's elbow can be extended and then it snaps back in a rather violent, rubbery fashion. These phenomena can be considered in terms of stretch reflexes, of which there are perhaps two, a tonic one and a phasic one, possibly depending upon two parts of the gamma efferent system, one more active in resistance to rapid mobilization, and another in resistance to slow passive manipulation. What the cerebellar and cerebral effects may be in the newborn, we do not know. The "flappability" of a limb in which it is more than normally movable when suddenly seized is seen chiefly with cerebellar disease, with other types of hypotonia, and of course in Syndenham's chorea. The mechanical resistance of the joints and tendons and the elastic quality of the muscles have a good deal to do with some aspects of neonatal tone, particularly the rebound after release and the range of motion of joints. To a large extent, the available range of motion and the resistance of tendons and joints depend upon rather simple mechanical factors, perhaps more than on neurological reflex arcs. The full-term baby who has been confined in utero and is rather cramped has a very great range of dorsiflexion of the foot so that the great toe can be touched to the tibia, whereas this is impossible in the premature baby (this difference is one of the more reliable distinctions between full-terms and prematures).

Some of the characteristic reflex findings in the normal newborn infant depend more on this background of tone than on differences within the central nervous system. For example, the absence of the triceps jerk in the normal full-term infant results purely and entirely from the predominant flexor tone of the upper limbs. If one deals with a premature baby, in whom the flexor tone is missing and the limb relatively extended, or if one deals with a newborn with upper brachial palsy, the triceps jerk is easily demonstrated. The spinal reflex arc is always there, but is covered up or suppressed by the prevailing pattern of tone.

In a spastic baby of 4 months in vertical suspension, one notes the fisting of the hands and particularly the extension and scissoring of the lower extremities. This depends primarily on descending vestibulospinal impulses activated in the vertical posture. Two of the standard neonatal automatisms are the *supporting reaction* of the lower limbs to bear weight, and the *placing reaction* in which the dorsum of the foot is brought up under the edge of the table and the foot then placed on the table top. The early diagnosis of spasticity in the less obvious cases may depend on the relative excellence of the *supporting reaction* (for which extensor hypertonus is an asset), and on the relative poorness of the *placing response* (in which the same extensor hypertonus is a liability). There is no difference in the spinal mechanisms of supporting and of placing, but rather in the background of tone on which they are executed. In the baby with a hypotonic type of cerebral palsy, which will later be followed by choreoathetosis or some other type of unwanted movement, the reverse is true; he is relatively flabby and he places better than he supports weight. This again depends more on the background of muscle tone than on any difference in two spinal reflex patterns, although we can nevertheless use it for diagnostic purposes.

The *supporting reaction* refers to the capacity of the baby to support part of his weight when suspended vertically with the examiner's hands under the axillae and his feet placed on a table top. It would appear that while some supporting reaction is encountered in practically all newborns, at 1 month of age it is rather less and up to 4 months it continues to diminish. One has the impression that one may be dealing with the algebraic sum of two curves, one of them falling and the other rising. A definite worsening of the ability to support weight with the lower extremities at some point does not reflect the loss of a neurological pattern which is later reacquired, but rather is the change from more or less automatic neonatal supporting based on hypertonus in semiflexion of the lower limbs to the subsequent emergence of a second type of supporting action in which we are dealing with a true reflex of complex nature and unknown locus, which involves active, full extension of the knee so as to lock it. (The newborn infant supports weight in a semicrouching position, with the hips and knees slightly flexed, but the child of 6 months supports weight by locking the knee fully extended.)

The normal infant, if he is born at full term, then changes from a rather hypertonic, compact newborn with the upper and lower extremities both in a considerable degree of flexion to a hypotonic infant at 2 to 4 months. One can speculate about the psychiatric implications of this change from a compact, somewhat hypertonic individual with the limbs drawn tightly against the trunk to the normal floppy infant of 2 to 4 months, in which the muscle tone is diminished compared to what it had been before and to what it will be later, with rather chaotic movement of the limbs. This comes about at a time when the awareness of the infant of his environment is the first evidence of what we often think of as cortical activity. There is much more reason to suspect neonatal cortical activity than often stated, a point to which I shall return, but this change from a compact, hypertonic infant to a floppy one, with relatively poor muscle tone and poor control of his movements, coming at about 2 to 4 months, with a loss or deterioration of many of the neonatal responses which the infant once had, occurs at the same time he is becoming more aware of his environment. He fixates on the mother with his eyes, smiles responsively, follows her around the room, and he is becoming more aware at the same time that he is becoming less able physically and more helpless.

POSTURE AND MOVEMENT

A second aspect of developmental neurology concerns posture and movement. I have used *muscle tone* in a broad sense, meaning not merely static tone at rest but the alteration of tone by spinal synergisms associated with movement and posture. Movement and posture, of course, should not be separated, as Sherrington pointed out long ago, stating that posture follows movement like a shadow and that every movement begins and ends in a posture. The most striking point in relation to development of spontaneous movement is that of differentiation of fine movement, associated with but not necessarily due to myelination of the pyramidal tract. The hand of a newborn infant is predominantly fisted. The statement that the hand is fisted most of the time is not true, as Cobb et al. (1964) have found by continuous observation of normal infants, but as the hand opens and the flexor tonus of the wrist and fingers disappears the infant is not able to make a full series of finger movements initially. At first the hand can only be opened or closed as a whole; later there is differentiation to permit individual finger movement, and the grasp, as we all know, evolves from grasp by the whole hand to that by thumb and two fingers, and finally to the pincer thumb-to-forefinger type of grasp. One cannot know whether the basis of this is myelination of the pyramidal tracts or whether the myelination is the consequence of use, but the infant does acquire better control of the rather limited set of movements which he has in the neonatal period; the movements become more differentiated, more discrete types of movement are possible, and there is also better modulation by sensory feedback.

Certain reflexes which we see in the newborn become more differentiated with age—the knee jerk, for example. The knee jerk of the neonate is relatively hyperactive compared with that of an adult or older child. It also includes contraction of the adductors of both hips. This crossed adductor spread is normal up to 8 to 10 months of age, although it persists or reemerges in spasticity; the spread of the knee jerk to include two adductor contractions is lost after 8 to 10 months of age in the normal baby, and represents a differentiation of the motor response. There is also differentiation of the sensory part of the reflex arc in some cases. The extensor plantar response or Babinski sign of the newborn is an example. The current thinking is that the basis of the positive Babinski sign is an overlap between the afferent sensory zone for the withdrawal response of the great toe and that for the withdrawal response of the lower limb as a whole. Stimulating the sole of the foot results in withdrawal of the limb with a dorsiflexion of the great toe and spread of the other toes.

The reaction to pricking the great toe itself is, of course, withdrawal of the great toe. The electromyographic studies which Kugelberg and others (1960) have done suggest that the basis of the positive Babinski response is an overlap of afferent zones so that the pricking or scratching of the lateral aspect of the sole of the foot in some way sets off the withdrawal response of the great toe, which in normal older children and adults is elicited only by pricking the ball of the great toe itself, resulting in its dorsiflexion. The lack of sensory differentiation gives us a normal overlap of the two responses in the newborn and even up to 2 to $2^1/2$ years of age. There is no necessary correlation, by the way, between the conversion of the plantar response and the ability to walk. In older persons with pyramidal lesions there is a corresponding loss of differentiation, a backward step which will be considered later.

Some movements of the newborn become more differentiated in both their motor and sensory phases as they get older. Integration, in contrast, takes place with certain others. In the automatic spinal stepping of a newborn or a baby up to 3 months, when one foot is in contact with the surface of a table and the trunk inclined slightly forward, the baby executes a train of automatic steps. This "stepping" is lost by 2 to 3 months of age in most cases, and it does not seem to reemerge until 6 to 8 months in many. In others it persists all the way through without any dissolution.

The spinal stepping of the newborn is quite unintentional; it does not depend upon efforts to get anywhere and it does not even depend upon position in space. If the baby is held comfortably with the feet against the wall, he will walk up the wall; or if the examiner is tall enough, the baby will walk across the ceiling upside-down. This depends chiefly upon pressure and upon proprioceptive impulses from the ankle joints.

In the placing response, the foot is drawn up against the undersurface of the table and the baby then flexes the limb and places the foot squarely on the table top. This is later followed by a mobilization of muscle tone upward so that the limb becomes more rigid, from the foot upward and eventually up the trunk, in a straightening reaction. The placing response is usually stated to be cortical. Rademacher (1931) so stated in his book *Das Stehen,* and this has been repeatedly passed on. However, we have only to think that the placing response, like stepping, is present in hydranencephaly (they may not be present in anencephaly, but most anencephalics are moribund by the time we get to see them). I have seen one case of complete transection of the spinal cord due to birth injury, in which a fairly adequate placing response was demonstrable. This is clearly another of the spinal mechanisms; almost all of the things which we see in the newborn are spinal or brainstem reflexes.

There is no timetable which can be set for the disappearance of this placing response. Unlike stepping, which is usually gone by 2 to 3 months and comes back later when standing support is possible (and therefore walking with support), the placing reaction is gradually covered up or integrated into voluntary activity without any age being normal for its disappearance. Palmar or plantar grasp (reflex grasping with the fingers and toes) of the newborn persists until 6 to 8 months, or perhaps a little longer during sleep and is then no longer obtainable as a reflex, but what this amounts to is that the spinal mechanism has been subjected to higher control without actually being lost. However, the forced grasping of an adult with a frontal lobe lesion is not the same as the grasp of a newborn, since the newborn grasps essentially as a reflex to traction against the fingers, whereas the grasping of an adult with frontal lobe lesion is better elicited to a moving stimulus; the adult will even grope after the finger if it touches his hand, or sometimes if he sees the examiner's hand near his.

In the incurvation response of the trunk, one of the most phylogenetically primitive of the neonatal reflexes, the running of a finger along the paravertebral gutter or the pinching of the skin above the pelvic brim, or a series of taps with the fingernail, results in the pelvis being swung toward the stimulated side. This is basically a withdrawal reflex of the vertebral column, which arches away from the finger. It is demonstrable even in salamander embryos of a fairly young age. This is retained only as an emergency response to noxious stimuli. A person of any age, if the stimulus is sufficiently forceful and unpleasant, will arch the vertebral column away from it as a withdrawal response. This is another way of alteration of neonatal automatism with increasing age, where the mechanism is retained as an emergency response but not in other circumstances.

In the traction response from the supine position, the baby has been lying on the back and is drawn up to the sitting position by the examiner's hands. Assistance from the shoulder muscle takes place, then a mobilization of tone along the trunk, and finally some recovery of the posture of the head. In the straightening reaction of the trunk, the baby is held by the examiner's hand across the abdomen and in response to manipulation of the feet there is a mobilization of tone to extend the trunk and eventually the neck, and the baby assumes the upright posture. Both the straightening reaction of the trunk and the traction response are really alterations of muscle tone and of the distribution of tone in response to various manipulations, and are perhaps not simple reflexes. Again, an age at which they disappear cannot be reliably stated. They are integrated into other activity, but certainly not subsequently demonstrable in this automatic fashion.

As infancy advances, certain other reflex movements of the newborn are not differentiated in either motor or sensory aspect, nor are they integrated into any seemingly useful pattern, but are in contrast completely suppressed. The Moro reflex is the best known of these. We know astonishingly little of the physiological basis of this, despite all the suggestions that this is a catching response to keep the monkey from falling from the tree. In the most reliable method of getting a Moro response, the infant is suspended with the examiner's hand under the head and back, and the head is allowed to fall back 20° or 30° in relationship to the trunk; then the familiar clasping movement is executed. This same response can be obtained in a diversity of ways: slapping the bed beside the infant (Moro's original method), jerking the baby by the feet, pulling out the hands and then letting go, or by a loud noise or by a light shone in the eyes in some cases, if the baby is slightly jittery. The common denominator is some movement of the head with reference to the trunk and if the test is carried out so that the infant is strapped to a board and allowed to fall back without it being startling enough to the muscles of the neck, no Moro takes place. Thus, the reaction is probably not vestibular. A baby with congenital absence of the vestibular function was studied in Sweden (Karlsson, 1962) and found to have a perfectly normal Moro response, so that this response probably originates from proprioceptive endings in the neck muscles or in the cervical vertebrae. It is known to all of us as the cardinal reflex movement of the newborn; except for the smaller prematures all normal newborns have it and its absence makes one worry about anoxia, hypoglycemia, excessive effect of maternal anesthesia, infection, metabolic errors, and a diversity of possible diagnoses, all having in common a depressed function of the central nervous system.

We have studied the dissolution of the Moro response in a group of 66 infants. By 1 month, a small number of newborns fail to show the Moro response; by 4 months 40 percent had lost it, but by 5 months a few still retained it, although by 6 months it was always gone. This indicates a sharper end point than do most studies of the evolution of reflex patterns. The difficulty with many published studies has been failure to see the infants frequently enough, failure to examine them by the most sophisticated level of people, and failure to make sure that the babies were normal in the first place. It does appear possible to say that no normal, full-term baby has a Moro after 6 months, but it very seldom reemerges in the presence of decerebrating conditions (quite in contrast to the tonic neck pattern). Further, the Moro is usually covered up and lost almost as quickly in abnormal babies as in normal. In another series of 130 infants with motor defects of various types, chiefly cerebral palsies, the Moro response was very seldom retained past the normal age for disappearance. There were only 9 out of the 130 who retained the Moro reflex after the age of 6 months and all of them had lost it by the age of 14 months.

The tonic neck pattern, in contrast, is very frequently retained too late, or frequently reemerges in the presence of neurological disease. A degree of tonic neck reflex is seen in normal babies, and the interpretation of how much of this to accept as normal at what age is one of the most difficult things to teach residents in pediatrics and neurology. The demonstration of abnormal tonic neck reflexes past the normal age is of key importance to differentiating what appears to be delayed development or regression due to organic neurological disease from what may be general psychomotor retardation from an emotional regression. The tonic neck reflex is not produced in any emotional way that I know of; it is not encountered with autistic children, and is seldom prolonged very much in general psychomotor retardation, certainly not past 9 to 10 months. In fig. 1 we see the sequence in normal infants. This is again the series of 66 normals examined monthly, and the tonic neck reflex was defined as definite for more than 30 seconds (that is, the

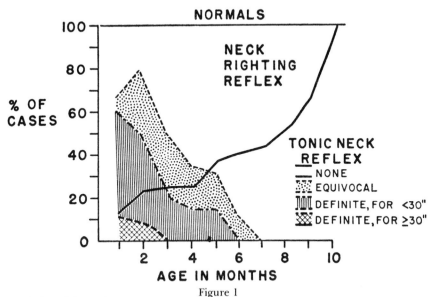

Figure 1

Evolution of the tonic neck reflex which is not striking in the majority of newborns but is most consistently demonstrable at the age of about 2 months but should not be encountered with normal infants after 7 months. In none of the normal infants was the tonic neck pattern imposable for an indefinite period (that is, the infant was always able to escape it by struggling).

baby did not get out of it sooner than 30 seconds), a definitely imposable pattern for less than 30 seconds, or an equivocal pattern, which was
really the examiner's impression that he was able to make the baby do
this some of the time, but not for 6 trials out of 10, which was considered the criterion of the definite imposable pattern. None of the normal babies had an indefinitely obligate tonic neck reflex, and they were
all able to get out of it sooner or later by struggling. This response has
a different sequence of evolution than some of the others; it is not
present in the majority of neonates, whether they are normal or not.
The tonic neck response reaches its peak at about 2 months when 80
percent have some imposable degree of it, and then falls off so that by
7 months none of the normal babies had it. The neck-righting response
appears and replaces it as the tonic neck disappears. The neck-righting
response consists in the examiner's turning the baby's head to one side,
after which the child will swing first the shoulders and the trunk and
pelvis toward that side so as to roll over on to the side.

The tonic neck reflex is abnormally imposable and abnormally obligate or retained too late in a large number of abnormal neurological
conditions. Tonic neck reflexes are more obligate and were retained
later in spastics than in normals, and also abnormally late in what might
be called dyskinetic cerebral palsy (athetosis, choreoathetosis, dystonia,
and the so-called athetoids). Persistence of a tonic neck reflex has no
differential diagnostic value between spasticity and athetosis as the future handicap. It does document, however, in the case of children
above 6 months of age that there is some specific motor abnormality. If
we think of this reflex as being produced by decerebration at the level
of the superior colliculus in animals, it amounts to a degree of motor
decerebration. The persistence of the tonic neck reflex in abnormally
imposable degree, or inescapability, or its persistence past the normal
age, even if escapable, indicates a specific motor deficit. Its disappearance is very slightly delayed in mentally retarded children who prove to
have no motor difficulty later on, but its persistence represents a delay
in maturation of posture and implies, if present past 6 to 9 months of
age, that there is probably (although not inevitably) going to be some
persistent motor disability, i.e., a cerebral palsy of some kind if not due
to progressive disease. Its reemergence after it has gone implies a degree of functional decerebration, but without necessarily and intellectual implications; the severe athetoid who is bright but who is confined
to a wheelchair at the age of 6 to 12 years, will often show a tonic neck
reflex which has no necessary correlation with intellectual function but
merely with motor disability and particularly with the lack of standing
balance.

In the case of spastics where the question is one of orthopedic surgical procedures on contractures in the lower extremities, one is often

able to say that in the presence of an obligate tonic neck reflex the child will not have standing balance even if operated upon, and that therefore the contemplated procedure might well be deferred until and unless he loses this hallmark of lack of standing balance.

Another automatism which is better studied during the later months of infancy is the Landau reflex. In Landau's original description this depends on the degree of extension of the neck, trunk, and legs, which the infant develops in horizontal suspension in space. The newborn, if held horizontally in this posture by the examiner's hands about the trunk, has the head below the horizontal and is slightly convex upward in the spine, even to 1 month of age. With increasing age the spine is straightened horizontally, the head is got above the horizontal, and finally the spine arches so as to be concave upward instead of convex. The Landau reflex is not in its essence the loss of this extension of neck and trunk when the examiner depresses the baby's head. (Whatever degree of extensor tone has been mobilized will be lost when the head is passively flexed.) It is not until 10 months of age, although most have it at 9, that the full response with head up and back arched is reached. (One of the big points that came out of our serial study was that the range of variation of normal in the evolution of all of these things was greater than had been expected. If one states that something like the thumb-to-forefinger grasp is supposed to be present at 9 months, we were interested to find that some infants of 5 to 6 months had it, although not many; a lot of them did at 7 months; and 12 months was the first age at which they all had it, if normal.)

Among infants with spastic cerebral palsies (this is equally true of the future athetoids), the sequence of evolution of the Landau posture in horizontal suspension is considerably slowed. This slowing of a sequence of evolution of neurological signs is one of the ways in which developmental neurology helps us diagnostically just as much as in the case of qualitative abnormality or the presence of something that should not be there, or the absence of something that should. Serial examination of infants with motor handicaps is essential in making a diagnosis and in predicting what their future course is likely to be. We may be surprised, in the case of spastics, that they all collapsed into the shape of an inverted letter U over the examiner's hand at 3 months; at 6 months a few of them had reached the normal neonatal ability, but at 6, 9, 12 months, etc., when they were already becoming spastic in the limbs with exaggerated reflexes, a stretch reflex, or even a tendency to contracture, the spastic infants were hypotonic in the trunk. The hypotonicity of the trunk and neck is very well brought out in this maneuver, and they were much later than the normals in getting the spine arched and the head up. This is essentially a delay in maturation of posture in the horizontal position, just as is the acquisition of standing balance (not the supporting of weight in which spasticity may be an asset).

In a general consideration of the diagnostic use of this kind of developmental neurology, we have to make several points. The reemergence of one of these abnormal signs, such as a tonic neck reflex, may be a particular characteristic of a motor dysfunction of organic nature. One may also see the reemergence of something like the palmar grasp, which is essentially deintegrated from the more complex patterns or removed from the voluntary control which it had; a different phenomenon from that of the reemergence of something which has been suppressed. A loss of differentiation is another possible abnormality, as in the Babinski sign. Finally, certain abnormal reflexes may reemerge, such as the crossed extension response seen with spinal cord transection, which is never normally demonstrable.

Prematures are somewhat different. The effect of intrauterine compression results in more limited dorsiflexibility of the feet and is the basis of the normal premature newborn's walking on the toes. Walking on the toes, an interesting phenomenon, is frequently seen in autistic children, but equally frequently in spastic children and in normal prematures; but in normal prematures it is purely on the basis of the distribution of tone and the range of extensibility of the joints, which I think has a mechanical basis in relatively slighter uterine compression.

The study of spontaneous fetal movements in abortuses and in prematures is extremely interesting. It has been suggested that the premature demonstrates to a considerable extent a series of evolutions of movement which the full-term "has to do over again" after being born. The very premature baby, or the early abortus if it lives for a few minutes, will often show flexion movements of the fingers as a whole. Later, in slightly older fetuses there may be movement of the fingers individually, or movement of the thumb, but never apposition of the thumb to the forefinger. We know that the newborn undergoes, if fullterm, a sequence of evolution of movement which is somewhat reminiscent of what the fetus is supposed to do in intrauterine life. I do not think that this is quite true. I should like to suggest that the flexor tone of the full-term newborn suppresses most of this and that the full-term infant cannot do anything with his fingers until he gets them out of the fist. Then, so to speak, he may have to learn over again the patterns of movement which he had in intrauterine life, but I do not know what the implications of this might be. We also know that the fetus makes a good many athetotic movements and that the movements of the premature of 7 months or so are quite often squirming and athetotic in character.

Some of the neonatal automatisms can be classified according to their degree of sophistication. (1) The incurvation of the trunk and the withdrawal to pinprick, which are spinal reflexes, are seen even in anencephalics if they are not moribund. (2) Even the smallest prematures have tendon jerks and response to sound and light, although the response to sound is highly variable even in full-terms. (3) Sucking and rooting, rotational nystagmus, the traction response, palmar and plantar grasp and the Moro are seen in the larger prematures, (4) but it is only the full-term who makes the normal creeping movement in the prone posture, who controls the head vertically, who makes a type of crossed extension movement to push the examiner's hand away if he is manipulating one foot. Placing and stepping and the straightening reaction of the trunk are characteristic only of the more vigorous full-terms. The sequence of evolution of these signs after premature birth depends more on total age than on anything else. The French school of André Thomas and his associates (Sainte-Anne Dargassies, 1955) believe that extrauterine life is closely equivalent to intrauterine in terms of maturation of reflex movement of the early infantile sort. That is, the baby born at 7 months, who has been alive for 1 month, is pretty much like an 8-month newborn. (The change from the smaller to the larger type of premature responses takes place at around $7^{1}/_{2}$ to 8 months.) Similarly the larger premature who is 8 months at delivery and is 1 month old is supposed to be about like the full-term neonate. I have not had the opportunity of working with a sufficient number of prematures to study this personally, but limited experience suggests that this is largely true.

SENSORIMOTOR MATURATION

Sensorimotor maturation is perhaps a better word than sensory maturation because sensation, as opposed to movements which we can see, is testable only in terms of either low level reflexes or of more complex higher level responses, or else in terms of a conscious answer which inevitably involves gnosis. We can test for perception of pinprick in terms of reflex withdrawal or crying, and we can test for response to touch in a newborn, if we are lucky, in terms of movement of the limb; but when we get to testing for touch as we do in an adult, we are asking for a conscious response, in which the patient says "now" each time he feels a bit of cotton.

Visual

Visual responses are the modality of sensation which is most easily studied in the newborn. A blink reflex to light is present in all but the smaller prematures or abnormally depressed, and this can be elicited even with the eyes closed unless they are already maximally closed as in crying. Pupillary constriction to light is of course also to be expected, but constriction of the pupil to light in the absence of following movements is not a criterion of cortical blindness in the newborn in the sense that it would be with older children or adults. The ability of the baby to follow his mother around the room and to smile responsively, at 6 to 8 weeks of age, is usually stated to be the first evidence of cortical function in early infancy. However, Gorman et al. (1957) have demonstrated that the opticokinetic nystagmus, which depends on following movements, can be elicited in normal full-term infants with a special apparatus which draws a striped canopy across the entire visual field. The explanation is probably that macular central vision is thus not required, or else that the following movements may in the case of newborns take place at a tectal or other subcortical level, just as is true with birds and certain animals. Also, following movements of the eyes may be demonstrated on one occasion or another if trials are repeated with sufficient patience, in the majority of normal full-terms if use is made of some device such as a plastic disc or ring about 4 inches in diameter. Curiously it has been generally experienced that a red test object is more successful than other colors (this may be early and surprising evidence of color vision in the neonate), and even that a red design roughly similar to a human face is the most successful of all.

There is a separate question of visual discrimination of patterns. Stirnimann reported as early as 1944 that young infants tend to look at patterned surfaces in preference to homogeneous ones. Fantz and his associates (1962) have shown that infants as young as 1 week of age tend to fixate on a striped stimulus more often than on a homogeneous grey one, and that this tendency is likely to precede the ability to demonstrate opticokinetic nystagmus, while Gorman et al. (1957) and others have estimated the visual acuity of the newborn at about 20/600. These findings suggest greater importance than has been generally supposed of the visual experiences of the very young infant in influencing his future interactions with his environment.[1] Various conditions and various apparatus in which the ill newborn or particularly the premature may be cared for should be of concern to psychiatrists, and the optimal of such conditions has not so far been adequately studied.

Acoustic

The response of the normal newborn to acoustic stimuli is much more variable than that to visual stimuli. Using a sufficiently loud handclap or noisemaker, one can obtain some evidence of hearing in the majority of normal newborns if repeated trials are made, but any apparent response is absent on numerous trials even with perfectly normal new-

1. See also Carpenter et al. (1970)

borns and a presumptive diagnosis of deafness cannot be made at this age. However, using a standard stimulus at 60 decibels, Benedetti and Cocciante (1959) obtained a cry, a blink, or other response from 80 percent of normal newborns when awake and from 90 percent while asleep. The percentages were significantly less among infants who had had anoxic births. Ten percent of normal infants showed a more exaggerated generalized response, including a Moro reflex, probably in response to movement of the head in relation to the neck and trunk as a startle reaction. The postnatal maturation of responses to auditory stimuli is also somewhat slower than that to visual stimuli. At 1 month or 2 of age, the normal infant inhibits his own activity in response to a sudden sound. This is the earliest evidence of hearing, aside from an occasional startle to a very loud sound, which is likely to impress the baby's mother. Subsequently, at 2 to 3 months, the normal baby turns his eyes toward a sudden interesting sound and at 3 to 4 months he may turn the head as well. Delay in maturation of the early infantile responses to visual and auditory stimuli often leads to an erroneous impression of blindness or deafness, but far more often turns out to be the result of general developmental retardation and to be followed by mental deficiency.

Olfactory

Peiper (1956) has presented evidence that normal newborns can respond to strong olfactory or gustatory stimuli, as evaluated in terms of facial expression. This is not too surprising, considering the generally accepted primitive phylogenetic nature of these special senses, but their importance in the maturation of the human infant remains obscure.

"SET" AND THE FOCUS OF ATTENTION

The sensory responses also depend a good deal on what one might call the "set" of the system. We know that some newborns are jittery and some are relatively depressed; a simple stimulus such as a tap on the forehead will make one infant jump off the table in a violent Moro response, and another will show practically no reaction at all. The same applies to reactions to light, to sound, to touch, and to vibration. This jitteriness or depression is not stimulus-specific in the newborn. There are occasional infants who are depressed and who also overreact to stimuli in the newborn period. This is the combination which often follows an anoxic birth (if not due to something like maple syrup urine disease) and which is followed by permanent neurological deficit more frequently than any other (Donovan and Paine, 1962). The variability between one examination and another of a normal baby is another example of the set of the nervous system. It is common for the resident to find one set of neurological signs at 9 o'clock, and for the attending physician to whom they are shown to find something entirely different at 11 o'clock. This usually does not mean that either was wrong, but that the baby had changed in the meantime.

The biggest point of evidence, I believe, for the existence of cortical, or at least of cerebral function, in the newborn is that there is a difference between a baby who has no brain, a baby who has a normal one, and one who has an abnormal brain. The hydroencephalic shows most neonatal automatisms in a peculiarly stereotyped, frequently exaggerated way so that one may even suspect the diagnosis without trans-illuminating the head. The abnormal infant generally is also less variable than the normal, and we are dealing with spinal and brainstem reflexes of a rather simple sort, without too much modification from above. The fact that greater variability exists in normal neonates does imply cerebral activity on the part of the newborn.

Another concept which is comparable to the question of "set" in the maturation of sensory function is what one might call *focus of attention,* or conversely, the development of some degree of cerebral inhibition. The normal 2-year-old who responds to every stimulus in an obligate fashion, going quickly from one to another, readily becoming over-stimulated and hyperactive, is not called the "terrible 2's" for nothing. He is quite reminiscent of the older "brain-damaged child" who is equally distractible and equally stimulus-bound. We do not know whether the development of cerebral inhibition or focus of attention depends on some frame of reference in the temporal lobe, or whether it is mediated through some descending sensory inhibition, which a larger amplitude of stimulus might break through.

The ability to respond to a minimal stimulus and particularly to discriminate between stimuli is known to increase with age. The ability to discriminate weight, size, shape, and texture, which require integration of sensory inputs and correlation with past experiences and conscious analysis, is one feature of sensory maturation. We know that the threshold of 2-point discrimination diminishes with increasing age. One can, of course, only test that in a child who knows 1 from 2 and is willing to tell, but even down to the age of 4 or occasionally 3, stereognosis and 2-point discrimination can be tested. We find that the degree of separation of the points on the fingertip or any other part of the body required for 2-point discrimination gets less as the child gets older. Stereognosis becomes possible to test and a larger number of objects or shades can be tested; tests of texture recognition also become possible. (These are actually tests of gnosis of an object since we test them with common objects rather than recognition of a geometric shape by matching, which would be a more elegant test.)

ELEMENTS IN MATURATION OF A CONCEPT OF OWN BODY

The maturation of a concept of his own body is an even more interesting aspect of sensory maturation in an infant. We know that the newborn infant can localize a stimulus on his body if he is touched or if he is pricked in some noxious way. He is able to a considerable degree to locate the stimulus with his hand as if to push you away, or with the foot in the case of the lower extremity. It would be hard to say that he has a concept of body image at this stage, but it is a rather complicated spinal reflex, if that is what it is, in which he is able to find the stimulated point and to bring the suitable limb into play to push the stimulus away.

In the case of nonnoxious stimuli about the face there is an interesting separation of a perioral zone where a tactile stimulus results in "rooting" and the mouth is brought toward the object, from a region more posterior, behind which a tactile stimulus on the cheek then makes the head withdraw to the opposite direction. These are not really associated with a concept of body image but are an interesting example of differentiation of the apparent areas of two low-level reflexes.

Another feature of sensory examination of young children, up to the age of 5 to 6, is the tendency for cephalad displacement or caudad extinction if simultaneous stimulation is carried out. If one stimulates the cheek and the hand simultaneously, it is quite common for preschool children to appreciate the stimulus only on the face. Similarly, if the hand and foot are stimulated, the phenomenon may be extinguished on the foot. The phenomenon is much more readily demonstrated if two stimuli are applied and the patient asked to tell when one is withdrawn. Actually one leaves them both in place, but the more caudal one is falsely reported as being extinguished fairly frequently. In normal children up to the age of 5 to 6, we see this caudad extinction to a degree that we would consider abnormal in older ones.

Some concept of body image must be present by the time the ability to play peekaboo is acquired at 10 months of age, and certainly by the time the infant can point to parts of his body on command, at $1^{1}/_2$ to $1^{3}/_4$ years. One of the most interesting aspects of study of this is in the drawings of young children.[2] Such drawings require not only intelligence, past experience, and visual-motor coordination, but also concepts of body image, spatial orientation, right versus left, etc. Drawing is one of the functions which is selectively depressed and proportioned to over-all intelligence in the presence of organic cerebral or particularly cortical syndromes. Thus, one should expect the drawings

2. A considerable collection of drawings of human figures and of houses by normal preschool children and of drawings by neurologically abnormal children of various ages was presented in the original lecture, but cannot be reproduced here.

of a human figure to be disproportionately poor and can anticipate that the Goodenough Draw-a-Man Test will give a lower score than the full-scale IQ on the Stanford Binet or WISC in a subject with an organic encephalopathy. Some such patients show disassembly of the parts of the whole figure. disproportionate size, or anomalous arrangement of the parts, rotation or reversal of figures, or other unusual features. However, the most common abnormality is the production of a drawing which is rather comparable to the normal product of a somewhat younger child. The most bizarre distortions of drawings which the physician encounters are obtained from children with schizophrenia or other severe emotional disturbances, and the interpretation of drawings requires a great deal of experience in this field and even then considerable caution.

SENSORIMOTOR EXPLORATION

The normal infant explores any object which comes his way with all sensory modalities at once. If an object makes a sound, he hears it, looks at it, reaches for it, and grasps it, followed by manipulation of it with the hands or with the mouth. What he sees is probably perceived all at once, or at least lightning-quickly. The exploration with the fingers is one of the most interesting angles. The ability to make individual finger movements, and to reach out after something with a sufficient concept of space to find it, makes possible the stereognostic or haptic exploration of space (see Bower, 1972). Much of what the infant learns depends on this, which is a slower sequential point-to-point type of exploration than mere grasp. When we test stereognosis in older children or adults, if the individual is given an object and is forced merely to squeeze it in the hand, he has difficulty in recognizing anything not fairly obvious from a limited set of possibilities previously shown. An adult or an older child given a coin or a bottle cap or a block or marble will move it about with the fingers. This is different from visual perception in that it involves point-to-point exploration and in some manner a sequential analysis. It depends also on proprioceptive and deep stimuli as well as on superficial cutaneous impulses. One might define haptic sensation as a combination of proprioceptive and exteroceptive (cutaneous) stimulation. The information which can be obtained from this is quite comparable to that from visual exploration, with the single exception that color is lacking (unless one believes that some people can feel color, as some of the magazines have suggested).

On the other hand, haptic sensory exploration gives us two additional bits of information not furnished visually, one of them being texture and the other weight. This kind of examination of an object (and I suggest an infant learns a large part of what he knows about objects by feel with his fingers or feel with his mouth) requires many abilities in the brain which are quite comparable to what is required for the understanding of language. It requires a short-term memory, perhaps at a subconscious level, of the different points of the cube which he has been feeling just as the series of phonemes heard in speech have to be stored in immediate memory. Many so-called aphasic children appear to have short-term immediate memories for either acoustic or visual stimuli. The processing of this point-to-point fingering of an object and the building up of a concept of a shape of the object, or identifying it with some invariable with which one has had previous experience, require short-term memory and also require a sequential analysis, just as the understanding of a spoken sentence requires not only the perception of the phonemes but their analysis in a sequence in time, and in a sequence in directed time. It requires a discrimination that A followed by B is not the same as B followed by A, or AB presented together. The number of "bits," to use the language of the cybernetic experts, only partially determines the amount of information which can be transmitted, and the amount of information transmitted is much greater if the bits acquire different meaning according to the sequence in which they are arranged. This ability for sequential analysis both in the understanding of speech and earlier in the exploration of the world by handling and fingering is an aspect of maturation of sensory function which deserves further exploration.

VOCAL COMMUNICATION

The acquisition of the ability to communicate is the last aspect of maturation of nervous function which I shall consider. The variability of the cry of the newborn is well known, and mothers of several children are familiar with the fact that each infant is different from every other in this respect as well as capable of producing different types of cry which soon acquire different meaning. Stereotyped crying, particularly if high-pitched, is characteristic of neurologically abnormal newborns, just as is other stereotyped activity. Neonatal crying is followed by a more or less automatic sequence of squealing, cooing, and subsequently the production of monosyllables and of bisyllabic babble. These double syllables such as "mama," "dada," and "bye-bye" appear at the age of 6 to 10 months and are often confused with true speech, although they occur in deaf children as well as in those who hear.

Absence of the sequence of automatic vocalizing is of some diagnostic importance since it is likely to be completely missing in severely autistic children and to be deficient or distorted in many developmental aphasias (Condon and Sander, 1974). It is well known that of the various phonemes, the consonants are normally acquired later than the vowels.

Certain consonants such as the two *th* sounds, *ch*, and *sh* are normally last acquired, possibly as late as 7 or 8 years in some normal children. These, together with *s* and *z* are those of highest frequency and most affected by high-frequency hearing losses, although it would be hard to prove whether hearing for high frequencies matures more slowly than that for low frequencies for children. The subsequent individual variations of speech are acquired later and are chiefly environmental (many travelers have remarked that very young children in the United States and in Great Britain speak a highly similar "childrenese" and acquire distinctive accents only later). The responses in a child to acoustic feedback of his own vocalization are undoubtedly important and warrant further study even though technically difficult and limited at present. We know that children differ in the earliest months of life in their response to pleasant or to menacing sounds, both of which produce diminished reactions in autistic and aphasic children. Normal children usually respond with pleasure to other persons' imitation of their own vocalizing, whereas it is often stated that autistic children cease vocalizing if they are doing so at all and that children with developmental aphasias are indifferent.

SUMMARY

I have attempted to consider some of the problems of what one can call developmental neurology in several areas: first, the evolution of the prevailing patterns of muscle tone and the changes in posture and movement which depend mainly on muscle tone and account for many of the things we call development in the very young infant; the acquisition of the ability to perform more or less undirected spontaneous movement and more complex sensorimotor responses. I have considered the differentiation of the sensory and of the motor components, of the way in which some of them are integrated into more complex movement, and others are suppressed. Curiously, the spinal ones are chiefly those that are integrated into other movement, and the higher ones at a brainstem level, such as the Moro and the tonic neck pattern, are suppressed or lost, although some of them may reemerge later under abnormal circumstances.

Much of the contribution of developmental neurology to diagnosis of the complaint of slow development or of distorted development in these young children depends upon recognition of the distortion of the sequence of normal evolution of one of these responses as compared with another, or on some qualitative abnormality of a particular response, or on a regression, a loss of something which was previously done. We are at a considerable disadvantage with this in the differential diagnosis of developmental defects of the nervous function in children because, first of all, we may be dealing with a distortion of the normal sequences of evolution by the presence of a chronic brain syndrome. One essence of child neurology is that the acquisition of an abnormality of the brain at a young age distorts normal sequences of development, rather than subtracting from a fully functioning system. If we are dealing with a progressive disease of the nervous system, whether a psychic one or an organic one, we are dealing with a battle between the normal process of maturation, the force of the infant's central nervous system to do more and to do better with increasing age, versus the dragging down by the disease process itself. It may be terribly difficult to decide whether the presence of a tonic neck reflex in a child of 6 to 8 months is due to a chronic, nonprogressive abnormality, producing a degree of motor decerebration, or whether we are dealing with some degenerative process such as Tay-Sachs disease which has begun just about the time the response ought normally to have been lost. The process of maturation [3] may win the battle for a while, and the downward force of the disease itself do so only subsequently, so that the progressive nature of progressive disease is far from obvious during a stage of advancing development.

The greatest difference between the neurology of adults and that of small children is this force of development and the need for judging everything against a sliding scale according to the child's age. The potential for recovery and the difficulty in diagnosis both rest on this, and therein lies much of its fascination.

3. Further details of the studies on maturation of postural reflexes in normal infants are contained in Paine et al. (1964).

5

THE STUDY OF INDIVIDUAL DIFFERENCES AND THE PROBLEM OF STATE

Sibylle K. Escalona, Ph.D.

For as long as there has been any systematic study of phenomena in nature, the variable of state has been recognized as crucially important. Even when scientists deal with systems other than living organisms, the state of the behaving system is known to modify its reactivity to stimuli. In biology, and even more in the psychological study of human behavior, the problem is especially complex. For it is more difficult to assess the precise state of the organism than it is to measure external stimuli or to assess the prevailing conditions in the field in which behavior occurs. A succinct formulation by Kurt Lewin (1936) defines how the state variable is necessarily part of any investigation of behavior: Behavior is a function of the state of the organism and of the total situation. By the latter is meant the forces acting upon the organism (stimuli) and the medium in which these forces act.

I have no intention of discussing the state variable in general. Instead I shall focus on the bedevilment created by these particular variables for those of us who attempt to study the behavior and development of very young children. The necessity to do so arose from day-by-day working experience and became especially urgent in relation to a program of research now in progress at the Albert Einstein College of Medicine. The effort is to delineate behavior characteristics of newborn babies, to recognize individual differences in the functioning of neonates, and eventually to explore the possible consequences of early infantile characteristics for the pattern and course of later development. We consider, as does almost everyone else in the same research area, that individual differences can have no factual definition or meaning except in the context of universal characteristics of neonatal functioning. At present our primary concern is an investigation on the psychophysiological level with close attentiveness to overt behavior. In much more

Reprinted from the *Journal,* 1 : 11–37, 1962.

preliminary and tentative fashion we have initiated observations on the purely behavioral level since there exist behavior differences which have no measurable neurophysiological correlates. In the present context these domestic preoccupations are mentioned merely in order to point to the very direct connection between the problem of individual differences and the problem of the state of the organism. Our experience confirmed that of all others. Whenever a group of healthy newborns is exposed to the same set of controlled stimulus conditions, their behavior in response is widely different. Yet each time we see one baby startle to a sound, while another merely flicks an eyelid; each time one baby alters his behavior with each new stimulus, while another appears to have a very limited repertoire of responses, we ask ourselves anew whether we are dealing with true differences among the babies in terms of the characteristics of their nervous systems, or whether they may be in a different state despite the fact that approximately the same period of time has elapsed since their last feeding. It might well be that one is more drowsy than the other, that one has a minor respiratory obstruction, or that one may already be reacting to internal events culminating in a bowel movement five minutes later.

It proves interesting to survey at least a portion of the available literature with an eye toward just this one thing: how did the researchers deal with the problem of state? How did their management of the problem limit or expand the range of phenomena that could be dealt with? What implications did it have for the generalizations that can legitimately be drawn from the data? It appears to me that fairly clearcut relationships can be traced between how the problem of state is handled and the kind of research results it is possible to obtain. The discussion to follow consists of two major parts, which are dealt with in alternating fashion rather than separately. One refers to some of the more representative ways in which child development researchers who operate within or close to a psychoanalytic frame of reference have dealt with the problem of state. The other concerns the manner in which the state variable has been dealt with by investigators whose approach is primarily in neurological terms. Specifically I shall refer to a portion of the program of Frances Graham and her associates (1956) and a portion of the research program by Prechtl and his associates (1958, 1959) in the Netherlands. Both these research groups were interested in determining the possible effects of birth injury or other brain damage upon later development. Both were therefore interested in studying the behavior of newborns and in defining differences between healthy and neurologically impaired neonates. These areas are selected for discussion because I have become convinced that the controls devised by the neurology group, and even more their studies of the effect of state upon behavior activation, are relevant to many of the psychological investigations now under way. Perhaps many of us have made too little use of information already available from other disciplines, and are thereby unnecessarily adding to the already extraordinary complexity of the task we set ourselves.

Most variables can be dealt with in any of five ways. They may be ignored, they may be circumvented, they may be controlled, they may be representatively included, and they may be studied in their own right. A survey of the relevant literature shows that all of these patterns have in fact been employed in developmental research insofar as the variable of state is concerned. Moreover, I believe that depending upon the problem under investigation and upon other factors, each of these methods can at times be appropriate. A design which circumvents the variable of state, at least for the initial assessment of subjects, has been used to good effect in much neurological and epidemiological research, and in some psychoanalytic studies as well. In these instances, investigators used as the independent variable not a measure obtained from the infant directly but a criterion extrinsic to the infant organism. Examples for such criteria are the birth weight of premature infants, the occurrence of prenatal or paranatal complications, and the like. Thus by studying groups of children one of which had normal birth weight whereas the other group consisted of prematures, it was possible to demonstrate that among premature babies, birth weight as such is associated with a greater incidence of defective or otherwise impaired functioning at later ages (Knobloch et al., 1956). The underlying principle is identical with that used by Spitz and his associates (1945b, 1946) in relation to the syndrome he called hospitalism. An external factor, namely, the circumstance that children were raised in a certain kind of institution, selected the experimental group, to be compared with a group of children who were raised in normal homes. Since the comparison was made in terms of the behavior and developmental characteristics of these children at later ages, the matter of state enters only in respect to the criterion measures. In both these investigations, nothing in particular was done about the state of the children at the time they gave the behavior responses which at later ages determined whether or not their behavior was considered to fall within the normal range. It was assumed that some children might be a little below par as compared to their usual state at the time of examination, whereas others might be in an optimal condition. There was no reason to believe that this distribution of state would be significantly different in the experimental group than in the control group. In both these investigations, the problem of state was circumvented at the start in that an external circumstance was used (rather than a direct assessment of the babies) in order to select subjects in relation to the independent variable. With respect to the evaluation of follow-up data, the state variable was expected to randomize.

A somewhat different approach in which the state variable is ignored is illustrated by Fries's pioneer study on congenital activity types (Fries and Woolf, 1953). As you know, here the infant's behavior did furnish the basis for a classification as to activity types, and behavior and developmental data later on were used to demonstrate that the groups at a later age still differed from one another as they had in terms of the original assessment of activity level. While the authors do not specifically discuss it, the rationale for such a procedure in an exploratory study is self-evident. It was assumed that activity levels would prove a determinant of such overriding importance that differences in state along with many other kinds of differences among these children would not obscure its effect. In other words, it was assumed that congenitally quiet babies would of course show varying degrees of activity when quiescent as compared to agitated states, but that through a great variety of states basically inactive babies would consistently differ from basically active ones. The data obtained in this study do not lend themselves to the statistical technique of calculating correlations, but the design of the Fries study is essentially a correlational one, and the significant comparison is between groups of very active, moderately active, and markedly inactive children, as is the case with the Spitz and also the Pasamanick studies (see Knobloch et al., 1956).

In my view, it is good research strategy to begin an investigation in this fashion provided it is hypothesized that one is dealing with very major factors. If the data confirm the investigator's hunch, a definite relationship will have been demonstrated. Additional and differently designed studies can then concern themselves with exploring the nature of the process involved, the limitations within which the lawful relationship will emerge, and all the rest of it. If results are equivocal or negative, it becomes necessary to refine the approach and to control numerous relevant variables, of which state is a very important one. As it happens, the activity study, and what subsequently happened in relation to this problem, is an excellent case in point. Other researchers who were impressed with the importance of the activity level variable have not been able to obtain results as consistent as those originally reported. Some interpret their findings to mean that activity level may remain constant but does not regularly do so. I would include myself in this category, and on such a basis the research problem is changed to that of defining the conditions under which activity level does and does not change. Some colleagues believe that until we have developed more exacting measures by which to determine neonatal activity level, we shall have no way of knowing whether or not this behavioral attribute has stability and significant consequences. Other investigators believe that the amount of activity an infant will show is almost entirely a function of state. Yet those who hold this view do not necessarily deny a relationship between early activity level and later patterns of adaptation. They would say instead that if during early infancy the child is predominantly in a state which facilitates high activity levels, this experience of having been active an unusually large proportion of time may play a role in determining the child's subsequent pattern of development. The point of importance here is that in exploratory studies concerned with variables believed to be of major importance, disregarding the state of the subjects at the time the crucial responses are made, need not interfere with obtaining significant results and may at times be strategic. When it comes to validating varieties of research, or when initial results cannot readily be repeated, or also when interest focuses upon the nature of the developmental processes involved rather than the fact of an antecedent, consequent relationship, then it becomes necessary to investigate and control the problem of state. A corollary of this generalization is to say that where a problem of this type is investigated without regard to state, negative results do not disprove the original hypothesis. If anyone wanted to and could show that there is no such thing as a congenital activity type which remains a characteristic of the organism throughout, this could be done only by perfectly controlling the state variable at the time of the original measurements and then demonstrating the absence of a relationship between high and low activity levels in infancy and any aspect of later development.

The great majority of current investigations do come to grips with the problem of state in one way or another. Before turning to a discussion of current efforts to measure individual differences and make sense of them in developmental terms, I would like to discuss those aspects of the neurologically oriented research which seem to me suggestive for our own future efforts.

Graham and her associates (1956) aimed to explore the consequences of birth injury for later development. In particular, they hoped to identify those among the traumatized newborns who are likely to show abnormalities later. Since the behavior of the newborn infants was to be the sole basis for differentiating traumatized infants from normal ones, a major part of the study was concerned with devising ways and means by which neonates showing impairment can be separated from those who do not. A rather elaborate scale or battery of test situations was developed. These tapped a variety of functions both in the primarily sensory and the primarily motor realm of behavior. The distinction between those observable aspects of behavior that specifically refer to the sensorium (vision, pain threshold) and those behavior data which involve motor responses in an important way (reflexes, motility) is important to our problem. There is evidence to suggest that the effect of momentary state upon behavior responses may be quite different for these two categories. For it turned out that state needs to be controlled in different ways and to different degrees when dealing with such responses as specific reflexes, as compared to the controls required when one is dealing with visual reactivity or pain threshold. In any case, Graham's work, as well as that of many others, focused upon learning *not* what is the neonate's most frequent and most typical mode of behaving, but with respect to each function what is his *capacity*. Therefore, she and her associates spent much time and thought in order to create conditions which would elicit optimal responses from their small subjects. They tried to make their determinations during a "constant state between waking and sleeping." Everyone who has tried to examine neonates knows that this is easier said than done.

Graham describes with admirable clarity just what she did to counteract conditions which tend to prevent optimal behavior integration on the part of the neonate. For instance, during the testing of pain thresholds it was first necessary to make certain that failure to respond was not a consequence of the babies' having gone soundly asleep while the experiment was in progress (by using data only after a series of positive responses had occurred); but beyond this, irritable babies or babies who were too active for the purpose were provided with a pacifier. It required a separate statistical check to determine that in the case of this particular variety of response the use of a pacifier did not alter the results. The researchers were careful not to apply the pain stimulus at a moment when the baby was sucking very actively. Rather they soothed the baby by giving him the pacifier and then stimulated while the baby was not avidly sucking. Yet when it came to some of the reflexes it turned out that the use of a pacifier was inadmissible. Attempts to make the baby more comfortable by this means did significantly alter the baby's responses, and other means of controlling or manipulating state had to be devised. For the reflexes and related motor responses it was essential that the baby be alert but not irritable if results were to indicate maximal capacity. In this situation Graham and her associates did what mothers do: they tried to soothe the babies by any and all means. When all their methods failed, they did what all of us have done, which is to send the baby back to the nursery. The most exacting among her tests was that of vision in the newborn; it requires the kind of combination between alertness, contentment, and wakefulness which occurs rarely and briefly in the day of the neonate. The investigators learned that one stands the best chance of achieving this by catching an infant just as he awakens and before he has had time to become irritable. Here again, when they were unsuccessful in this and babies remained too drowsy, the researchers tried everything they knew how to do which would alert the baby yet not make him irritable or active. (Incidentally, in their experience, the best method is to hold the baby in a vertical position either upright or upside down.) If I take time to describe some of these details, it is because accumulating experience suggests that the validity and the reliability of behavioral measures in early infancy depend upon just such minutiae. We associate scientific accuracy with rigid control of stimulus conditions and with highly standardized methods of procedure. For behavior measures in neonates I would like to suggest that validity, and therefore also reliability, require operations beyond the usual experimental controls. In order that the baby's condition and the actual stimulus input conform to what is intended, it is necessary to engage in highly flexible manipulations which help to create the one and only condition under which the stimulus ought to be applied.

For the sake of later comparisons, let me briefly summarize what I think Graham and her associates did about state, though only the more important aspects are mentioned here. She did not use a constant interval since the last feeding, which in the past has frequently been held to control state sufficiently. Nor did she use broad categorizations of state, such as are still to be found in much of the literature where babies are categorized as being either awake or asleep, either awake and not crying, or awake and crying, and as either wet or dry. Rather she attempted to define the infant's state by the criterion of how the infant responded to known stimulus conditions. Whenever possible, she intervened and so manipulated her subject as to bring about the behavior which she held to indicate the existence of the desired state. (This may sound like circular reasoning, but as long as state variables are defined by response behaviors not identical with the responses to be measured this is not the case.)

In this study it appears to me that we see complete congruence between the research design, the aims of the research, and the manner in which the problem of state at the neonatal level was dealt with. This is again a study of group differences and is essentially correlational in design. All Graham meant to demonstrate was that among children who during the first days of life manifest certain kinds of behavioral deviations, the incidence of a somewhat abnormal, or at least a relatively lower, level of intellectual functioning will be greater than it is for children who as neonates are able to do everything that one could reasonably expect of them. To judge by some preliminary communications she will be successful in so doing. Hers is a midposition between the approach exemplified by the work of Pasamanick's group (see Knobloch et al., 1956) and a still more individualized and process-oriented approach yet to be described.

It is apparent that many of the behaviors that are included in Graham's assessment of neurological status are identical with behaviors in which we are interested as a possible source of temperamental differences. It follows that if she found these state variables important even when the discrimination to be made was between pathological and normal groups, how much more important must it be for us to control the effects of state on these same behaviors, since within the normal range we cannot expect differences of equal magnitude. This is indeed the burden of my song, but I want to mention a few additional types of control of state that came to my attention primarily through the work of Prechtl and his associates (1958, 1959). This group also was concerned with the problem of selecting at the neonatal level those varieties of neurological impairment which are associated with defective or other deviant development later on. In this investigation indices of birth trauma also were derived from the behavior of the infant himself, and again the state of the organism at the time the measurement was made was viewed as a primary problem. Necessarily these investigators were also interested in obtaining an indication of the neonate's optimal capacity, not the regularity and the most typical behavior manifestations. Thus the Prechtl group used all of the controls for state that have already been mentioned in connection with Graham's work. In some respects, however, the group in the Netherlands went beyond these and thereby enlarged one's notion of what all may be denoted under the general concept of state. I believe it is not accidental that such an inclusion of additional component state variables occurs in the context of a theoretical orientation both somewhat different from that of the Graham group and somewhat broader. For this group, the clinical aim of identifying significantly traumatized infants is interwoven with theoretical interests which the senior author describes as ethoneurological. That is to say, both the factual knowledge and the conceptualizations developed by ethologists are brought to bear upon the ontogeny of human behavior in an effort to illuminate the fundamental nature of the developmental process. One way of highlighting both the differences and similarities between these two essentially neurological pieces of research is to compare the programmatic outline of the research plan as formulated by each. Both groups felt it necessary to describe neonatal behavior in as many of its sensory and motor aspects as possible. In order to make the initial assessment meaningful in the maturational context, both research groups required developmental norms covering neonatal behavior from day 1 onward. That is, with respect to the behaviors in which they were interested, it was clear that the behavior of a normal 1-day-old and a deviant 6-day-old may appear to be identical, and if differences are to be elicited, maturational level must be equated as much as possible. The Graham group made this initial assessment and the development of day-by-day norms in essentially a quantitative manner. (It is true, however, that often the quantum consisted of a number registering a qualitative attribute of behavior.) The Prechtl group subdivided their activities into first a qualitative analysis of newborn behavior and subsequently the development of a method of quantification which, as it happens, is in many ways comparable to that developed by Graham. At this point we come to a temporary parting of the ways. By the time developmental norms had been obtained for the neonatal period and a quantitative scale had been developed, the Graham group was ready to launch their instrument and test its efficacy through follow-up studies. The Prechtl group, on the other hand, used their quantitative methods first in order to study the variations within and among infants that arise in relation to various physiological states. Only after this had been done did they proceed with follow-up studies in order to compare children who had shown evidence of neurological impairment soon after birth with those who had not.

In the following characterization of Prechtl's approach to the problem of state, I draw from an extensive study of rooting behavior and from a mimeographed summary of the larger investigation which has already been referred to (Prechtl, 1958; Prechtl and Dijkstra, 1959).

In this investigation an effort was made to keep the state variable constant by testing babies within the hour before their next scheduled feeding, provided they were neither irritable nor asleep. However, this was the point of departure for controlling state rather than the end point. All of the babies whose behavior was used in constructing the quantitative scale, and certainly all of the babies to whom it was applied in a first effort at validation, were given extensive neurological examinations. These were given to all children, whether they were regarded as traumatized or normal, and included an impressive array of clinical indicators of neonatal well-being (reflexes, tonus, athetoid movements, etc.). For the test of the quantitative scale only those subjects were used who, by this additional criterion of neurological examination, were *at the identical stage of development.* In other words, regardless of whether a baby happened to be 2 days or 4 days old, his performance on the impairment scale was evaluated against the baseline of maturational level, not chronological age in extrauterine terms.

In this connection, I wish to call attention to the fact that up to this point I have spoken of state as though it were necessarily limited to fluctuating physiological conditions. Actually, maturation and development also change the condition of the organism with time, only not as rapidly as is the case with hunger, irritability, or any other physiological variable of that order. Logically, more structural and stable characteristics of the nervous system and the entire organism that change as a function of age should be held separate from individual characteristics for the same reasons as the more rapid fluctuations ordinarily considered under the heading of state. In other words, when what one is studying happens to be individual differences, I believe that maturational level itself can be regarded as a state variable.

In addition to equating the babies for maturational states, the Prechtl group also required that their neonates be in an awake and alert condition. While exploring the effects of state, a large amount of data was actually accumulated but not used in applying the predictive scale. However, as a great service to the rest of us, these other data concerning the systematic effects of state variables were reported separately. Thus alterations in the baby's behavior thought to reflect his condition at the time rather than the essential attributes of the organism are transformed from a source of error to a source of relevant systematic information.

By way of examples I refer to a few of the direct relationships between the state of the infant and his response to specific stimuli that were demonstrated by Prechtl's group. In his very painstaking work on rooting behavior, one of the obvious states requiring detailed investigation was that of hunger. In accordance with what has been reported by many others, it was found that for most responses hunger lowers thresholds while drowsiness raises them. It is often overlooked but clearly demonstrated in Prechtl's study that while this general effect holds for many aspects of infantile behavior, it does not apply to all. For instance, that component of rooting which consists of a protrusion of the lips in response to touch of the mouth area works in an opposite direction. That is to say, drowsiness facilitates the emergence of the response, and fully awake babies give it less regularly, less strongly, and upon relatively more intense stimulation. While we have no time to speculate upon this interesting exception to a fairly general principle of infantile behavior, I cannot forego mentioning that some of the work at our laboratory also shows that babies' responses to tactile stimulation of the lip depart from the usual pattern of reactivity to a great variety of other stimuli, including tactile ones to other body zones. The implication of an observation of this nature is that whenever we wish to use a specific activation as an experimental datum, it is necessary first to determine not merely that the baby is in a generally optimal state. Beyond this, it is necessary to define the particular condition that constitutes an optimal state for the emergence of the particular response in question.

An altogether different kind of state variable is introduced into the picture by observations reported by Prechtl in relation to rooting responses other than lip protrusion. It seems that when the response in question involves larger movements of the body, the baby's precise position is of greater importance than most of us have reckoned with. As is known, babies will very early turn their heads toward the stimulated side in response to tactile or thermal stimulation of the cheek, and under appropriate conditions the lips will then close upon the nipple or any suitable object. If the baby is in the supine with his head already turned toward the side that is to be stimulated, it was found that the head-turning response is relatively weak and latency is longer. However, if in the supine the baby's head also is turned opposite from the side to which stimulation is applied, the head-turning response will be quicker to come and more vigorous. Clinical investigations, especially if they occur in a psychoanalytic framework, are likely to be interested in the vigorousness and efficiency with which newborn babies manage to get themselves next to food. It is quite plausible that certain extremely important adaptations during infantile life may be facilitated by really well-functioning rooting responses. Yet it is clear from what has just been said that one might get a wrong estimate of the relative vigor and efficiency of rooting behavior in the neonate if one standardized the situation in every way but failed to pay attention to the position of the head and, as it turns out, the arm as well. For if the arm on the stimulated side is in a headward position, the response tends to be relatively stronger. If the arm on that same side is placed in a downward position, the head-turning response is weaker. It may be that for many of the behavior activations which are of interest to students of individual difference, a whole new dimension of state problems needs to be considered, namely, the baby's initial position. Once this has come to one's attention, it seems embarrassingly obvious, for we know that reflexes can be elicited properly only from specified initial positions. The interesting fact is that when it comes to psychologically oriented investigations, we seem to have to learn the same thing all over again as it applies to the particular phenomenon that interests us at the moment.

One last example of the kind of thing I have in mind is mentioned simply because it exemplifies the great variety of events and conditions that properly belong with the state variable if we are talking about neonatal behavior. Again with respect the head-turning response, and therefore presumably many other responses as well, it was found that if a baby in a suitable general state is made to startle before the stimulation to the cheek is applied, the resulting response on the baby's part will tend to be stronger than otherwise. An arousal, such as is provided by a startle, seems to facilitate the emergence of subsequent responses to specific stimulation immediately afterward. Presumably, this would be true whether the startle was experimentally induced or spontaneous, and hence one of the extra things that one might have to look out for is the length of the interval since the newborn has produced a generalized arousal response. Again it is not surprising to learn that a more massive activation of the startle variety will so alter the state of the nervous system for some time to come as to alter the baby's response to the next stimulus. The trick is to find out under what conditions and for what kinds of behavior neglect of these sorts of state variables will actually vitiate results.

I now turn to a consideration of developmental research which is conceived within a psychoanalytic frame of reference. There has been an increasing amount of interest and activity in this field, which is not yet completely reflected in the literature. A great many of the important studies now in existence have published only tentative and preliminary reports. Since the problem of state becomes a pressing one only after one is involved with the immediate problem of data collection, it is probable that published formulations as to what investigators are doing about state variables lag behind actual practices and current thinking. Certainly, my thinking has been guided at least as much by what I know of the work going on in various centers as by what I have read. The purpose of this discussion is to present a somewhat schematic overview of the various ways in which the state problem can be dealt with in developmental research. In citing examples drawn from various projects now under way, I may describe procedures that have since been changed and that are not representative for the investigation in question. Actual examples are interwoven with hypothetical ones, and I hope it will be understood that I am not engaged in a description of the research scene, but merely in the clarification of some methodological issues.

Psychoanalytically oriented speculation about relationships between very early behavior characteristics and subsequent patterns of personality development can be grouped into several different types or categories. The differences are a matter of emphasis rather than of principle, and a number of studies combine more than one of the approaches I am about to mention. One line of inquiry might be characterized in an oversimplified fashion somewhat as follows. Beginning at birth each organism possesses a certain number of structural or physiological properties, reflected by certain behavior characteristics, and these are so much an intrinsic part of the individual that they will continue to be present throughout all the changes that come about with growth, maturation, and diverse experience. The basic notion here is that something that is present at birth will also be present throughout childhood and into maturity. Some aspects of behavior that have been speculated about in this way are: activity level, sensory thresholds, a more generalized characteristic variously described as vigor or zest, and tempo. There are a good many documented instances which demonstrate that a particular child remained very much like himself, so to speak, with respect to one or several behavior attributes. I am not aware, however, that any research group has yet succeeded in demonstrating that there is any one of these or other early behavior characteristics that in general tend to remain stable. For example, a recent attempt (Escalona and Heider, 1959) to verify predictions based on infancy observations proved more instructive in pointing to patterns of substantial change than in pointing to behavioral stability, though the latter was encountered in some children with respect to some behavior characteristics. From acquaintance with the raw data obtained in the Yale Child Development Study, I would venture the opinion that those results justify a very similar overall conclusion.

If one were to attempt a study of behavior consistency or stability in this sense, it is by no means obvious how the state variable had best be treated. It is possible to think about these dimensions of infantile behavior, which may or may not be constant, both in terms of capacity and in terms of typical or most frequent modes of responding. If the variable under consideration were such a thing as intensity of reactivity or vigor, one could formulate one's expectation either way. One could say that what will differentiate neonates from one another is the maximum vigor and intensity of which they are capable. The unspoken implication would be that those who are capable of the highest levels of intensity or vigor in responsiveness will tend to be vigorously responsive in general. On the other hand, it is just as plausible to assume that in response to very strong stimuli most healthy babies will reach very similar levels of intensity in their response. They might differ from one another not in terms of maximum capacity, but in terms of the readiness for vigorous reactivity in response to moderate stimulus intensities. If the first of these hypotheses were to be tested, all the controls previously mentioned in order to assure an optimal state for vigorous responsiveness would be appropriate. Since vigor and intensity become manifest through bodily responses, this would include not only those aspects of state having to do with hunger, drowsiness, and the like, but also those details that have to do with body position prior to stimulation, the occurrence of startles, and the like. Assuming that all of these were taken care of and a series of babies had been tested under conditions which permitted emergence of the most vigorous responsiveness of which they are capable, it would of course still be necessary to demonstrate that during the neonatal period at least, this was a constant attribute of the baby. That is to say, one would have to assure oneself that those babies who were high on the continuum of vigor and intensity on day 1 and 2 continued to be high on the same continuum on day 4, 5, and 6. With the single exception of an unpublished doctoral dissertation by Brownfield, I have not been able to find in the literature a conclusive demonstration of the stability of individual differences within the neonatal range. The nearest thing to it is some work by Bridger and Reiser (1959) who demonstrated that certain aspects of responsiveness in terms of heart rate stay significantly the same for a period of two days. Another study in our laboratory is designed to test the consistency of certain behavioral attributes throughout the neonatal period (Birns, 1965). Provided one is ingenious enough to find meaningful and objective criteria for relative vigor and intensity of response at later age groups, the test of this particular hypothesis would offer no further difficulty. If, however, one entertained the notion that neonates differ from one another not so much in terms of the extremes of behavior, but rather in terms of how much energy is typically mobilized under more ordinary and frequent conditions of stimulation, the state variable will offer greater difficulty. It is clearly impossible to run a sizable number of subjects through the entire range of possible stimulating conditions from minimal to maximal and to repeat this on a sufficient number of successive days to establish constancy during the neonatal period. Yet, if the problem is to be dealt with properly, I see nothing for it but to assess the relative vigor of the baby's responsiveness in a variety of states and with varying kinds and degrees of stimulation.

This latter approach, though in a less experimental manner than here proposed and with infants beyond the neonatal level, is in fact being applied, or has been applied, by a number of research groups. Examples might include the longitudinal study carried on under the direction of Pavenstedt, the work at Denver, the Yale study, and the earlier study of infant behavior in Topeka (Escalona et al., 1952). Despite considerable variation among these studies, all of them have in common that the same baby was seen in a variety of states and under a great many different conditions of stimulation. The hope was that certain behavioral tendencies which are brought into any situation by the baby would manifest themselves under a great many different circumstances. Provided the number of units of observation is large enough, it is perfectly conceivable that among a group of infant subjects, everyone might at times be seen to be minimally responsive, everyone might at times be seen to be maximally responsive, and yet there might be impressive and significant differences in terms of frequency distribution which would place some babies at the high end of the continuum, others at the low end, and others in the medium range.

I will use this same example for yet another alternative way of dealing with the state variable on the assumption that what one wishes to search for is an outstanding individual characteristic by way of a behavior tendency, not a difference in capacity. This would consist of applying a principle which has proven itself sound research strategy at older age levels when behavior, to be sure, has already received more stable organization. With respect to vigor or any other variable of this kind, we do not at present know whether the baby's reactivity to any one of a few stimulating conditions, and in any one or a few states, is or is not representative of his behavior under other conditions and in other states. If we knew that a neonate who is awake and alert and responds to a moderately loud sound with a massive body activation is also a neonate who tends to respond strongly and with relatively large segments of his body to most stimulations that come his way, it would be safe to determine what kind of a baby he is (with respect to vigorous bodily activity) from testing him in this and only this situation. In other words, an extensive pilot investigation might show that certain combinations of the infant's state and the type of stimulation applied intercorrelate so highly with his responses in a great variety of other situations in which we are interested, that it would be safe and sound to use only these selected experimental conditions for an assessment of the baby. As far as I can see, this is entirely an empirical question. The amount of work required for the demonstration of the existence of such representative situations is so overwhelming that I would hate to see anyone attempt it unless and until we are very sure indeed that the behavior variable under study is one of profound significance for psychological development.

Another kind of hypothesis, probably more representative of current psychoanalytic thinking, is that some of these same behavioral differences to be found during the neonatal period do not represent a permanent characteristic of the organism, but foreshadow differences in the pattern of later personality functioning. To speak schematically again, one might be interested in activity level or perceptual sensitivity or some other neonatal variable not because one believed that the child's perceptual discrimination or activity level will remain the same, but because one believes that this variable may affect the development of other ego functions. For instance, high activity level in infancy may speculatively be associated with such developmental characteristics as low frustration tolerance, a late and difficult acquisition of the capacity for thought and abstraction, or a relatively greater amount of ambivalence and turbulence in early object relations. Since at the moment we are discussing only how clearly to define and measure early individual differences, the problem of state could be met in much the same way in this context as was enumerated above. Again one would have to decide whether one is talking about difference of capacity or differences in the most frequent and representative pattern of activation and response. However, in this second and more interesting variety of hypothesis formation, the assessment of single responses under highly specific circumstances seems less appropriate. If we think that certain ways of responding as a newborn predispose toward certain patterns of ego development, it must be because we think that these primary and given behavior propensities exert an influence on the baby's experience. If it were true that the more excitable baby is likely to have a more tenuous relationship to the mother and therefore to be more vulnerable to separation anxiety at age 1 or 2 years, it is because we speculate that his infantile experience as a whole will contain more disruptions, more frequent as well as more intense disequilibrium, less dependable regularity, and perhaps less straightforward direct need gratification than would be the case were he less excitable. What we are really interested in is what his earliest behavior has to tell us about the quality of his experience later on, rather than the initial behavior characteristics themselves. A reasonable approximation of the state of affairs might be to say that the more we are interested in the developmental processes that may be facilitated or inhibited by the absence or presence of certain organismic characteristics, the more it is necessary to pay attention to the relationship between the baby's state and the baby's responsiveness.

A third kind of approach to the problem of individual differences in relation to later development is suggested by a number of tentative observations. I refer to the probability that a significant difference among babies may consist of the degree to which their behavior is altered by state variables. There are babies whose behavior appears to vary relatively little and others who show enormous variability. For instance, to the stimulus of an air puff or a sound, some babies will respond with a startle and only a startle as their sole mode of response. At times this may be mild and incomplete and at other times strong and complete, but the difference will remain one of degree. In response to the same stimuli, other babies will now blink, now merely move their fingers or their toes, now grimace, now jerk one foot or one arm, now squirm, or engage in slow flexion, and at still other times respond with a startle. Thus in the last-mentioned case, one observes a far greater variability as a function of the baby's state. Or again, in a pilot study done at our laboratories by Mrs. Birns, it turned out that when babies were given the cold-pressor test in the usual fashion, and were given the same test while a pacifier was in their mouth, many babies responded much less strongly to this stimulus with the pacifier than they did without. Yet there were some babies whose response while they had the pacifier was hardly different from their response without it. Or, to mention a third and very provocative tentative result, it is possible that differences in motility in the awake and the asleep condition have predictive significance. Grace Heider (1966) has analyzed the Topeka infancy data in relation to repeated studies of the same children during preschool and early school years. Through informal communication, I have learned that there appears to be a higher correlation between a discrepancy between sleeping and waking motility in infancy and some aspects of later adaptation than there is between single behavior characteristics such as general activity level and later adaptation characteristics and later patterns of behavior. In particular, those children who as infants were exceedingly active when awake but became very nearly motionless when asleep differ as school-age children from those who as infants showed a large amount of movement both when awake and when asleep. In terms of psychoanalytic conceptions about the function of sleep in the psychic economy, this type of individual difference in early infancy might prove a most rewarding area of investigation. In studies which would focus on this problem, it is apparent that a major aspect of the assessment of individual differences early in life would concern itself not so much with the absolute level or kind of response in any given state, but rather with possible consistencies and discrepancies in the baby's responsiveness through various states.

There are a host of interesting studies of individual differences which circumvent many of the difficulties connected with the assessment of behavior and which rather hope also to circumvent many if not all problems that have to do with the infant's state. I mean the many investigations in which the assessment of the neonate or young infant is made on a psychophysiological level, with or without concomitant observation of behavior. Richmond and his associates (1955, 1959) have gone far in this direction, as has Bridger at our laboratory, and a good many others as well. Here, as in the other approaches, it has not been difficult to establish that very young subjects can be relied upon to differ from one another in their autonomic responses to standard stimuli. The history of the psychophysiological approach to the study of individual differences is instructive. Leaving aside much of the earlier work without which no one would have known what differences to look for and how to measure them, the more recent course might be described as follows. To begin with, we are all very enthusiastic to learn that heart rates, respiratory rates, and many other similar variables show a wide variability among infants and seem to indicate real differences in the functioning of the nervous system at an early age. Then many laboratories began to find it difficult to reproduce their own results or to confirm those obtained by others. Painstaking work by many people in many places made one aware of the complexity of the problem and the technical nicety and statistical sophistication required in order to obtain valid data. As technical implementation became more perfect, and purer measures were obtained, it became difficult to establish a sensible relationship between the intensity of the stimulus and the level of response given by the babies. For the same baby at different times and also among babies, a stimulus of the same intensity was shown to elicit a moderate response sometimes, a very strong response at other times, and a minimal or even a negative one at yet other times. By negative response I mean that heart rate would decrease after the same stimulation which ordinarily leads to an increase.

Based on earlier work of Lacey et al. (1953), which has come to be known as the "law of initial value," Bridger was able to devise a statistical technique which allowed the orderly and lawful nature of these autonomic responses to become apparent. The law of initial value rests on the idea of the importance of state, though, in my judgment, it by no means resolves the entire problem. The principle is that the magnitude of a response needs to be evaluated against the level of functioning that existed immediately prior to the stimulus. Thus if a baby who at the moment has a high heart rate is given a relatively strong stimulus, the increase in response to the stimulus will be small. If the same baby is given the same stimulus at a time when his heart rate happens to be low, the increase in heart rate in response to the stimulus will be large. It has been possible to demonstrate individual differences in autonomic responsivity among neonates once the prestimulus level of autonomic activity is properly accounted for.

There has been a good deal of speculation about the ways in which differences in the functioning of the nervous system measurable by psychophysiological methods may prove meaningful in relation to subsequent development and functioning on a psychological level. There has not yet been a satisfactory study to demonstrate that any of these autonomic variables remain constant during the neonatal period. Assuming that this is in the process of being taken care of in various laboratories, there remains the systematic problem of whether autonomic level prior to stimulation is a sufficient description of the baby's state at the time. Somewhat paradoxically, the reason why prestimulus value alone does not meet the case consists of the very fact that there *are* individual differences on the physiological level. Sufficient information is on hand to know that, for instance, some babies will have a heart rate of 150 while quite aroused and crying, whereas other babies may be peacefully asleep with the same heart rate. For some the maximum capacity is well over 200, others may never go above 160 no matter how agitated they are. If one were to take differences in reactivity to a stimulus at the same basal rate of say 150 as an index of meaningful difference between these two babies and their two nervous systems, one would automatically build in an assumption that might be difficult to substantiate. Who is to say whether a baby who at a given heart rate is somewhere near his maximal rate and who is in a state of considerable arousal can be compared to a baby who at that same heart rate is functioning somewhere near the midpoint of his range and who is not particularly aroused. In psychological terms, the major reason for our interest in these autonomic functions is the reasonable assumption that we are tapping centrally important pathways or mechanisms for the management of excitation—in other words, that we are dealing with focal homeostatic processes. If it is true that many aspects of psychic organization and the homeostatic aspects of psychological phenomena develop through a process of differentiation from the matrix of biological functioning, then it would interest us most how the organism copes with various degrees of arousal and excitation—and this is information not to be had from a mere equation for prestimulus levels.

Little consideration has so far been given to possible ways of dealing with the state problem in investigations which lean upon systematic behavior observation more than upon the experimental method. In most instances, such studies are longitudinal ones, a circumstance which makes it easier to determine the presence of reliable individual differences. If a given subject is relatively lazy while under observation as a neonate and if on many, many other occasions throughout childhood it proves relatively difficult to arouse and excite him, we know wherein he differs from his more energetic peers. At the same time the demonstration of individual characteristics by relying on consistencies over a span of months or years makes it more difficult to know what determined the characteristic in question. While a neonate could not have been greatly affected by his experience with the world about, whatever behavior the child develops later is very certain to be at least in part a consequence of the pattern of existence provided for him by the important figures in his life. Most longitudinal studies of a psychological nature attempt to differentiate between behavior propensities which the child carries into any situation and those behavior characteristics which develop in response to his experience. There is no systematic way of differentiating between these determinants, and some of us believe that a clean separation between the two is not only impractical but theoretically meaningless. However, there remain a number of alternatives as to how studies that are primarily observational in nature can deal with the problem of state. For this portion of the discussion, I think of studies such as the one conducted at Boston University, the work of the Yale group primarily under the direction of Ernst Kris and Katherine Wolf, the psychological part of the program at the Child Research Council in Denver under the direction of John Benjamin. An earlier study by Leitch and myself on the variability of behavior among normal infants also belongs in this category, though it was limited to a cross-sectional appraisal.

What have all of us done about state? The Yale study included a fairly intensive assessment at the neonatal level and, so far as I can see, the problem of state was partly dealt with by exclusion and partly by sheer frequency of observation. The grueling schedule required several observations during each 24-hour period on each of the first several days of life. Whatever the babies happened to be doing was observed, provided they were not involved in some routine manipulation such as feeding. Whatever happened was grist for the mills; and while the response to touch and a sudden change of illumination was usually included, the approach was not at all experimental. What actually happened was that most of the babies most of the time were asleep or drowsy and most of the babies were also occasionally seen while hungry or otherwise mildly active. A situation of this kind facilitates the recognition of certain behavior differences and precludes the detection of others. Since in these babies the process of arousal was seldom studied, what emerged at the neonatal level were primarily differences in postural behavior and motility. If certain postures and types of movement are predominant in the behavior of a certain baby during, for example, six out of eight neonatal observations, while the same postures and types of movement are infrequent or absent in eight out of eight observations on another baby, it is reasonable to conclude that an individual difference with respect to these dimensions of behavior did in fact exist. What cannot be known about neonates studied in this fashion is the degree to which the same differences would still be manifest in other states. Nor can it be known what differences might exist in the activation patterns of these babies, in their sensory discriminations, or in their capacity to respond to soothing or need-gratifying interventions. It is equally true that where neonatal assessments are concerned primarily with the infant's way of responding to excitatory stimuli, such differences as do exist in postural behavior and motility do not readily emerge.

When this same observational approach is brought to bear on infants rather than on neonates, the range of states covered by the observations will, of course, increase. In the Topeka study, as in the frequent observations of the children during the first year of life in the Yale study, as in all the others I have mentioned, the underlying expectation is as follows: if differences between the children exist, and if they are the kind of differences that make a difference, this fact is certain to emerge from multiple observation over a range of states. In the Topeka study, for instance, babies were observed for a period of four hours. In the life of a young baby, four hours include varying degrees of hunger, the eating situation, fatigue and sleeping, and a very large number of different stimulus conditions during the waking periods. The only way of dealing with the problem of state is retrospectively to break the behavior flow into meaningful episodes which consist of behavioral and contextural indications of state in combination with known stimulus conditions and known behavior resultants. This mode of data collection and data analysis again facilitates the recognition of some among the existing individual differences and makes it next to impossible to recognize other equally important ones. For instance, throughout the range of states and situations a certain baby may be conspicuous for the fact that vision seems of predominant importance. He may tend to regard, follow, and gaze with absorption in many situations which from other babies tend to produce primarily body activations, vocalizations, or physiognomic changes. The same baby might also show a greater reactivity in response to visual stimuli than do many of his peers. It is reasonable to infer that this baby as an individual was characterized by the fact that vision played a dominant role in the totality of his experience. The same applies to any aspect of behavior that has an opportunity to manifest itself in response to widely different situations. Yet it is clear that many relevant problems cannot be approached by the method of multiple observations through ranges of state. For one thing, no two children are ever compared under identical circumstances. Two hungry babies or two sleeping babies are not really in the same state, and the naturally occurring succession of external stimulation is different on each and every occasion. In addition, observations of this kind cannot be trusted to reveal either the capacity or the available range of behavior. Instead, it is the frequency distributions in terms of the direction, kind, and relative intensity of responsive behaviors that delineate individual differences.

Considerations of the kind presented in this paper do not lend themselves to either conclusion or summary. Instead I shall briefly enumerate those systematic relationships between the treatment of the state variable and the hoped-for research results that have most impressed me. Modern psychoanalytic ego psychology is interested in the possibility that biological properties of the organism present at birth foreshadow developmental and hence characterological patterns of development. Within the same theoretical framework, it is equally important to search for characteristic patterns of functioning which are largely determined by physiological factors, and which can often be studied by psychophysiological methods. In this latter case, the search is for the identification of vital biopsychological processes which determine the quality and content of early experience and must play a formative role for all later development. The considerations advanced in this paper lead me to believe that these two types of research question require different modes of dealing with the problem of state. In the first case, what is required is either a measurement of capacity and hence optimal state conditions for the response in question, or a function which is demonstrably independent of state. In the second case, what is required is an investigation of the variable effects of different physiological states upon each of the behaviors thought to constitute a source of individual difference. Moreover, whenever we use the behavior of newborns to a known stimulus condition as an index, cognizance and control of state variables include a broader range of circumstance than has usually been included in psychologically oriented studies. I am referring to such things as exact maturational level, body position, preceding excitations, and the like. I am also more impressed than formerly with the necessity of going to greater length than we have usually done in establishing the stability of individual difference throughout the neonatal period. As I tried to describe earlier, any effort to do so again involves first and foremost a systematic control of state variables.

When our studies extend beyond the neonatal level the logical issues remain much the same, but the methodological approaches to the problem increase in number and complexity. Depending upon the main focus of the research problem, the specific aspects of behavior under scrutiny, the number of subjects, and other factors, it is possible to go all the way from allowing the variable of state to randomize in large populations through the inclusion of a range of specified states to the inclusion of any and all states that happen to occur with careful investigation of specific interactions between the state of the organism and the behavior in question. And lastly, though not unrelated to what has gone before, it appears to me that any effort to establish causal or at least antecedent consequent relationships requires that state be kept as constant as possible. If so, this type of study is difficult to combine with an investigation of the nature or the mechanisms involved in the developmental process. On the other hand, if the major interest is to investigate the chain of events which pattern experience and the course of development, state must be allowed to vary, and at this moment I see no way of sufficiently controlling the multiple state variables in order to make research be conclusive in the sense of fully validating a developmental hypothesis.

6

INDIVIDUAL DIFFERENCES AT BIRTH

Implications for Mother-Infant Relationship and Later Development

Anneliese F. Korner, Ph.D. and Rose Grobstein, A.B.

In the last 20 years an increasing number of investigators have become interested in research with infants. While the majority of the studies appearing in the literature deal with the effect of early experience and of maternal deprivation, there has been a steady increase of investigations concerned with the primary endowment with which infants are born. Underlying many of the studies of neonates is the hypothesis that contained in the individual differences at birth may be the rudiments of later characterological and psychosomatic dispositions.

In "Analysis Terminable and Interminable" Freud (1937) stated that "each individual ego is endowed from the beginning with its own peculiar dispositions and tendencies." Hartmann (1950b) expanded on this, linking individual differences in the primary ego apparatuses to later choice of defense and by implication to choice of illness. Lustman (1956) demonstrated differential sensitivity of the erogenous zones among neonates and discussed the ramification of these for potential fixations or arrests in psychosexual development. Fries and Woolf (1953) in their observations of what they termed "congenital activity types" were among the first investigators who tried to capture certain variations in primary ego endowment and to relate these to later personality development. Escalona et al. (1952) and Birns (1965) have investigated individual differences in sensory sensitivity among infants. A host of investigators have studied, and currently are studying, variations in autonomic reactivity among newborns, hoping to detect the physiological antecedents to different types of affect management and the precursors of choices of psychosomatic disease (e.g., Richmond and Lustman, 1955; Bridger and Reiser, 1959; Lipton et al., 1961). Thomas

Reprinted from the *Journal*, 6 : 676–690, 1967.

et al. (1963), through longitudinal contact with parents, demonstrated primary reaction patterns in children, identifiable in early infancy and persistent through later stages of life.

Our own study of the organismic differences among the newborn is governed by several predictive hypotheses (Korner, 1964). We share Hartmann's (1950b) supposition that there may exist individual differences at birth not only in the primary ego apparatuses but also in the "core of differentiation between the ego and the id." These variations may throw an individual cast on the manner in which a child will deal with each maturational task. What may be involved here is not only an inherent difference in the unfolding of his functions, but also differences in experiencing and perceiving universal childhood events.

We also hypothesized that if mutuality between mother and child is to develop, the infant's individuality must evoke differences in mothering (Korner, 1965). Thus, it is not only the mother's conscious and unconscious attitudes, her style, and her child-rearing practices which may shape the mother-infant relationship, but also the infant's own maturational rates, his particular styles of perceiving and experiencing, and what these evoke in maternal response.

THE VARIABLES

The following are some of the variables we have chosen to study. Since this choice evolved from preliminary observation, the description of the variables already contains a discussion of the contrasting ways in which infants behave with regard to these variables.

1. Like many other investigators (Bell, 1960; Birns, 1965; Escalona et al., 1952; Wolff, 1959), we are interested in the neonate's response to visual, auditory, textural, and tactile stimuli. Differences in the readiness to respond to these external stimuli reflect varying degrees of autonomy from the pressures of internal stimuli and a greater or lesser need of a stimulus barrier. We hypothesize that availability to sensory stimuli coupled with the synthesizing capacities to keep from being overwhelmed will affect the rate and depth of both ideational and interpersonal development.

2. Babies vary in the clarity with which they convey that they are hungry or tired. With some, there is no doubt; others convey their internal state much less distinctly. This variable is particularly pertinent to our topic since distinctness of internal state may affect a variety of ego functions as well as the mother-infant relationship. We hypothesize that this variable as well as the variable of self-consistency may influence the infant's capacity to communicate, anticipate, and discriminate. It is easy to see that a baby who is unpredictable and/or unclear in communicating his needs will be confusing to his mother in her caretaking

efforts—a factor that may threaten her self-confidence and beginning feelings of mother-infant mutuality. Also, indistinctness of *experiencing* various internal states may delay the formation of internal sets of expectations and the discrimination between external and internal reality, possibly predisposing to later regression in this discrimination.

3. Many of our observations are directed to the effects of hunger on behavior. Since every organism has to cope with hunger over a lifespan, the study of its effects may reveal particularly enduring reaction patterns. One aspect of this problem is the degree to which hunger tension will disorganize the behavior of a given infant. Peter Wolff (1966) hypothesized that up to a point hunger tension improves hand-mouth coordination, but when it becomes too intense, coordination breaks down. Quite likely, individual differences exist in the point in time and the degree to which the infants' behavior dedifferentiates. Early and/or strong vulnerability to dedifferentiation of behavior with hunger may be the earliest manifestation of a vulnerability to regression under drive tension.

4. Our observations also suggested that there are individual differences at birth in psychosexual disposition. For example, some babies mouth constantly, irrespective of hunger; others do not. We have seen baby boys who have a great many erections and others who do not have a single one over a 9-hour observation period. There are also differences in the quality of mouthing. Some babies are primarily sucking or tonguing, others are chewing. Some infants are spitters, others never spit. Some suck with vigor, others are more passive. In Erikson's terms (1950a), the infant's mouthing may be primarily incorporative, retentive, eliminative, or intrusive in character. The question we are asking is whether an early zone or mode reliance may reflect a lasting and distinctive drive quality. If it does, this may predispose some children more than others to psychosexual fixations.

5. The variable which may involve some of the most central attributes of the infant's later development is the manner in which he defends against overstimulation. This does not imply that defense mechanisms in the psychoanalytic sense are used from birth, but that there exist in each child rudiments which will make the adoption of certain defense mechanisms much more likely than others.

We had the first inkling of differences in dealing with overstimulation when watching various infants during ophthalmological examinations. In this procedure, the physician looks at the eyegrounds by shining a light into the baby's eye after the nurse restrains him and offers her finger with a sterile nipple as a pacifier. Some babies suck more strenuously when the eye examination begins, others stop completely. Urination and defecation evoke crying in some and alerting in others. Some babies respond to the touch of a soft cloth by crying more vigorously, while others quiet. It is as if some infants can deal with excessive stimulation only by diffuse motor discharge, while others respond through motor inhibition and by dealing with one sensation at a time.

These are extreme positions on a continuum of reactions involving perhaps enduring differences in an individual's neurophysiological processes. We can think of many situations in later stages of life where this dichotomy of dealing with intense stimulation exists. For example, some people welcome the distractions of music during dental treatment; others will tolerate no such distraction, needing to stick to the task at hand. Some deal with the impact of stress by seeking the diversion of a movie or a drink; others need to stick with the problem until they achieve a modicum of mastery.

We suspect that babies who consistently freeze in the face of overstimulation may differ radically in their development from babies who persistently respond through motor discharge under similar conditions. The former may adopt more readily cognitive control principles and defenses designed to ward off, to sift, and to make manageable incoming stimuli. Leveling, sharpening, and focusing come to mind as cognitive control principles (Gardner et al., 1959), repression, isolation, rationalization as defense mechanisms. By contrast, one would expect the individuals who consistently react through motor discharge to seek tension reduction through displacement behavior, acting out, and hypermotility. In the cognitive sphere, these individuals may more readily become scanners; they also may never develop as sharp a distinction between seeing and doing or between feeling and acting as their more self-dosing peers. At the same time, novel stimuli may be welcomed and sought after by this group, whereas they may be experienced as painful and may be reduced to a minimum by the other.

The above are examples of some of the variables we are studying. There are others, described in a previous paper (Korner, 1964). In addition, we are gathering data on variations in irritability, soothability, the quality and quantity of motion and sleep patterns. We are also recording individual differences in the proneness toward reflex smiling, in hand-mouth dominance, and in the capacity for self-induced tension reduction.

SAMPLE

The sample of this study consists of 40 bottle-fed 3-day-old neonates. To determine whether parity influences the neonate's behavior as reported by some investigators (Weller and Bell, 1965; Korner and Grobstein, 1966), the sample consists of 10 firstborn and 10 later-born males and 10 firstborn and 10 later-born females. Since it is easy to find individual differences which are not an expression of the infant's behavioral individuality but are an artifact of pre- or postnatal complications, only completely normal, healthy, full-term babies are included in this study. Stringent selection criteria were developed to screen for prenatal maternal health, duration of labor, maternal analgesic dose, mode of delivery, and condition of the infant at birth and thereafter.

METHODS

In order to collect data on each of the variables outlined above and on all other variables we are studying, each baby is observed for 9 hours. During the first 5 hours which are interrupted by a feeding, the observations are free from any experimental interventions. After the next feeding, sensory stimulation experiments are scheduled. These include response to touch, texture, light, sound, and to multiple simultaneous stimuli. They also include trials of visual pursuit of objects.

Standard procedures were developed to insure that the behavioral variations observed are a function of the child's individuality rather than a product of varying conditions of observation. Thus, illumination, temperature, and the position of the baby in which the various observations are made are held constant. The infants are observed dressed in a shirt and without diapers. Since response to sensory stimulation differs in kind and intensity with each state of arousal, to achieve comparability among infants, we do each experiment in the same state of arousal in all infants. (See Escalona's discussion [chap. 5] of the need to control for state of arousal.) In monitoring the states of arousal of deep sleep, irregular sleep, drowsing, alert inactivity, waking activity and crying, we use Wolff's behavioral criteria (1966).

In order to allow for recovery from the birth process and to minimize, at the same time, the effects of differential maternal handling, the observations are made on the third postnatal day. In an effort to avoid diurnal variations, all babies are seen at the same time of day. Since we are very much interested in the effect of hunger tension on a variety of behaviors, our most detailed observations are made in the half hours immediately before and after a feeding and at midpoint. These are the intervals when most of the sensory stimulation experiments are scheduled and when detailed running records are kept of a multitude of behaviors during the first 5 hours of observation which are free from experimental interventions. For example, we record the frequency and duration of various states of arousal and, in the context of these, the incidence of periodic spontaneous discharges as described by Wolff (1966). In recording these we are interested in the individual variations of reflex smiles, erections, startles, and reflex sucks. Also included in these observations are individual manifestations of rapid eye movement during sleep as well as any behavior reflecting zone or mode expression.

During the period free from experimental interventions, we also use a movie camera to record periodic time samples of the infant's behavior. A timer attached to the camera automatically turns the camera on and off, thus taking identical and unselected behavior samples for each child. In this process, we take 1,000 feet of film on each baby spread over a 5-hour period and are accumulating a bank of behavior data on the neonate which can be used by us and other investigators for any number of investigative purposes. The movies provide a permanent and objective record of a multitude of behaviors which, in their frequency and sequence, would be difficult to capture even by multiple observers. Analysis of these behavior samples which are identical in length and in the interval since the last feeding for each child will permit a quantitative comparison among the babies in the variable studied.

With the help of a computer attachment to our projector, we were able to make the analysis of the film data manageable. We can analyze 16, 32, 48, and 96 frame units at a time and in several speeds. In order to avoid subtle changes in frame of reference over time, observer reliabilities of the film data are checked periodically throughout. The reliabilities of scoring the film data are satisfactory. In blocks of 24 ratings on 32 frame units, the average disagreement between score-rescore is less than one in the various dimensions analyzed so far. Responses to the sensory stimulation experiments are recorded by two observers with observer agreements ranging from 86 to 100 percent in the various behavior categories.

Case Illustrations of Contrasting Neonates

We shall now present observations on individual neonates and illustrate how these may affect the prospective mother-infant relationship and later development.

Our first example involves the incidence of reflex smiling. Reflex smiles occur in the newborn usually during irregular sleep, sometimes during drowsing, and only very occasionally during alert inactivity. Reflex smiles range from being faint and barely visible to full-fledged, broad grins. We find marked differences among babies in the incidence of reflex smiling. For example, Baby Girl 5 did not reflex smile a single time during a 3-hour observation period. By contrast, Baby Girl 13 was seen to do this 11 times in the same period, and she smiled so broadly that she bared her gums. If we think in Piaget's (1936) terms, we might predict that, by virtue of having practiced the smiling schema a great deal, the infants given to frequent reflex smiles may also become the earlier social smilers. In one follow-up which we have done, this proved to be the case. We hope to check this hypothesis more systematically at a later time. One thing is certain, judging from our own reaction, even though a reflex smile is not a social smile, it definitely evokes a social response. If anything, a mother will react more strongly to this event than the observers. Thus, a mother who happens to have a baby given to a great deal of reflex smiling may, from the start, socially interact with her infant on more numerous occasions, socially stimulating the infant in turn.

We note very marked differences in the frequency and length of visual alertness episodes in our subjects. For example, Baby Girl 13 had 8 sustained episodes of this kind in a 3-hour period. She readily focused her eyes on a moving object, pursuing it 180 degrees. She also did a lot of reflex smiling and this was noted in one instance when her eyes focused on the moving ring. By contrast, Baby Girl 5 was visually alert at no time during the same period, with the result that the visual pursuit experiments could not even be attempted. The reason we attach such importance to these differences is that visual prehension is one of the very few means at the neonate's disposal to make contact and to take in the environment. The neonate capable of sustained alertness may thus have earlier and more frequent opportunities to learn and to get acquainted with his mother and his environment.

In another study (Korner and Grobstein, 1966), we noted that visual alertness, which occurs spontaneously only on rare occasions even in the most alert newborn, can be induced almost invariably when a crying baby is picked up and put to the shoulder. One of the implications of our findings is that the newborn picked up for crying will have many more opportunities to scan the environment than the infant left crying in his crib. Considering only the opportunities or visual experiences, Baby 5 may need the experience of being picked up more acutely than Baby 13, who was capable of providing visual experiences for herself. We have here a good example of how organismic and environmental factors combine to create differences in the impact of universal childhood experiences. A baby who alerts infrequently and who shows other signs of high sensory thresholds may show the effect of maternal neglect much more acutely than an infant who is more receptive to environmental stimuli.

We note marked variations in the soothability of our subjects. When picked up, Baby Boy 15 stopped crying in 3 out of 3 trials after only one or two whimpers. After he was put down, the soothing effects lasted for a short period in 2 out of the 3 trials. Baby Girl 1, by contrast, stopped crying only in 1 out of 3 trials, persisted in crying for a long time while on the shoulder, and showed no soothing effects after being put down. The impact of an infant who is difficult to soothe as compared with a baby who is easy to comfort must have differential effects on a mother's feelings of competence and relatedness to her infant. In addition, babies vary in their readiness to make postural adjustments to the person holding them. Baby Boy 15 was cuddly when held to the shoulder; Baby Girl 1 was stiff. From observations of this kind, we suspect that babies, from the start, may differ in the degree to which they avail themselves of others for purposes of tension reduction, which may, in turn, influence the intensity and depth of their interpersonal development.

The contrasts between Babies 9 and 15 may highlight markedly different distributions in ego and drive endowment in two infants. Baby Boy 15 had a great many penile erections throughout the 9-hour observation period. His erections occurred after urination as often as before, in many different states of arousal, and were sustained over long periods of time. One may, of course, question the instinctual drive specificity of neonatal erections and prefer to think of this phenomenon as a nonspecific discharge, equivalent and interchangeable with other spontaneous discharges such as startles and reflex sucks (Wolff, 1966), or as a tensional manifestation (Halverson, 1940). The question still remains why some male infants primarily use this particular channel of discharge or tension release, while others use different channels. Also, even if neonatal erections do not represent an expression of a drive derivative, the experience of an infant who has a lot of penile erections must be different from the child who does not. In all likelihood, his penis will become cathected earlier and more strongly. In the case of Baby 15, the high incidence of erections was coupled with other indications suggesting that he might be more heavily endowed on the instinctual than the ego side. For example, when he tried to establish hand-mouth contact, it was his mouth which searched for the hand, and not the hand for the mouth. To date, our observations suggest that more commonly babies seek hand-mouth contact with the hand taking the initiative. Also, Baby 15's coordination in hand-mouth contacting was very poor. He was thus less well developed than his peers in what could be described as one of the earliest executive ego functions. Furthermore, he was not particularly sensitive to sensory stimuli. This suggests that this boy may have less autonomy from the pressures of internal stimuli than some of his age-mates who are more responsive to external stimuli.

Baby Boy 9 was the opposite of Baby Boy 15 in all of the characteristics described. He did not have a single erection during the entire 9-hour observation period. In his case, the hand was searching for the mouth and very successfully so. He was an expert and sustained thumb and fist sucker, and he was capable, unlike most neonates, to coordinate both his hands to his mouth. Altogether, passive-receptive functions were much less developed than active ones. For example, his auditory receptivity was limited. By contrast, he looked around very actively and frequently. He behaved like no other child we have seen to date when he was offered a sterile nipple. On several occasions he ejected it and cried. He apparently could not accept an object in his mouth when he was given one, while at the same time striving avidly to incorporate one by himself. If we have captured enduring characteristics of these two children, what might this mean for their later development? One might predict that the 3-day-old "do-it-yourselfer" might renounce the sway of the pleasure principle much earlier than his more instinctively endowed peer. Also, depending on their respective mother's position regarding instinctual and mastery strivings, Baby 15 may engender pride, alarm, awe or aversion, while Baby 9 may please his mother with his skills or disappoint her for depriving her of gratifying him.

Our observations suggest that the fate of an individual's oral strivings may depend on additional factors to the ones most commonly stressed in the literature. We find confirmation that there are great variations in the *intensity* of the oral drive. These are expressed in the differences in frequency and persistence of oral activities. We also observe differences in the *quality* of oral behavior. This quality may lend direction to later organ mode choice. Certainly the mother's style of dealing with her own orality, her way of feeding and weaning the infant, will leave an impact on the child's oral disposition. But, in addition to these commonly stressed factors, there may be organismic propensities in the infant which have no direct connection with oral behavior but may, in combination with oral activities, influence the infant's oral strivings. For example, the quality and quantity of an infant's motor activity may have a direct bearing on the degree to which the mouth becomes cathected. Observation suggests that a diffusely active baby very rarely succeeds in establishing hand-mouth contact, in contrast to the more slowly moving and better coordinated infants. Observation also suggests that babies who will not remain in the supine position, preferring to lie on their sides, will have little difficulty reaching their thumbs. At the same time, we note that success in hand-mouth contact often leads to further success: that the mouth having become cathected through self-stimulation will be easier to find on subsequent trials. It should be stressed that these hypotheses were derived from observation of single children in whom this association of behaviors was noted. Our film data will help us test statistically how generally true these interrelationships are.

FOLLOW-UP CONSIDERATIONS

The methodological and conceptual problems involved in longitudinal follow-up have been well described by Bell (1959–60), Escalona et al.

(1952), Stone and Onqué (1959), Thomas et al. (1963), and Wenar and Wenar (1963). The following are some of the pitfalls involved in prospective studies: frequently, masses of data are collected, which, by virtue of their bulk, are difficult to analyze and contain but little relevant information regarding the hypotheses in question. All too often the search for continuities between early and later development is too literal and underestimates the unpredictable permutations of the developmental process. By contrast, it can also happen that continuities are obscured by inappropriate choices of conceptual and methodological approaches designed to find the links between early and later development.

One fact emerges very clearly in any consideration of follow-up work: optimal research strategies vary with the developmental phenomenon to be followed. For example, in the case of the study here described, the observations made during the newborn period have both long- and short-range implications. The infant's proneness to smiling, his soothability and irritability, the clearness with which he communicates his need state should have immediate, though subtle effects on the mother-infant relationship. The subtle and reciprocal influences between the infant's organismic characteristics and the mother's handling can be captured only by very closely spaced follow-up observations immediately after discharge from the newborn nursery. The same is true if one wishes to study the developmental process involved in the gradual transformation of neonatal behaviors into the behaviors of early infancy. By contrast, low or high sensory thresholds, the tendency to freeze or discharge through motor pathways in the face of overstimulation, or to regress under the pressures of need tension are apt to influence the quality of many long-range developmental acquisitions. If one chooses to study these long-range influences, closely spaced, truly longitudinal follow-up from birth is not the strategy of choice and can become, in fact, an unsurmountable encumbrance. The solution for this kind of follow-up lies in the formulation of predictive hypotheses of the ways in which neonatal characteristics may manifest themselves in later development, very much as we have tried to do in this study through the choice of our variables. Since the concern is with the *persistence* of certain characteristics, it would be strategic to follow only those infants who shortly after birth show a given trait with unusual clarity and strength. This is based on the assumption that the development of an infant with an average disposition, growing up in an "average expectable environment" (Hartmann, 1939), will proceed fairly unremarkably. All one would be able to witness in such a case would be the products of a successful amalgamation between the child's original tendencies and his environmental influences. This is apt to be less true in infants who are strongly endowed in one direction or another since the persistency of a trait, or the derivative of a trait, may largely depend on its original strength. If the object of a follow-up is to trace the consistencies in individual development, the results of intermittent evaluations may be more poignant than truly longitudinal contact. These evaluations will be most productive when timed to coincide with developmental phases in which the predicted behavioral traits are apt to be clearly in evidence.[1]

1. For a more recent and complete overview of the author's work on individual differences in newborns, see Korner (1971, 1974).

7

INFANT-CARETAKER INTERACTIONS

Stephen L. Bennett, M.D.

Current early child development research has been concerned not only with neonatal capacities and responses such as learning, perceptual discrimination, and autonomic reactivity, but also with varieties of handling which in interaction can result in experiences of great difference, what Escalona (1968) calls "specific patterns of experience."

One distinctive characteristic of the newborn is the rhythm and organization of the arousal and inhibitory systems. This is expressed in behavior as the sleep-wakefulness-hunger cycle. One segment of this cycle, alertness, or the alert inactive state, is of special interest because visual discrimination (Fantz, 1967) is dependent on its presence. It has been demonstrated (Lipsitt, 1967) that the newborn is capable of simple learning processes, most likely during the alert state. From the view of interaction, this state serves as a powerful stimulus to the mother (Brazelton, 1962), who can enlarge or diminish it by arousing or calming techniques.

In a beginning study of the development of alertness (Bennett, 1968), the characteristics of arousal, inhibition (Birns, 1965, Birns et al., 1965), and attentiveness (Wolff, 1965) were studied in 16 3-day-old infants. These characteristics were responded to by the mother in ways that were influenced both by the infant's behavior and by the mother's personality and socioeconomic background. Maternal apathy and depression can result in no face-to-face encounter, no play, and even in a total absence of visual stimulation. On the other hand, maternal ebullience and skill in handling can lead to extraordinarily complex combinations of arousal and calming. These in turn can create a striking involvement between mother and infant during the first weeks. This has to be seen in order to grasp what happens. Experienced mothers and baby nurses have skills which are not in the repertoire of the usual child development worker; that is, by rocking, tickling, singing to, and stroking the infant's face, they can produce a state of aroused vigilance

Reprinted from the *Journal*, 10 : 321–335, 1971.

evidenced by an intensely animated expression. Cultural and economic factors play a role in determining what states are sponsored. For example, the mother with many children in a small apartment is more apt to stress pacification, while the mother with help and adequate room can afford to use arousal techniques and encourage early play.

The purpose of this paper is to describe some observations and reflections that followed from a study of 10 infants during the first weeks of life. Studying the infant's alert state and his ability to fix and follow visually (literally looking him in the eyes) suggested that this state could be appraised in terms of the early roots of affectual and social responses. These elements are often studied at the time of the beginning of the smile reflex at 2 months. What at first appeared to be tangential observation led, on further consideration, to some thoughts on the relation between newborn characteristics and perception of differences by the caretaker.

METHOD

The spirit and setting for this study were essential for the results and ideas that followed. The earlier studies were carried out on 3-day-old infants who were to leave the hospital the next day. They were observed in the newborn nursery during the busy morning hours. There were several reasons for this: the infants were then more apt to be alert; there was a similarity to home conditions, a wish for training in later home observations plus a personal bias against studies in isolation. With 3-day-olds it was possible to sit in the corner by a crib and watch inconspicuously.

With a second group of infants a very different situation was encountered. These were babies awaiting adoption, the so-called "boarders." The second time I arrived to view a boarder, I was greeted by a baby nurse with, "Here's Daddy come to play," and the infant was handed to me. My first play was lumpish, but with practice in the manipulation of states I obtained a feel for maternal handling. For example, the amount of rocking necessary to maintain alertness in an irritable baby can be rated. One technique used was to place the infant on my lap, to catch the reflection of my face in his pupil, and then to try to obtain fixation. A second method was to move my head to see if there was following. Special attention was paid to facial expressions and any excitations that suggested affect.

It was during observations of 10 boarders seen twice a week for the first month of life that I gradually became aware of, or rather stopped ignoring, an interesting phenomenon—that each of these infants had acquired a unique personality. By this I mean that if one listened to the chatter and talk of the baby nurses, the light banter about the infants, and especially to the singing, scolding, and soothing words during changing, bathing, feeding, and play, each baby emerged with his own special story. This stream of talk was offered with lightness, ease, and lack of self-consciousness. By comparison the mother's talk to her 3-day-old infant was similar but sparse and restrained, lacking the openness of the nurses' words. The same kind of talk by the baby nurses also touched the 3-day-old infants. However, unless there was something extraordinary about a newborn, there was insufficient time during the usual 4-day hospital stay for a story to be elaborated.

The categories of cues that were the source of these associations are of some interest. Features and body configuration, hands and hair were anatomical cues. It was striking how a rich and full head of hair could attract attention to one infant in a busy nursery. Feeding behavior was another source of personality construction with emphasis on such traits as greed, piggishness, and cooperation.

The characteristics of sleep and wakefulness were picked up by mothers at 3 days of age in observations such as, "He's lazy, he likes to sleep a lot," and, "He's a smart baby, he looks at me."

THREE PERSONALITY SKETCHES

Three black infants were chosen for description here because their stay overlapped and hence they were frequently compared. I shall examine the special characteristics of the infants' alert state during the first several weeks of life, since this was the original focus of the study. Those cues and characteristics which were actually responded to and commented on by the caretakers will be emphasized. These perceptions were elaborated into a unique personality, which in turn influenced subsequent perception of the infant's behavior. This in turn had real consequences of the greatest importance for the handling and care offered the child.

Smith

Baby boy Smith was a sturdy and handsome infant. At the age of 3 days he showed characteristics which he maintained throughout: long periods of alertness without much fussing, an easy arousal, awakening without a cry, and easy calming. These characteristics were viewed as indicative of a basic good nature, and a solid and happy temperament.

It was difficult to obtain fixation and following in a small arc when the baby was 10 days old; one could do so only in quiet periods. From the beginning, the staff felt that he made a quick and sociable engagement to others. At first this was due to his easily obtained alertness, rather than to ease of visual contact.

One characteristic seen clearly at 10 days was his ability to maintain alertness even with a high activity level. This combination of sustained alertness and high activity was his most striking characteristic and the one that attracted the most attention; it was interpreted as exuberance, a high-spirited and zestful approach to the world. His cry was robust, full, and infrequent; the staff regarded it as a spunky and rightful demand, and it was responded to well.

When he was 13 days old, fixation and following in a wide arc could be obtained easily by anyone who came in contact with him. It was this appearance of good visual contact that led the staff to engage with him so quickly. Out of this vis-à-vis arose an empathic relationship with several of the nurses and an increase in their care and interest; at the same time the elaborateness of the stories told about him increased as well. At times when he was not in direct visual contact with the nurses his wide eyes and active search movement suggested a quality of high intelligence.

At 17 days, there was "affect" present. By this I mean that during the alert state when he was engaged visually as well as by singing, tickling, and rocking, facial expressions appeared which had not been present earlier and which in an adult would have been associated with affect. One such expression involved opening his mouth and pursing his lips. These, together with the wide eyes, suggested a greeting and acknowledgment of the viewer's presence. These expressions grew more varied as time went on and appeared responsible for another jump in the interest and imagination expended on him.

Although these observations were continued into the second month, the characteristics described above were the basis for the associations about him. In this child and the others it was by the second week that the "personality" blossomed.

The basic personality given Smitty, as he was quickly nicknamed, was friendliness and good nature. Early the most frequent comment was, "He's a very smart baby." Although his patience was appreciated, he was respected because if his appropriate demands were not met, he could become loud and assertive. It was stated that he was all boy and would undoubtedly be successful with the girls. One comment made in the second week was, "Oh, Smitty, you've been out with girls all night, you bad boy, you naughty boy." This talk was accompanied by hugging, kissing, and comments that he loved to be loved.

The amount of care he received was considerable for a busy nursery. He would be carried about while simple chores were performed and during discussions and shift changes would usually be held on someone's lap.

Brown

Baby girl Brown had a round face with fat cheeks and strikingly rich curly black hair. When first seen at 5 days, she showed clear and easily elicited alertness. Spontaneous search movements, fixation, and following were all quickly obtained. Her facial expressions were for the most part bland, but there were periods of evident vigilance which were usually interpreted as brightness. During drowsiness there were clear smiles; these appeared to be the smiles occurring in the drowsy REM state described by Emde and Koenig (1969). These smiles were more striking in this infant than in most others and were seen by most observers as evidence of warmth and sociability.

Brown had the ability to sustain alertness for long periods. Her activity level was below average. In the main, she cried with hunger, but she was easily pacified. During most of the morning a glance in her direction would encounter her profuse hair, her wide full eyes, and her motionless body.

Observations at 8 and 12 days did not reveal much change. At 15 days an expressiveness was present which was not merely a consequence of increased vigilance, but which emerged from a greater variety of more active facial movements, especially involving the mouth. There were bursts of activity with arm-waving during which her face was more animated. Comments made about her at 15 days were, "She's a lovely baby and has a nice personality." "She's very contented, not like Jones [to be described], ugh!" "She has a lot of expression to her face and you can get her to smile." "When she wakes up, she's quiet; I don't like babies that cry as soon as they awake."

At 18 days, the facial mobility was noted chiefly during her bursts of excitability. During one 5-minute period of full alertness with no evidence of REMs, three smiles were present, plus one pleasant animated look and a coo.

Her main characteristics were a regularity of states and low activity level. The staff viewed this as evidence of a calm and even temper, as well as niceness and femininity. There were cries, but they were not urgent except with hunger; and this was interpreted as modesty and consideration. Except for the smiles, her facial expressions were sparse compared to the other babies.

The "personality" that emerged was that of a simple feminine girl who was not sexy or flirtatious. There was a modesty and good taste about the reasonableness of her demands. There were various opinions about the vividness of her personality: some felt that she was just nice, while others saw some sparkle. The common view was that she would be lucky to get Smitty.

The amount of handling she received was average. She was hugged and cuddled at times of bathing, feeding, and changing, and variably at other times depending on who felt she was cute. This child had an early capacity for visual engagement, but did not receive much face-to-face contact. It should be noted that in a busy nursery there was not often time for this special type of play.

Jones

Baby boy Jones, born the same day as Brown (both were 5 weeks younger than Smith), was lean and well-built. At 5 days it was noted that he was easy to awaken but would not remain alert unless jiggled and rocked. There was questionable fixation. When tickled he would quickly become aroused and his trunk would writhe and his limbs flail. There were many wry facial expressions during drowsiness.

By 8 days, Jones had developed a stable, alert state. His activity level was average, but there were bouts of excitation during which the wry facial expressions were seen. A smile was observed during drowsiness. No fixation was obtained.

At 15 days, the child displayed a general irritability. Crying was frequent. He was unable to maintain alertness without intervention. After a half minute of activity with limb-thrashing, the trunk would stiffen and he would begin to cry unless some sort of pacification was initiated. The amount of rocking required was small and for the most part if he was merely held he remained calm. A type of body movement that most observers found to be unpleasant was a sudden stiffening of his trunk; this was often interpreted as a rejection. This response to physical contact appears to be one of the types described by Schaffer and Emerson (1964a). Fixation and following were obtainable, but visual engagement alone did not sustain alertness, as it did in other infants. During bursts of excitation there were responses that could be called affect, an increased activity level, plus facial expression that communicated emotion. The look involved widening of the eyes and expansion of the cheeks, an expression of perplexity which was not pleasant to look at.

A staff attitude appeared during the second week which became outspoken by 15 days. It amounted to: this is a disagreeable child. "He's irritable and tightens up and gets purple so he doesn't get held as much. I think that in 20 years you'll find that he is brain-damaged."

One time when I came to examine him the joking comment was, "Don't you dare wake him up; if you do, you can take him home with you." While Jones was being commented on, Smitty was being held and alertly maintained visual contact with the nurse's face. "Hi, fresh face, we'll give you peas and carrots. Jones is not the nice baby, Smitty is. I know it's not a nice thing to say about Jones, but it's as if he knows he's not wanted in the world."

At 18 days, the above-described behavior and the corresponding staff attitudes toward him continued. In the comments about him his perceived personality took on vividness and fixity. Though he was seen as pained and unhappy, he alienated himself from sympathy by what was interpreted as his attitude of open rejection and disagreeableness.

By his greed, defiance, and unreasonable rages he made himself an outcast. He was considered a controversial figure by the staff, and the force of his sorrow and rage provoked pity and guilt.

Interplay

To demonstrate the imagined personalities, let me describe a half-hour morning period which catches the interplay between the 3 infants as well as the differences in care.

Brown and Jones were 18 days and Smith was 56 days old. When I entered the nursery I was greeted with, "Jones is waiting for you; I'm not going near that spastic kid." He was in the treatment room because of his crying and Smith was being played with in the nurses' station while a discussion was under way as to what solid foods to feed him. "Look at Smitty, he's full of beans, he needs a steak. Do you hear that Jones in there, he should be dumped somewhere." After 15 minutes of play with Smith, the conversation again turned to Jones and someone went in and picked him up, and the crying stopped immediately. "Now that's what I call a spoiled baby." He was put down after a minute, the crying resumed, and the comment was "Oh, come off it." Another nurse teased, "All she wants to do is play with the quiet baby and not the crying one." Later, commenting on Brown who had been quietly staring with wide eyes, "Look at that doll Brown; Smitty and she have been making goo-goo eyes at each other." At the end of 30 minutes Smith had been played with the entire time, Jones had been picked up for a minute, and Brown had been talked to one time.

Reappraisal

The openness and the expressiveness of the attitudes toward Jones led to a reevaluation of the techniques used to handle him. At the end of a half hour of discussion, the staff felt that he required more soothing, and plans were made to send for a rocking chair. The very fact that it could be said of him, "If you don't behave yourself, I'll break your head," made it possible to identify this child's behavior and make appropriate changes. If it were not for this openness, he would be just one more crying baby in a nursery of 20 of them. It was the fabricated personality that caught the essential features of his arousal system and made it possible to plan a thoughtful approach.

At 22 days, a grim facial expression was again observed. After I held Jones for over an hour with gentle rocking, his face became less tense, several times there was truly a coo with an associated affect that was almost positive. A question that the staff posed continually was whether such soothing would spoil him.

At 29 days, for the first time Jones was observed to be awake and not crying. Wakefulness was tolerated for 15 minutes without a cry. The facial expression was more mobile and, although not pleasant, did not have the previous pained look. Comments were made that he had changed, that he enjoyed attention now, and was more responsive and cried less. When he was held, his eyes engaged and his cheeks stroked, his face appeared to relax; this, together with his wide eyes, produced an impression of mild positive affect.

Departure

An epilogue came the following week after all 3 babies had been placed in foster homes by the Welfare Department. Smitty's brightness and charm were missed, but it was felt that this would carry him through wherever he went. Brown was not mentioned, and there was an expression of relief at the peace and quiet that came on Jones's leaving. His fate was felt to be dependent on the patience and forbearance of the foster mother.

DISCUSSION

There is a human propensity to create anthropomorphic fantasies, to endow animals, nature, and intrapsychic structures with human characteristics. Bibring et al. (1961) have described the changing maternal fantasies and defenses which become fluid and later stabilize during the crises of pregnancy and delivery. From the standpoint of a theoretical view of infancy, the baby nurses and most mothers are Kleinians in the sense that they attribute to the newborn qualities of sexuality, rage, greed, and sophisticated object ties. It was these fantasies, the imagined beginning of a unique individual, which created for the baby nurses the framework within which subtle engagements could be made. If there were no fantasies, there was no "personality" and the care offered could only be rigid and routine.

Our concern here is what are the cues out of which the story is fashioned? The baby nurses, who had no previous investment in the infant, took a physiognomic approach and picked up certain signals which would otherwise be hard to pinpoint. Better than anyone else, Darwin (1873) describes the facial configurations which signal emotion in animals, human infants, and adults. Current communication theory (Ruesch, 1956) elaborates on the cues other than verbal that are important in human exchanges.

Of all the baby's cues, the most compelling were offered by his eyes. Wide bright eyes, especially with search movements, were seen as signs of intelligence and curiosity. A subtle movement that empathically produces a sense of social recognition is a sudden widening of the eyes. This is usually part of an orienting reflex (Lynn, 1966), but seems nevertheless to send the message of "what is it." There is a special quality of brightness of the eyes which can be seen during vis-à-vis and other more aroused periods of alertness. This, together with the widening of the eyes, communicates a sense of relationship with the infant during the first month, a sequence which is as striking as the smile reflex of a few weeks later. Darwin describes this well: "A bright and sparkling eye is as characteristic of a pleased or amused state of mind, as is the retraction of the corners of the mouth and the upper lip with the wrinkles thus produced."

The specific interaction of eye-to-eye contact between mother and infant has been reviewed by Robson (1967). He points out that the strangeness about the new infant diminishes with vis-à-vis. This is how the mother can begin to love the new creature well before the striking engagement of the social smile occurs. Of 16 infant and mother pairs studied (Bennett, 1968) only 4 displayed clear attempts by the mother to establish eye contact. These were the same mothers who used arousing techniques specifically to encourage alertness and who also played with their infants after a feeding. This early vis-à-vis has two consequences. One is that the presentation of what Wolff (1965) calls an "interesting, nonperemptory visual stimulus" can prolong alertness. As Rheingold (1961) comments, the human face is the most interesting stimulus available. From personal observations of some bare ghetto dwellings, I would add that it may be about the only one. In the early weeks there appear to be some social and affectlike responses as well. These occur almost exclusively during the aroused state, best obtained by long visual engagement and accompanying auditory and visual stimuli. It is important to note that these expressions are subtle, transient, and not easily seen unless there is close visual contact.

One compelling set of cues arises from mouth movements. Viewed from a distance, these movements appeared to be chewing or rooting. When experienced directly, however, or if the caretaker-infant interaction is closely observed, they appear to be approach or greeting responses. They occur occasionally during neutral, unengaged alert states. In the main, they are evident during visual stimulation, especially in the state of arousal caretakers can engender when they engage an infant with tickling, rocking, and singing. At this time the infant will open his mouth, circle and purse his lips, and sustain this for several seconds. This is often accompanied by tongue thrusts as well as body quivers and small thrusts of the head forward. The latter is most easily noted if the infant's head is held with the hand cupping the neck so that tensing of the neck muscles can be felt even without visible movement. These responses, especially when accompanied by the widening of the eyes, are as compelling as the social smile at 6 weeks. Peiper (1963) makes brief reference to this type of mouth movement in what appear to be older infants. It can be clearly seen at 2 and 3 days in some infants, and the caretaker will often be drawn into this facial play and mimic the infant's movements. A systematic study of these responses is planned with emphasis on their ontogenesis and state relations. This pursing of the lips with the accompanying head thrusts along with head and extremity movements during social engagement have a similarity to gaping in birds (Tinbergen, 1951). (This comment has previously been made about the early smile by Freedman, 1964.)

Other striking cues at about 2 weeks (Stechler and Latz, 1966) were certain affectlike expressions which can occur as part of the aroused behavior accompanying vis-à-vis. These may portray pleasure or displeasure. The Stechler and Latz study described the pleasurable affect of a home-reared infant at 10 days and a ward infant at 15. A difference was also noted between the infants studied here in respect to the time of occurrence and the type of these affectlike expressions. A speculative question is: do these differences have some relation to the amount of visual stimulation, i.e., are these early milestones influenced by previous handling? So far the expressions I have seen have included the looooning of the face into a grinlike pleasurable glow, plus a tight frownlike expression.

Activity level has a clear effect on the way the infant is perceived because the same facial expression is seen differently depending on the associated degree of arousal. The difference in the way Smith and Brown were viewed by the staff was largely influenced by the activity level.

There are a variety of facial expressions which can be seen during the early REM state (Roffwarg et al., 1966). This raises the question of their relationship to configurations which occur during alertness. A systematic study of such expressions, notably the smile and frown, has been undertaken by Emde and Koenig (1969a, 1969b). They describe the smile that occurs during the drowsy REM state and point out that it is usually interpreted by the caretaker as a social response, especially when it is noted right after a feeding.

The process of development involves an interaction between a genetically determined ontogenetic schedule and the experiential moldings of caretakers. Ultimately this leads to stable characteristics in the mother-child relationship. One approach to the understanding of this complex process is based on studying short time periods (Wenar and Wenar, 1963). There are directions and themes in development (Bell, 1968). For example, it should be possible to pick out mother-child pairs where the thrust of change comes at a specific time from one side or from the other. One source of confusion is to assume that early individual differences of "temperament" are genetically based (Thomas et al., 1963). It is precisely some of these varieties of temperament that evolve out of the complex mother-child interchange during the first weeks.

That frequently used model of social transactions, the two-way feedback system (Miller et al., 1960), can also be used in the first weeks of life. Separate phases of this system have been described in the last several years. There appear to be individual differences in the early alert inactive state (Korner, 1964; Wolff, 1965), but no large-scale series has been presented. Any increase in alertness necessarily increases availability to external stimulation. Activity level also can determine the amount of stimulation (Schaffer, 1966). Stechler and Latz (1966) have described milestones in the ontogenesis of attention and arousal during the first several weeks. Carpenter and Stechler (1967) offer evidence that by the second week an infant can discriminate the mother's face from a mannikin; they suggest that an internal representation had developed. The different physiological states within alertness have been emphasized by Lewis et al. (1966) for older infants and by Stechler et al. (1966) for newborns.

Early maternal behavior has a clear impact on visual and arousal systems (White and Castle, 1964; Korner and Grobstein, 1966; Moss and Robson, 1967). The state of the infant in turn affects maternal handling (Levy, 1958; Moss, 1967). As Wolff (1965) points out, meaningful encounters with the environment are one of the critical factors which maintain alertness in infancy. Sander et al. (1970) describe a correlation between maternal handling and the infant's broad rhythms of sleep and wakefulness within the first 10 days. Wolff (1963b) has caught the details of these early processes with charm and subtlety in his description of the first weeks of an infant in a Boston Irish family. Mother-child pairs which end in pathology, due in part to deviant handling of arousal systems, have been described by Fish (chap. 15) and Brody (1967). The larger biological implications of these themes of organization and specificity have been considered by Weiss (1970).

Gewirtz (1968) has asserted that the main importance of these early behaviors, especially facial expressions, may be their effect on the caretakers who make the major decisions about the infant. He suggests that infants in foster care should be taught "charm," i.e., that positive social responses should be conditioned. Although concerned with later responses such as smiling and vocalizations, this could apply as readily to the behaviors described in this paper.

SUMMARY

Early characteristics of the infant's state include alertness, visual behavior, activity level, and facial movements. These may suggest affect and approach responses, and thus serve as cues which allow the caretaker to construct a fantasy about the infant's "personality." In the infants described here, this construct was clearly apparent by the second week. It served either to facilitate the complex interchange and feedback which can occur between child and caretaker, or to impede it. Some early infant characteristics can be modified by the care offered: for example, alertness can be inhibited or augmented. During a given small time segment the initiative for a specific system can be taken by either caretaker or child; usually it comes about through an interaction of the two. It is out of this complex process that an early and unique style and temperament can develop.

8

THE MOTHER'S ROLE IN INFANT DEVELOPMENT

A Review

Marion Blank, Ph.D.

Mother-child interaction has been a subject of considerable interest for many years. It is generally accepted that mothering affects the child's development. However, there is considerable controversy about which patterns of mothering influence the child and what processes are involved. Because of the difficulties in human mother-child research, it is not possible at present to offer any definite answers to these problems. However, a review of the major ideas pursued to date seems valuable both: (1) to evaluate the theories that have been proposed, (2) to indicate the lines for future research.

THE QUESTION OF BIOLOGICAL ENDOWMENT

Any discussion of mother-child interaction inevitably raises questions about the role of constitutional differences in development. This problem, however, cannot be effectively considered in this paper since there are, at present, no adequate techniques for determining a person's basic endowment. Even within a few days after birth, the infant's behavior may be influenced by caretaking practices (Marquis, 1941). To overcome this difficulty, measurements have been made shortly after birth. However, behavior, even at birth, may be determined by prenatal environmental factors, such as maternal stress (Sontag, 1940, 1941).

Innate abilities are important at any stage of development since they can be assumed to exert a continuing influence on behavior. It is extremely difficult, however, to define significant patterns of innate functioning in the newborn. In comparison to an infant of a few months, a neonate's behavior is severely limited. As a result, it is difficult to select

Reprinted from the *Journal,* 3 : 89–105, 1964.

indices of behavior which are forerunners of more complex actions, or even which correlate with later behavior. The infant's developmental level at birth, emphasized as a possible factor in later performance, has yielded negative results in predicting sensorimotor functioning (Shirley, 1933; Bayley, 1949; Campbell and Weech, 1941). In the few studies in which there have been follow-ups of other measures such as physical development and activity level, these measures have not been effective in satisfactorily differentiating infants after a few months (Weech and Campbell, 1941; Campbell and Weech, 1941; Fries, 1944).

These data do not reject the influence of innate patterns in later behavior. They do indicate, however, that at present the "basic equipment" of the child must be viewed as an undefined factor in most work concerned with environmental influences in infant development.

Although mother-infant studies have been hampered by these problems, the main limitations on research in this area have come from two other sources: (1) the assumption that sensorimotor development is governed almost solely by maturation, and (2) the inadequacies in measurements of maternal behavior. Both trends deserve further elaboration since they indicate the pitfalls which have hampered progress in this field.

MATURATION AND SENSORIMOTOR DEVELOPMENT

Although there have been numerous studies concerned with the effects of maternal care on the "psychological well-being" of the infant (e.g., colic, sleep disturbances), there has been little research on the environmental influences on sensorimotor development. For years, the significant correlations between IQs of parents and older children influenced much of infant testing. For example, attempts were made to correlate the baby's developmental scores with socioeconomic variables since these are indicative of parental IQ (Bayley and Jones, 1937). The failure to obtain correlations with either the child's own later IQ or with various measures of social status led to the conclusion that differences in rates of development were unrelated to later intellectual ability and were due almost solely to maturation. This conclusion had the effect of limiting research on environmental influences in infancy. For example, Sontag et al. (1958), in studying environmental factors and patterns of mental growth, excluded children under 3 years because "it seems reasonable to suppose that learnings in the first few years of life are relatively more dependent upon physiological and maturational factors" (p. 138).

This conclusion also stemmed from the generally negative results of the studies on direct training of skills in infancy (Gesell, 1954; Landreth, 1958). From these studies, it was concluded that the developmental sequence proceeds independently of environmental pressures. This work, however, assumed a direct cause and effect relationship between specific training and the development of particular skills. As a result, less direct stimulation, which might have been relevant to the skills tested, was not denied to the controls (Fowler, 1962). Therefore, before rejecting the hypothesis of environmental influences, more adequate controls of environmental stimulation must be applied. Significantly, there have been some recent reports of alterations in the developmental sequence when environmental conditions were markedly restricted (Dennis, 1960; Hindley, 1957).

The uniformity of the developmental sequence in unrelated spheres (e.g., prehension, locomotion) is cited as additional evidence of the negligible role of environment on sensorimotor development (Shirley, 1933). However, McCarthy's (1960) findings of the interdependence of achievements in such apparently unrelated spheres as locomotion and vocalization suggest that the uniformity of the sequence may not be completely autonomous. It should also be noted that later intelligence reveals a marked uniformity in the sequence of its stages (Piaget, 1936; Inhelder, 1953; Zazzo, 1953). Numerous studies indicate that this uniformity does not preclude the influence of environmental factors (Sontag et al., 1958; Skodak and Skeels, 1949; Kent and Davis, 1957; Mundy, 1957).

In addition, maturation does not fully explain such specific phenomena in infant behavior as the slow rate of development in institutionalized children (Dennis, 1960; Goldfarb, 1945), the variability in an infant's developmental quotients even within the infancy period (Bayley, 1949; Shirley, 1933; Campbell and Weech, 1941), and alterations in the developmental sequence when marked environmental restrictions exist (Dennis, 1960; Hindley, 1957).

These data indicate that even such basic development as sensorimotor functioning may be influenced by the environment. There are numerous environmental factors which can affect an infant's development (e.g., prematurity, illness, sensory deprivation). However, because of her central role in the infant's life, emphasis can justly be placed on the significance of the mother or mother figure. Therefore, a major problem is to understand more fully the effects the mother may have on the infant's development. In order to achieve this, it is necessary to determine how maternal behavior can be assessed.

MEASUREMENT OF MATERNAL BEHAVIOR

The lack of an adequate theoretical model has been a major feature of mother-child research. Although theories of personality development, particularly psychoanalysis, have influenced work in this area, the broad clinical hypotheses of psychoanalytic theory cannot be readily subjected to controlled experimental investigation (Ainsworth and Bowlby, 1954; Escalona, 1958). The selection of indices of maternal behavior for study has therefore lacked a clear rationale. Initial efforts were directed mainly at relating specifc and discrete child care practices (e.g., breast feeding) with particular behavior in the child (e.g., oral activity). As the review by Orlansky (1949) showed, these attempts have yielded negative results.

With the failure of this approach, studies of mothering began to include maternal attitudes as more sensitive indicators of significant environmental factors. Attitudes, although perhaps more relevant than readily defined variables such as economic status, are difficult to assess. Many studies, as a result, have been marked by "inadequately defined measuring tools; the use of ambiguous or ethically loaded concepts; the use of nonrepresentative groups with resulting overgeneralizations" (Plutchik and Kronovet, 1959, p. 174).

In an effort to overcome some of these difficulties, scales of maternal behavior have been developed (Schaefer, 1959; Schaefer and Bell, 1958; Schaefer et al., 1959; Champney, 1941a, 1941b). Although these scales represent an improved attempt to measure rather complex interpersonal behaviors, they still have many limitations. For example, several of these scales (Champney, 1941a, 1941b; Schaefer and Bell, 1958) were constructed on an *a priori* basis of what the investigators thought likely to be relevant rather than on the basis of direct observations of mother-child interaction. This method has the potential disadvantages of omitting significant factors, as well as including irrelevant variables. The most common failing has been the latter, namely, making the scales overly comprehensive since they are frequently used in longitudinal studies where it is deemed desirable that the same scale be applicable to children of all ages. For example, many commonly used scales include items concerning the content of what the mother says to the child, even though this is probably not relevant to mothering situations with young infants.

Implicit in this criticism is the hypothesis that the developmental capacities of the child will determine, in part, the relevance of different parental behaviors. That is, the child's ability to perceive and thus be influenced by particular parental behaviors will depend upon his developmental level. In addition, it is suggested that because of children's changing capacities and interests with age, as the child grows older, the same parental behaviors will exert different types and degrees of influence.

Well-documented studies of normative behavior (Gesell, 1954; Shirley, 1933; Piaget, 1936, 1945) demonstrate qualitatively different abilities in children at different ages. It is only reasonable to hypothesize that different environmental factors will be relevant to these changing capacities of the child. The variations with age in the preferred modalities of sensation—e.g., visual, tactile (Werner, 1948)—are further evidence for the concept that environmental influences vary according to the age of the child. For example, whereas physical sensations such as warmth and light are of particular importance in infancy, opportunities for socialization and freedom of movement dominate the interests and activities of toddlers. Even within the same age period, the various areas of development in the child (e.g., perception, emotion, motor) can be seen to be influenced by different environmental factors (Yarrow, 1961).

These data have important implications for the study of parent-child interactions. The commonly discussed "good" mother-child relationship implies, in part, a search for continuing, stable parental characteristics (patience, encouragement, tenderness) which enable the mother to cope with the child. If, as hypothesized, different parental behaviors are relevant at different periods, a mother, even though maintaining stable characteristics, may handle a child appropriately at one age and not at another. Conversely, a mother who shows significant changes in behavior over time may be an able parent if the changes are adapted to the developmental characteristics of the child. In opposition to this hypothesis, it might be argued that certain basic qualities are necessary to children of all ages (e.g., love) even though these qualities have to be demonstrated in different ways according to the child's age (e.g., an infant will require bodily contact, a 10-year-old will require verbal reassurance). It remains to be demonstrated whether there is any correlation between varying manifestations of these basic underlying qualities.

Coleman et al. (1953) presented a similar position in a discussion of four clinical examples of mother-child interaction. They particularly emphasize the need for parents to adapt to the changing circumstances presented by a developing child. Although they stress the importance of recognizing changes in parental attitudes even within the infancy period, they do not define precisely how these changes in attitudes are reflected in parental behavior, nor do they propose a scheme by which this could be determined.

Before such a scheme could be offered, it would be necessary first to define which parental behaviors are significant at different ages. The data outlined above do not offer a precise answer to this problem. They do suggest, however, that significant environmental factors, including parental behavior, can be determined if the mother-child situation is analyzed into component parts according to both the child's developmental level and the area of his behavior under investigation. Thus, the significant environmental variables should be defined separately for each major developmental stage of the child. Using this orientation, the literature dealing with the mother-infant relationship will be surveyed to indicate what maternal behaviors are most significant to the child during the sensorimotor stage of development. This period was selected since sensorimotor ability involves the child's initial development of the skills essential for his adaptation to his surroundings.

The Maternal Role

So far, the major evidence that maternal care can significantly influence human infant development has come from situations of maternal deprivation (e.g., institutions). Though the extent of the damage may have been overestimated (Dennis, 1960; Bowlby, 1958b), numerous studies confirm the detrimental effects of maternal deprivation on many aspects of development (Dennis, 1960; Pringle and Bossio, 1958; Pringle and Tanner, 1958; Goldfarb, 1945).

What remains much less clear is the interpretation placed upon these results. For many years, the emphasis was placed upon the importance of a warm, loving maternal figure as being essential for normal development in the infant (Bowlby, 1951; Spitz, 1945b, 1946; Ribble, 1943). More recently, this explanation has been challenged and the detrimental effects of institutionalization in infancy have been attributed to the lack of adequate stimulation (O'Connor, 1956; Casler, 1961; Yarrow, 1961). Work from the animal sphere particularly has been cited in support of this view.

Thus, quite different interpretations are offered to explain the same phenomena. Of course, these views may not be mutually exclusive; that is, a warm, loving mother may be found to be one who provides the optimum physical care and stimulation of the child. This, however, remains to be demonstrated. In addition, most attempts to analyze significant features of accepting mothers have stressed the attitudes of the mother toward the child, as opposed to her physical stimulation of him (Brody, 1956; Coleman et al., 1953). In trying to settle these issues, it should be noted that both of these theories emphasize that the infant's physiological state makes certain requirements for normal development and that failure to fulfill these requirements leads to retardation or arrest of development. Therefore, in evaluating these theories, it is essential first to determine the effects on infant behavior of changes in the specific environmental variables deemed important by each theory.

Unfortunately, there have been few studies which have tried to define or manipulate the environmental variables which may be significant for the human infant. Commonly, unusual situations (e.g., institutions) have been relied upon to suggest ways in which major differences in caretaking practices affect the child. These studies, although not definitive, offer valuable leads for further research. For example, a study comparing premature and maturely born infants (Drillien, 1959) indicated that maternal competence is a major influence in infant development. It was found that, by 2 years of age, prematurely born singletons reared in the most favorable environmental conditions, with particular emphasis on maternal efficiency, were nearly equal to the maturely born children in both weight and height. Drillien also reports that although premature infants achieved lower developmental scores at 2 years than did the maturely born, these differences were "not nearly so obvious" (1959, p. 39) when the maternal care was good. Efficiency of maternal care referred solely to the adequacy of the physical care given to the child in such areas as cleanliness, feeding habits, and management of training problems. It might be argued that the most efficient mothers took better care of themselves during the pregnancy and so gave birth to the potentially healthiest children. However, some mothers showed changes in efficiency with time so that they were differentially adequate with the same child at different ages. In addition, the adequacy of the care given to different children in the family varied noticeably in that a mother was competent with one child and not with another. Before accepting these results as definitive, it is necessary to analyze more carefully the factors involved in competence of maternal care. It may be that competent care is highly correlated with other variables (e.g., attentiveness) which may facilitate development. Nevertheless, Drillien's findings reinforce the need to study finite aspects of maternal care as opposed to emphasizing solely the general relationship between the mother and child.

Studies of different cultures are also relevant to understanding mother-child interaction since they offer an opportunity to observe the effects of widely differing child-rearing practices. In a study of almost 800 infants, Arai et al. (1958) relate the departure of Japanese children from the Gesell norms to methods of child care which exist in Japan. For example, they ascribe the initially slow motor development of Japanese infants to methods of handling which give limited attention to the child and which include clothing that restricts movement. Significantly, there is a spurt in motor development at 20 weeks, about the age when the baby is no longer frequently alone in the cradle, but is instead carried on the mother's back for most of the day. Thus, in addition to the generally accepted importance of attention, physical freedom may be a significant environmental variable in infancy.

This conclusion is supported by a study of Williams and Scott (1953). They found that some groups of black infants were accelerated in gross motor behavior not because of racial characteristics, but rather because of their handling in areas related to physical movement. Advanced motor development was found among the black infants from low socioeconomic groups where contact with adults and freedom of movement were relatively unrestricted. By contrast, in the upper socioeconomic groups, where these conditions did not exist, black infants displayed significantly lower levels of motor development. Other practices which also correlated with socioeconomic class, but which seem independent of motor ability (e.g., breast feeding) did not correlate with motor scores, suggesting that the methods of handling physical activity directly facilitated or inhibited the child's motor development.

Rheingold (1960) made one of the first attempts to isolate discrete behavioral effects of "natural" versus atypical environments in her observations of the caretaking activities administered to a small sample of 3-month-old infants raised in their own homes in comparison to infants raised in institutions. Only minimal differences were found. However, there was an indication that because of the "caretaking practices," hand activities were somewhat restricted in the institutionalized group. These differences, although slight, may be significant since they occurred as early as 3 months and affected the important developmental area of prehension. For example, the hand activities of the institutionalized children may have been restricted by the lack of toys and other objects which are more readily available to home-reared children. Thus, one source of the growing variation found between home- and institution-reared infants may result from differences in the particular stimuli (in this case, objects) which are available to each type of child.

In spite of the differences in hand activities, important questions are raised by the absence of differences in other areas of behavior in this study. Deleterious effects of institutionalization on infant behavior at somewhat older ages have been commonly reported (Dennis, 1960; Goldfarb, 1945; Spitz, 1945b, 1946). The age differences of the samples in these studies suggest that child care practices have an increasingly important influence on the child's development as he grows older. Findings by Tsumori and Inage (1958) support this hypothesis. In this study, the relationships between maternal care and the infant's developmental scores were not significant at 2 months. By 6 months, however, the child's rating on social development was significantly correlated with variables such as contact with the mother. It appears that as the infant grows older, his developing capacities make him both more sensitive to, and more dependent upon, the type of care he receives.

The increasing influence of maternal care as the child grows older is given further support by an earlier study of Rheingold (1956). She found significant increases in vocalizations and social responsiveness in institutionalized 6-month-old infants when a consistent mother figure attended to them several hours a day for a period of only 8 weeks. Interestingly, although the experimenter placed no pressure on the babies to achieve skills, the experimental group began to show consistently, but not significantly higher performance on tests of postural control and on the Cattell Infant Scale.

These data indicate that the child's behavior is affected by stimulation provided by the mother. It should be noted, however, that in all these studies, the children were allowed some opportunity to develop a relationship with an adult human. Inevitably, the question is raised: could a machine, albeit complicated, adequately reproduce a mother's behavior, at least for the infancy period, or must the infant develop an attachment to a human person for normal development? The need for a relationship with humans, at least by the end of the infancy period (i.e., 2 years), is shown in the observations of psychotic children whose disturbed behavior is strongly associated with an inability to relate to people (Ritvo and Provence, 1953). However, because of the extreme complexity of this illness, it is not possible at present to determine the causal relationships between their interpersonal difficulties and their deficient cognitive functioning.

While the studies cited above do not clarify the importance of a relationship with a human caretaker, they do indicate that at least one vital aspect of the maternal role is the stimulation the mother provides. In addition, they indicate not simply that maternal care influences the child, but rather that specific aspects of maternal behavior affect particular developments in the child, including his learning of sensorimotor skills. A vital question raised by these findings is whether these effects are specific (i.e., affect circumscribed areas of the child's behavior) or general (i.e., affect several areas of his behavior). If the effects are general, it would imply an equivalence among different maternal behaviors; in other words, any one maternal behavior could affect many areas in the child; and conversely, the same effect could be achieved by a number of different behaviors. As a result, the amount, rather than the particular kind, of stimulation might be most significant. In the following section, some considerations relevant to this problem will be discussed.

THE GENERAL AND SPECIFIC EFFECTS OF MATERNAL BEHAVIOR

Several of the studies cited above support the hypothesis of specificity of the effects of maternal behavior (e.g., physical freedom and locomotor development, adequacy of care and rate of physical growth). By contrast, Casler (1961), in reviewing the literature on maternal deprivation, interprets the data to support the hypothesis of the general effects of stimulation. Consistent with this interpretation are studies such as those of Ainsworth (1959) and Geber and Dean (1957), who found that the amount of attention given to the child (e.g., number of hours with the parent) was extremely important in many areas of development (e.g., security displayed with strangers, developmental quotients of the children). Attention, however, is a diffuse concept. More adequate controls on the discrete environmental variables involved in attention are needed before these results can be confirmed.

Nevertheless, it is possible that both the general and specific effects hypotheses are valid. For example, on the basis of animal experimentation, it has been hypothesized that stimuli may have both a general arousal quality and specific effects (Hebb, 1949; Thompson, 1955; Cooper and Zubek, 1958). However, the specific effects of stimulation are said to occur only if the infant has been generally aroused because of the presence of numerous other stimuli. This interpretation may account in part for the significance of a mother figure, since the large variability and flexibility of her behavior allow her to provide simultaneously numerous forms of stimulation to the child. The varied stimuli afforded by her presence not only may arouse the child, but through this arousal cause him to respond more to his environment. Since an infant, during the sensorimotor stage, can learn only by doing, his activity in response to stimulation may enable him to acquire new behaviors. Interestingly, in line with these considerations, Rheingold (1956), in the study cited earlier, suggests that changes in the institutionalized infants who were given more attention were not caused by the increased caretaking itself, but rather that it led them to develop the direct act of "attending." She suggests, therefore, that the increased care did not directly teach the infants skills, but caused them to respond to and utilize their environment more fully.

These factors may be relevant to the lack of alertness of institutionalized children which was reported by Goldfarb (1945). The low level of stimulation usually available may have caused these infants to become generally unresponsive to their environments. As a result, even when stimulation is made available, they may not respond to it. Therefore, in addition to the absence of conditions necessary for normal development, the retardation of these children may be compounded by their developing a mode of functioning which is not conducive to learning, even when appropriate stimuli are made available. Thus, an essential factor is not only the availability of stimulation, but also the rate and manner in which the stimulation is presented to the infant. For example, overly long intervals between stimulation may lead an infant to become generally unresponsive to his environment.

These factors have important implications for attempts to alter behavioral patterns of infants. They suggest that a child cannot readily integrate radical changes with his normal functioning, even when these new conditions are of a supposedly stimulating or beneficial nature. Goldfarb (1945), for example, has found that institution-reared infants did not show significant improvement in functioning even after living in foster homes for several months. On the basis of such data, permanent damage, particularly in the language sphere, has been emphasized as occurring with increasing length of stay in institutions. These data are extremely important because of their implications for the role of early experience on later behavior. Thus, the permanence of the effects of child-rearing practices is a major problem, and some of the more recent evidence bearing on this issue will be presented below.

Permanence of the Effects of Caretaking

Rabin (1958) found that despite somewhat retarded development in infancy, *kibbutz* children showed normal development in later childhood. Since these children are reared from birth in institutionlike nurseries, this finding suggests that the retardation associated with institutionalization need not be permanent. Several factors limit the interpretation of these results; for example, cross-sectional rather than longitudinal samples were used, and the deprivation was not as extreme as that of an institution. However, the group situation which became available to these children at about nursery school age seemed to facilitate their intellectual growth. Thus, it appears that intellectual deficit of a nonsevere type can be overcome if appropriate stimulation is made available.

The lack of permanent effects of maternal care is also indicated in a study by Rheingold (1956). She found that additional nursing care given to institutionalized 6-month-old infants produced significant effects in the infants at the time. A follow-up of these infants at 20 months, however, revealed that these differences were not maintained (Rheingold and Bayley, 1959). It appears, particularly in infancy, that the effects of a particular regime administered for only a short period are not maintained indefinitely.

It is implicit in these results that caretaking regimes must be relatively consistent over long periods of time if the infant is to establish and maintain particular patterns of behavior. A study by Schaffer and Callender (1959) on the reactions of infants to hospitalization reinforces this conclusion. They found that infants under 7 months, when hospitalized, suffered from "perceptual monotony." This is consistent with data above which show the very young infant's need for sensory stimulation to allow normal development. By contrast, infants over 7 months showed marked disruption in behavior which the authors attribute to a general negativism caused by the separation from the mother. However, despite the continued absence of the mother, these infants showed a gradual resumption of normal functioning after several weeks, without the accompanying apathy described by Spitz (1945b, 1946). It appears that relatively normal behavior was possible in the hospital setting once the infants had become accustomed to their new surroundings. Thus, relative consistency in the environment seems essential for the infant to develop stable responses. It is apparent that the mother provides one of the major sources of consistency in the child's environment. However, to determine if the loss of the mother is the crucial feature, it is necessary to compare the reactions of hospitalized infants with those infants who have remained at home, but who have been left by their mothers for a prolonged period.

The implication from these data on consistency is that children need time to adapt to any environmental change, whether of a beneficial or harmful nature. Therefore, in evaluating both the permanence of retardation and the effects of enriched environments on institutionalized children, the length of time after environmental change must be more carefully analyzed.

SUMMARY

In spite of the acknowledged importance of the mother figure, the difficulties in assessing her role have interfered with understanding the ways in which she influences the child. In particular, a major problem has been that the mother-child situation has been treated as a single unit, ignoring the fact that the child is a constantly developing organism. I have suggested that a meaningful analysis of the mother-child situation must recognize that the significant factors in parental care vary according to the child's developmental capacities and interests. This approach emphasizes studying the immediate effects of caretaking practices as opposed to their possible long-term consequences. Following this orientation, the literature was surveyed to suggest some of the significant environmental factors that influence the sensorimotor development of the infant.

The retarded development of physically normal institutionalized children indicates that stimuli normally available to the average infant facilitate the rate of sensorimotor development. The evidence also suggests that this stimulation becomes increasingly important for the infant as he grows older.

Many types of stimuli show similar effects on infants' behavior. In addition to these general effects, specific effects are also indicated. For example, freedom of movement appears to facilitate locomotor development. Therefore, the quality of the stimulation as opposed solely to the quantity of stimulation appears to have significant effects on the infant's development.

An important sensorimotor development is the achievement of stable responses. This stability is dependent upon a consistent environment (see also Blank, 1964). Because he becomes so dependent upon his particular environment, the infant has difficulty in adapting to marked changes in his milieu. The implication of these factors is discussed with particular reference to studies of enriched environments in childhood and the permanence of the effects of child-rearing practices.

9

STYLES AND GAMES IN INFANCY

Justin D. Call, M.D. and Marianne Marschak, Ph.D.

We shall attempt to describe and interpret a somewhat elusive aspect of the interaction between parent and child in the period of mental development from birth through age 3 or 4. We wish to direct attention, not to whether the infant and young child gets fed or not at the right time with the right substances or gratified sufficiently, but to the parent's style of handling the infant and to the spontaneous games which grow out of the parent-child interaction. In a previous communication (Call, 1964) the pertinence of the mother's feeding style, particularly her manner of holding the infant, the presentation of the breast or bottle, and the speed and consistency of her actions with the infant have been detailed and have been found to be crucial and specific to the infant's earliest sensorimotor adaptations to the feeding situation.

What we wish to illustrate in this presentation is a particular aspect of ego development and learning in the infant which does not crucially depend on either gratification or frustration of needs and wishes but is a part of the child's relationship to the mother in a less "vital" connection.

We are referring to the very elements of the mother-child relation, in particular its reciprocity, which seem to defy the requirements of classical experimental control and which nevertheless form the essence of that which makes such a relationship a human one and without which the relationship becomes mechanical and nonhuman. Spitz's paper on the inanimate object (1963) touches upon this subject. He observes that *reciprocity* is the major criterion by which the infant determines if an object is human or nonhuman, contrasting, for example, the nonreciprocating toy doll with the reciprocating human face.

Another study (Marschak and Call, 1965) on normal and autistic 3- and 4-year-old boys in interaction with their parents provided some insight into this reciprocity in normal and severely disturbed children. The normal child replicated the parents' behavior and participated

---

Reprinted from the *Journal*, 5 : 193–210, 1966.

with the parent in the task situation more often, and parent and child were more capable of prolonged (15 seconds or longer) attentiveness to each other than were the autistic child and parent. The normal child remembered and spontaneously initiated an activity previously modeled by the parent. Mutual affective interaction was typical of the normal child and parent. All these forms of reciprocity were rarely observed in the autistic child and his parent unit, which was, however, characterized by other more primitive forms of reciprocity.

For example, in the above study, David, an autistic child, responded to his mother's smiling and squeaking rendition of the sound task (which he and his mother seemed to enjoy) by smiling and squeaking. When his father pronounced the same sound series in a matter-of-fact adult way, David remained mute and his facial expressions did not change. Another disturbed child responded by smiling and playful bunting to the mother's play overture. The child's movements and giggling seemed to anticipate the joint experience of foreheads touching. The mother facilitated his participation by regressing to a level where her voice sounded like that of a small child.

From these research experiences the heuristic value of the concept of style in infant care has emerged and has allowed more meaningful description of some of the more subtle but pertinent aspects of the interaction between parent and child.

Ernst Kris (1951) has suggested that direct observations of the child's development have the greatest value in pointing up areas of maturational development and are less helpful in making clear areas of ego development which emerge from the sphere of conflict. We hypothesize that if the mother's characteristic style of care and the infant's characteristic style of response to the care are taken into account, the sphere of conflict may become more accessible to direct observation.

Style, a conception elaborated by Max Weber (1921) for a theory of society and adapted by Erikson (1950a) to psychoanalytic theory, refers to modes of action, the manner in which an act is performed. We may first think of a motor act, then of processes of communication, and finally of ways of thinking. We may speak eventually of a life style of an individual apart from the style of his culture or his historical period. Style, as applied to the mother's care, characterizes not that which (or what) is done to, for, or with the infant but rather how this process takes place.

Sylvia Brody (1958) described a mother who was having trouble breast feeding her 1-month-old infant. The infant would fall asleep at the breast and when removed would wake up crying. On being put to the breast again, the same cycle would recur. No doubt later the mother would have stated that the breast feeding was unsuccessful because the infant did not respond. Brody suggested that the mother look at and talk with the baby. This proved to be a much more effective form of stimulation than physical stimulation had been and resulted in successful nursing.

Ogden and MacKieth (1955) have called attention to the importance of fully protractile nipples for successful nursing. Mavis Gunther (1961) has observed that if the shape of the nipple is marginal, such that the infant is unable to get the "full feeling" of nipple and areola on the palate and in the mouth, the infant will not suck vigorously. She has been successful in helping mothers position the infant more optimally so as to compensate for an inadequate stimulus configuration. Gunther has also observed that if the nasal air passage is blocked during nursing either by the infant's upper lip or by the mother's breast, the infant "fights" the mother with his fists and will show this behavior subsequently when placed in the nursing position! Again the importance of correct positioning of the infant at the breast to arrange for an optimal air-way along with appropriate attachment is demonstrated. Luis Feder (1964) has suggested that "an extra factor of time is needed to nourish the hungers (oral, tactual, and other sensory needs associated with feeding) with sufficient contemplation and relationships with the stimulus object . . . in order to foster adequate partial incorporation." Here we refer to the process of holding and feeding rather than simply to whether the infant was held or not held for feeding—to the mother's style of feeding. Thus by style is meant that which is characteristic, distinctive, special, in reference to the infant's care or the infant's responses. The concept of style forces the investigator to look at a series or a configuration of events as well as at repetitive patterns of interpersonal behavior.

To observe and analyze the mother's play is useful for two reasons. The mother's play, in particular the specific games between child and mother, shows the mother's style quite distinctly. Moreover, as the child develops, these games become modified and thus present a means of evaluating the developmental process (Call and Liverman, 1963). Anthony (1964) reports how in working therapeutically with a little girl a "moon game," originally a part of the relationship with the mother, was made available to the therapist and used to understand and resolve some of the basic issues of the neurosis.

Motion picture photography has been utilized as one of the means by which these processes of care and interaction have been analyzed. A follow-up of earlier work and a sampling of some newer data from our ongoing research will now be presented.

First, let us contrast feeding styles in two breast-feeding mothers. Peter was the first mother's fifth child. The mother had been successful in nursing all of her others and was very skillful at inserting a large amount of nipple, areola, and breast into the infant's mouth. This infant had learned to anticipate the insertion of the mother's breast at the eighth feeding and when placed in the feeding position opened his mouth widely in order to accommodate the mother's active insertion of nipple, areola, and breast. Follow-up 3 months later showed that the infant opened his mouth widely when the tongue blade was slowly advanced to the mouth as he had done earlier with the breast. By contrast, Danny's mother was always somewhat slow in advancing the infant to the breast, and in this process the infant, once having established the cue that the breast was imminent from the mother's holding position, would turn his head from side to side and, very often, even after grabbing hold of the nipple, continued turning his head from side to side. This often led to the "wrong side rooting." This pattern persisted for some months. Danny's mother was very interested in her infant and loved to observe and watch him. She usually spent 45 minutes to an hour with each feeding and when she weaned her infant at 7 months, she became somewhat depressed. Later we found that there was a close identification of herself with the infant which was based upon her own history of parental loss in infancy.

At 3 years, we studied the interaction of Danny and his parents as one of the normal children in the sample of the study referred to previously (Marschak and Call, 1965) using a series of tasks which the parent is given to perform with the child (see also Marschak, 1960). In the peekaboo game, in contrast to most mothers who hide their faces behind their hands and peek through their fingers at the child, Danny's mother hid her face for a relatively long period of time behind a sheet of paper. This behavior reminded one of her feeding style, of her slowness in lifting Danny to the nipple. Both situations reflected some manipulativeness and her objective factual interest, which were, however, coupled with an intense involvement with the child. Danny "learned" the mother's hesitancy, one component of her total style, via the mechanism of identification. Danny's mother reinforced his learning by handing him a sheet of paper. He followed her nonverbal cue and held the paper over his face. His imitation could be considered to be an early form of identification. In the same task, the father held the paper over his face very briefly. This had an exhilarating effect upon Danny and he responded with greater animation than with the mother.

In the separation task, when Danny's mother left the room, Danny was at first fixed to his chair and his upper body turned to the door. He was a good boy, as mother told him to be. Except for placing a cup which the mother had given him neatly on the sink counter, he remained seated for about one and a half minutes, then went to the door to bring back the mother. The closeness of the mother's attachment to the child, apparent since his neonatal period, must have been a crucial experiential factor in his ego formation and accounted partly for his immobilization during the separation task. One might say that without mother, Danny could not act. With her, he could act only within her defined limits.

Danny was shown to be emotionally less "fused" with his father than with his mother. During the separation task in the father's session, he displayed freedom of movement and initiative. He got up on his chair, stepped on father's chair, and shuttled back and forth. He was able to overcome his disillusionment (about father leaving) by inventing a game which had such diverse components as motor and fantasy activity, the creation of a father surrogate (the chair), and achievement of superiority over the father (being taller than father).

During the free play with clay in the mother's session Danny seemed initially interested in the clay, touched it, and made a doughnut as his mother suggested. By that time, his mother had spread her fingers, held out her dirty hands away from her body, and was unable to use them. Danny then became quite anxious, extended his hands, and wanted them washed off. The clay situation points out an area of significant difficulty between mother and child. Danny's mother had been unable to toilet train him. She had difficulty with both of her sons in this regard, being very anxious and consistently unable to structure the training situation, her fear being that her boys would rebel against training, which they indeed did. Deeper understanding of the mother's anxiety and indecisiveness revealed that she feared she would make them resent being trained. She herself had experienced a demanding, harsh training from her grandmother who had assumed responsibility for this after her parents were divorced when she was 2. She had resented the training, could not show it, and feared her children would feel the same way. This was intimately bound up with her fear of loss of love and being abandoned by grandmother if she complained or resisted openly. Here is a conflictual element of the mother's ego being reflected in the child via identificatory imitation. This learning differs by the degree of reversibility from the more transient learning of the mother's peekaboo style which he only initiated upon a direct cue.

In the behavioral interaction during the pat-a-cake game, the similarity of the mother's and father's version of the game was striking. The father's movements were, however, more expansive and his facial expressions less controlled. This difference was mirrored by Danny. The same expansive and free behavior was seen in a spontaneous whirling game which the father initiated with Danny.

CONTRASTING GAMES IN TWO MOTHER-INFANT PAIRS

In the hospital (age 2 days) Dale's head had been adequately supported with the infant close to the mother's body. At home the mother's holding position left the head relatively unsupported and unstable with the infant at some distance from her body. At 4½ weeks a serious estrangement between the parents and between the mother and her baby took place. She no longer was able to maintain support, either physical or psychological, of the infant. When the baby was 5½ weeks old, his mother initiated a game which consisted of brushing the bottle nipple over the infant's mouth several times quickly, then drawing it out of reach. Of this the mother said, "It's no fun [for the mother] when he doesn't snap for it." At 2 months of age Dale was observed to consistently turn his head and body away from the mother while being held for feeding in the mother's left arm. The baby was fed by the father about one third of the time and was held in his right arm. When held by the father, the baby always turned toward the father, looking in his face. All of the positive social responses in the first 8 months were directed toward the father and when the infant was brought to the unfamiliar clinic setting, he always turned away from the mother and toward the stranger. No stranger or separation anxiety was observed during the first year.

In contrast, the mother of Susan allowed her infant to participate in finding, latching onto, and holding onto the nipple, only shifting her position to reasonable proximity of the infant's mouth. This led to increasing skill on the part of the baby in finding, holding onto, letting go of, and finding the nipple again, first by means of rooting activity and later by kinesthetic and visual cues. Baby Susan developed a game consisting of hyperextension of the head over the mother's lap. This game grew out of the autonomy of head activity, which the mother allowed and encouraged during intervals in nursing, while at the same time providing adequate support and optimum position of head and body. At free moments in nursing, Susan loved to assume this hyperextended position and look at the world upside down, often turning her head from side to side. The mother had designated this as "her game."

COMMENT

A careful review of these early patterns of interaction between parent and child reveals the high degree to which the infant's reflex activities, especially his rooting behavior, head movements, and other orienting behaviors such as flexion and extension may be influenced by the style of care offered by the parent. Benjamin and Tennes (1958) reported a case of pathological head nodding in an infant. The nodding was in the up-and-down direction. When this infant was 2 weeks old, his mother was noted to stimulate his lip in an up-and-down motion with the bottle nipple, like that of Dale's turning to the side in response to his mother's stimulation of his lips with the nipple in the side-to-side direction. The differences in responsiveness of Danny to mother and father and the consistency of his mother's early feeding style with her later style of care for Danny illustrates further the early imitative behavior in the infant as a reflection of the caring style of the parent. Similar early imitative patterns have been cited by Brazelton and Young (1964) and Benjamin (1963). While no attempt is being made here to claim an exclusively experiential origin of all of the infant's adaptive behavior, the hypothesis suggested is that the style of care offered by the parent provides a relational matrix which underlies the development of synthetic processes in the ego. These in turn determine the infant's capacity for making identifications with the parents and others in his environment.

DISCUSSION

What we wish to emphasize here is the importance of the reciprocity of maternal and infant's reactions, the accommodation of mother and infant to each other's style of relating, their games which reflect these styles most completely. We have also touched on some early mechanisms of identification which may operate, initially, in game contacts.

The games which grow out of mutual enjoyment and which serve both instinctual and ego needs, particulary in the infant, have come to light. These games of infancy which provide the opportunity for mastery and for gaining bodily and social autonomy are as important for ego development as they are for tension reduction. Since they develop spontaneously between mother and infant, they can be regarded as a precipitant, a condensation, or the essence of that relationship. They also provide for the infant an opportunity to do actively that which he experiences passively. This prepares the way for mastery of the environment—first of the mother herself in the holding position, and then of the larger environment.

One may also detect in these games the opportunity the infant's ego has in shifting back and forth between primary and secondary process levels of functioning. They provide opportunities for regression in the service of the ego and for advancing ego functions. They are not unlike the transitional phenomena to which Winnicott (1953) has addressed himself, an area of intermediate functioning between the self and the object.

The infant's games, style, and play illustrate the interrelationship of ego functions derived from apparatuses of primary autonomy and ego functions which emerge from conflict and gain secondary autonomy as described by Hartmann (1939) and Rapaport (1960a). For example, the traditional game, peekaboo, can be looked upon as an activity in which the infant acquires "competence" in using his vision as White

(1960) would suggest. Such competence and use may be understood as the development of an apparatus of primary autonomy. On the other hand, the peekaboo game can be looked upon as a way the infant has of actively mastering anxiety aroused when the mother is not present, i.e., mastery of object loss. This allows him to establish more firmly the visual memory traces of mother's face when mother's face is not in the visual field. The motivation for this arises from instinctual sources. This "establishing more firmly" means that a time-abiding structure is being established in the ego. This ego structure, built on the basis of conflict (i.e., regarding fear of object loss), gains secondary autonomy as elements of conflict are resolved through mastery. Both primary and secondary autonomous functions interdigitate to set up that which becomes structuralized in the ego.

These games form the basis for what becomes the infant's style in dealing with both his instinctual life and the outer environment. Such styles may form the basis for ways of relating to people, methods of adaptation, as well as learning modes and cognitive styles (Gardner et al., 1959). They are developed through processes of mutual participation and imitation, involving both the parent and the child. These various styles, attitudes, and patterns of infant play form the very matrix of the ego into which specific content in the form of information, memory, skills, language, modes of adaptation, and identifications gain their peculiarly individualistic coloring. They may persist through old age, as Berezin (1964) has suggested.

Infants who experience physical care without reciprocity with the human being offering such care, or infants who have inconsistent mothering, or those with multiple mothering experience are likely to show developmental deviations such as marasmus, rumination, autism, and depression because of the lack of opportunity to identify with a steady, reciprocating, caring person whose style becomes consistently manifest in the life of the infant. Such infants and children show many autoerotic and bizarre patterns of motor and sensory functioning, delayed speech, and deficient capacity for abstract thinking (Provence and Lipton, 1962). These deviations can be understood as resulting from use of their own bodily functions as identificatory models instead of persons. What other ingredients determine the formation of these specific syndromes and separate one from another requires further study.

It may seem that we have talked around the point, or have been too vague in what we have said, or that the data have not been specifically focused. All of these statements are true, but they all serve to emphasize the point we are trying to make, namely, that there is a diffuse gluey substance in the ego which holds everything else together and gives it character.

Perhaps what we have described will have greater meaning if we suggest that this "gluey substance" be related to synthetic processes in the ego which retain and synthesize "abandoned object-cathexes" and "the history of those object-choices" to which Freud (1923) referred in one of his more comprehensive statements on identification:

> When it happens that a person has to give up a sexual object, there quite often ensues an alteration of his ego which can only be described as a setting up of the object inside the ego, as it occurs in melancholia; the exact nature of this substitution is as yet unknown to us. It may be that by this introjection, which is a kind of regression to the mechanism of the oral phase, the ego makes it easier for the object to be given up or renders that process possible. It may be that this identification is the sole condition under which the id can give up its objects. At any rate, the process, especially in the early phases of development, is a very frequent one, and it makes it possible to suppose that the character of the ego is a precipitate of abandoned object-cathexes and that it contains the history of those object-choices . . . the effects of the first identifications made in earliest childhood will be general and lasting [pp. 29, 31].

10

A MICROANALYSIS OF MOTHER-INFANT INTERACTION

Behavior Regulating Social Contact Between a Mother and Her 3½-Month-Old Twins

Daniel N. Stern, M.D.

When observing a mother and infant together, one rapidly gathers many impressions of the relationship: that the mother is "hostile" or "loving" or "controlling" or "responsive," and so on. Similarly, one gathers impressions about the interactive process: that the pair has "worked out" a smooth and easy interactive pattern, or a difficult one that characteristically gets "stuck" at certain interactive points. Many of the events leading to these impressions are age- or task-specific, others are more pervasive. It is generally agreed that the mother-infant relationship plays a large role in influencing the developing personality. Yet it remains unclear exactly which interactive events affect which emerging infant social behaviors with what short- and long-run consequences. Maternal "controlling" behavior, for example, is an abstract statement about the mother which can have no conceivable meaning to an infant. However, some cluster of maternal behaviors repeatedly occurring in some time relationship to specific infant behaviors underlies the impression of "control" and forms a very real part of the infant's experience. Unless we know the specific maternal and infant behaviors involved, we remain at a level of generalization which is no longer proving fruitful. This study attempts to identify some of the specific interactions between defined maternal and infant behaviors in the anticipation that such further detailed knowledge will advance our understanding of the mother-infant relationship and its impact on the development of specific mental functions and operations.

Using a method frame-by-frame film analysis, we have studied in detail an example of "controlling" and "overstimulating" maternal behav-

Reprinted from the *Journal*, 10 : 501–517, 1971.

ior. We have attempted to identify some of the specific infant behaviors which are significantly influenced by, and in turn influence, such an interaction. We have conceptualized and analyzed this interaction in terms of the behaviors of mother and infant which maintain, terminate, avoid, and initiate social contact and stimulation.

Behaviors belonging to the visual system have been chosen for study for several reasons. The visual system is of immense and obvious importance in regulating social behavior. This is especially so for the infant in the first half year of life. By the third month of life, visual behavior is uniquely qualified to perform subtle instant-by-instant regulation of social contact. Visual fixation and pursuit reflexes operate at birth and rapidly reach the adult level of function (Greenman, 1963). An infant's visual accommodative performance achieves an adult level by 3 to 3½ months (White et al., 1964). During the first several months, visual motor behavior (eye movement, eye closure, and head turning) is the only motor system (besides sucking) over which the infant has substantial voluntary control, and it is the only "on-off" perceptual system (Robson, 1967). Through eye closure and head turning, the infant has considerable control over perceptual input, and in a social situation this means control over the amount of visual contact. This control exists long before he has the motor capability of approaching or escaping physically from objects. Even "visually directed reaching" as an executive mode is not fully developed until almost 5 months (White et al., 1964).

Visual contact and the facing position between mother and infant are cardinal attachment behaviors which not only are under mature voluntary control early, but are increasingly thought to play a dominant role in forming the early mother-infant tie (Rheingold, 1961; Robson, 1967; Moss and Robson, 1970). True eye-to-eye contact, beginning at about 6 weeks, has a dramatic effect on mothers, making them feel related to a more responsive person and thus greatly enhancing their interaction with the infant (Wolff, 1963a). Conversely, at this point, infant refusals of eye-to-eye contact begin to be deeply felt by mothers. The face-to-face position is necessary for the normal emergence of the smiling response (Spitz and Wolf, 1946; Ahrens, 1954).

Just as looking, facing, or turning toward makes contact, not looking or facing away breaks contact. Infant gaze aversion and head turning away are thought to be active acts of avoidance which begin as early as the second week of life (Stechler and Latz, 1966; Stechler and Carpenter, 1967).

Eye-to-eye contact and facing positions play significant roles in the social behavior of animals and man (Lorenz, 1953). In human adults, positional body shifts and eye-gaze behavior follow predictable patterns that signal shifts in a dyadic flow (Goffman, 1963; Scheflen, 1965; Kendon, 1967). Head aversion and avoidance of the face-to-face position is one of the most "characteristic and persistent" behaviors of autistic children (Hutt and Ounsted, 1966). Whether or not people face or look at one another, when and for how long they do, and in what manner they look or avoid looking, is obviously of great importance. This is especially so in the preverbal child whose social behavior and comprehension rest exclusively on nonverbal cues.

METHODOLOGY

Subjects and Data Selection

A characteristic social interaction lasting 7 minutes between a 25-year-old primiparous mother and her 3¹/₂-month-old fraternal twin sons was chosen for detailed study. The twins, Mark, the firstborn, and Fred, were in separate infant seats facing the mother, who sat on the floor playing with them. Both infants were calm and alert at the onset of the interaction. After 7 minutes Fred was upset and the mother's efforts to soothe or distract were unsuccessful, in fact worsened the situation.

The clinical impression was that the mother was "controlling," "overstimulating," and "insensitive," in that she imposed the degree and amount of social contact she wanted, at the time she wanted it, with little sensitivity to the infant's wants and responsiveness to her behavior. This impression pertained mainly to her interaction with Fred. Her intrusions with Mark were fewer, shorter, and less intense. He remained calm.

This type of interaction, which was repeatedly observed during each visit, was chosen because: (1) it was highly characteristic of both mother-Fred and mother-Mark interactions; (2) the mother's behavior with Fred conformed to a global classification of maternal behavior of clinical interest; and (3) the mother-Mark interaction occurred at the same time and place as the mother-Fred interaction and each thus provided a basis of comparison for the other.

Clinically we might attribute part of the difference in the interactions to the fact that this mother had some ambivalence toward her husband and about having twins. Her ambivalence appears to have split, with the positive feelings resting more with Mark, whom she identified with herself, and the negative feelings resting more with Fred, the twin "more like father." However, the purpose of this study was not to infer how or why different interactions evolve, but rather to study the structure of the interactive process. For this, we wanted two interactions which "felt" different clinically, and had psychodynamic reasons to be different. We did not know, however, the nature of the differences upon which our impressions rested. Finding the nature of the differences, in terms of interactive events, was the goal of the study.

Data Collection

A portable television camera recorded all activity between mother and infants during three consecutive morning hours in the home. When the study was begun, the infants were 3 months old. Home visits were made initially twice a week for 3 weeks, then every other month through the infants' ninth month, then every 3 months through their fifteenth month. The experimenter interacted as little as possible with mother and child and when possible left the room after focusing the camera. During the infants' naps the mother talked freely to the experimenter in an unstructured interview situation.

Data Reduction and Scoring

Selected portions of the television tapes were kinescoped (converted to 16 mm. motion pictures) and consecutive numbers were printed on each frame of the film. The films were viewed with a hand-operated "movie viewer" which projects the image on a small gridded screen so that the speed and size of any motion can be quantified. The movie viewer allows the experimenter to go back and forth over any number of frames, at any speed, as often as necessary to determine exactly the frame ($1/24$ sec.) in which a motion starts and stops (Condon and Ogston, 1967). A sound reader placed next to the viewer reproduced the sound track on each frame.

The following motions were scored on a time-flow record with an entry for each frame: (1) Infant head motions. These were limited by the infant seat to rotational turns side to side or up and down. The direction of head turn relative to the mother's face was noted. For a $3^{1}/_{2}$-month-old infant, eye-gaze direction is generally synonymous with head-facing direction. Nonetheless, since we could not accurately determine visual fixation from the film, we report only face directions and head turns. (2) and (3) Rotational and nonrotational movements of the mother's head, with notation of direction relative to the infant's face, i.e., turning or moving toward or away from the infant. A third category, "other," included movements that were neither toward nor away from the infant. (4) Motions of the mother's upper extremities with notation of direction toward and away or "other" relative to the infant's face. The mother and infant behaviors were scored separately without reference to the record of the other member. With this scoring method it could be determined every $1/24$ of a second whether or not there was movement of either member, and whether or not the movements were toward or away from the other member. In addition, the face position of each partner relative to the other was on record.

Interrater Reliability

Two trained observers had 96% agreement as to whether a motion occurred or not, and a 95% agreement as to the direction of the motion. The mean error between observers on the starting and stopping of motions was 0.73 frames with a standard error of ±0.86 frames.

RESULTS

Patterns of Making and Breaking Face-to-Face Contact

If the mother and each twin are treated as a separate dyad, there are two dyads: Mother-Mark and Mother-Fred. (The interaction is really a triad, but the infants in this study directed almost no behavior toward one another.) The members of each dyad can engage in four possible dyadic face positions: both facing each other; neither facing; only one or the other facing. We then asked how much face-to-face contact occurs and who is mainly responsible for initiating it and terminating it? How much avoidance of contact occurs and who is responsible for initiating and maintaining it?

Table 1 shows for each dyad what member of the pair terminates which dyadic face position after how much time. The major differences between the two dyads are:

(a) Mark holds the face-to-face position 5 times longer than Fred (5.3 seconds for Mark and 1.1 seconds for Fred).

(b) When Mark and mother are facing each other, either of them is equally likely to terminate the mutual position and look away (55% ter-

Table 1

Dyadic Face Positions: Percent Terminated by Mother, and by Infant: and Duration of Face Position Held Before Termination

DYADIC FACE POSITION		TWIN	Number of Times Position Occurred	% OF POSITION TERMINATIONS		AVERAGE DURATION OF POSITION	
MOTHER	INFANT			Made by Infant	Made by Mother	Before Infant Terminates	Before Mother Terminates
MOTHER FACING	Infant Facing	FRED	49	90	10	1.1secs	9.7secs
		MARK	22	55	45	5.3	6.3
	Infant Facing Away	FRED	59	71	29	2.3	5.8
		MARK	23	22	78	7.1	2.0
MOTHER FACING AWAY	Infant Facing	FRED	33	67	33	1.5	3.0
		MARK	15	53	47	2.7	3.1
	Infant Facing Away	FRED	38	74	26	2.5	7.0
		MARK	24	29	71	14.7	6.0

minated by Mark and 45% by mother). Fred, on the other hand, terminates the face-to-face position with mother 9 times more often than she
does (90% Fred, 10% mother).

(c) When mother is facing Mark, and he is faced away, he will remain
faced away relatively long (7.1 sec.) and the mother will terminate the
position 78% of the time by turning away from him. Fred will not
remain faced away as long (2.3 sec.), and the dyadic face position of
mother facing and Fred away is terminated 71% of the time by Fred
turning back to face the mother, rather than by her turning away as in
Mark's case.

(d) The duration of Mark's facing mother and facing away is dependent on whether or not she is facing him. His behavior changes when
her face position changes. Fred is less discriminative of her behavior.
How long he faces her and faces away is little influenced by her face
position.

In general, Fred can neither stay face to face with mother for long,
nor remain faced away from her for long. Mark stays with her longer
and remains away longer.

Aspects of these facing patterns appear to be stable features of each
infant's social behavior. Table 2 shows that the average duration of the
face-to-face position held by Mark is consistently longer than that held
by Fred. This difference is maintained in interactions with mother at 3,
6, 9, and 14 months, with different strangers at 6, 9, and 14 months,
and with father. The absolute duration of the face-to-face position held
by each infant varies very widely, and depends on the interactant, his
position relative to the infant, the activity engaged in, and the speed
and proximity of attempts to achieve face-to-face contact. Nonetheless,
the difference between the two infants remains in all the interactions
observed, even though the behavior directed at them was roughly similar.

We cannot determine to what extent these characteristic differences
reflect differences in genetic factors (differential thresholds for stimulus intensity, individual scanning patterns, etc.) or result from accommodation to observed differential maternal behavior.

Table 2

Duration (in Seconds) the Infants Hold the Face-to-Face Position Before
Turning Away, at Different Ages and with Different Interactants

PARTNER	Mother	Mother	Mother	Father	#1 Experimenter	Mother	#2 Experimenter	Mother	#3 Experimenter
INFANT AGE	3 Mos. 15 Days	3 Mos. 17 Days	$6\frac{1}{2}$ Mos.	$6\frac{1}{2}$ Mos.	$6\frac{1}{2}$ Mos.	9 Mos.	9 Mos.	14 Mos.	14 Mos.
FRED	1.1	7.1	1.5	1.3	1.3	0.5	1.3	1.0	4.1
MARK	5.3	37.1	6.2	7.8	12.3	4.4	2.8	2.6	7.6

Pair-Specific Contact Terminating Behaviors

How does the infant cue the mother to terminate contact with him? This mother requires different social "cutoff" behaviors from the different twins. If the mother turns to Mark and finds him turned even slightly away, facing elsewhere, she will not approach. After looking at him for an average of 2 seconds, she will turn away from him. If she turns to Fred and finds him turned away, however, she will make further approaches to capture his full attention, rather than turn away. Simple face aversion by Mark acts on the mother as a signal to avoid further contact and to leave him alone. The same signal by Fred brings the opposite. Nonetheless, Fred, too, can make the mother turn away from him. To do so, however, he must avert his face to past 45 degrees away from her and then execute fairly definitive and extreme head turns further away. Fred must utilize different behaviors from Mark to produce the same maternal response.

Differences in Infant Responsivity to Maternal Motions

At $3^1/_2$ months infants can turn their heads rapidly and often. During the 7 minutes of this interaction Fred averaged 1.73 head turns/sec. and Mark 1.34/sec. During periods of greater activity each infant maintained rates around 3 head turns/sec. for many seconds. The changes in head and body motion that accompany adult speech are even faster (Condon and Ogston, 1967). The average duration of each infant head turn was $^1/_4$ sec.; 80% of the head turns fell between $^1/_8$ and $^1/_2$ seconds in duration.

In the course of repeated viewing of short film segments, frame by frame, we noticed a striking and unexpected temporal relatedness between individual infant head movements and the ongoing maternal movements. Initially, infant head movements passed unnoticed unless a head turn altered the dyadic face position. We assumed that these small head movements, when attended to at all, were unrelated to the mother's behavior except indirectly as a function of the infant's activity or arousal level.

With repeated viewing, however, we received the impression that split-second infant head turns away from the mother occurred predominantly when she was approaching the infant, and head turns toward the mother occurred with her withdrawals from the infants' visual field. Two such sequences drawn from the film are shown in figure 1. These behaviors do not require the infant to be facing or looking directly at the mother's behavior. Most, in fact, occur with the infant faced partially away and viewing mother peripherally.

To test the impression that mother and infant execute approximately simultaneous movements conforming to a mutual approach-withdrawal pattern, and to compare each mother-infant dyad with respect to these behaviors, the following analyses were performed.

(a) *The effect of the direction of maternal motion on the direction of infant head turning.* Across each numbered frame we determined whether the infant was turning his head toward or away from the mother. Similarly, across each frame we separately determined whether the mother was moving toward or away from the infant. Knowing the probability for

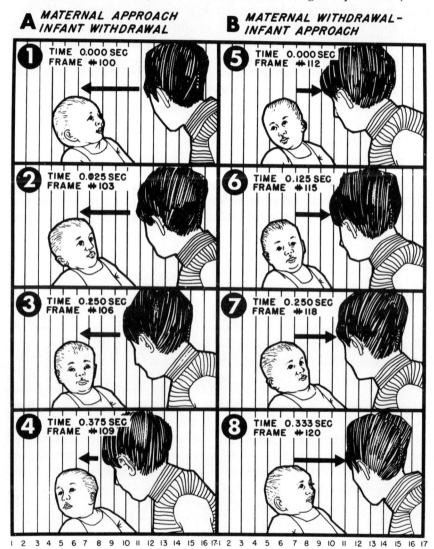

Figure 1

Mutual approach-withdrawal pattern between mother and Fred, age 3½ months, drawn from the film

any given moment that the infant would be turning toward or away from the mother, and the probability for any given moment that the mother would be moving toward or away from the infant, we ascertained whether the observed frequency of mother moving toward the infant, and infant turning away from mother, and vice versa, occurring in the same frame is greater than the frequency expected by chance. Figure 2 (top) demonstrates that this is the case. A mutual approach-withdrawal pattern is present (all periods when the mother is touching the infants and conceivably restricting or causing infant motion were excluded from this analysis).

(b) *Who is initiating the mutual approach-withdrawal pattern?* To demonstrate that these correlations were indeed based upon small units of movement, and to determine if one or the other member of the pair were consistently following and thus reacting to the other, we serially lagged in time the correlation between mother and infant behavior. The direction of infant motion occurring in a given frame was correlated with the direction of maternal motion occurring 0, 6, 12, 24, and 36 frames earlier and later than the frame in which the infant motion occurred (i.e., 0, $1/4$, $1/2$, 1, and $1 1/2$ seconds earlier and later). The maximum correlation between "mother toward-infant away" and "mother away-infant toward" occurs at simultaneous pairing of mother and infant behavior and when mother is leading the interaction by $1/4$ second. This is graphed in figure 3. We had anticipated that if the relationship between the direction of mother and infant motion were indeed built upon the association between individual infant head movements and individual maternal motions, the significance of correlation between these behaviors would rapidly fall off as they were separated in time. Mother and infant behaviors separated in time by as little as 1 to $1 1/2$ seconds are uncorrelated.

Statistically, the mother is more often the initiator of the mutual pattern; but the pattern can be initiated by either. The very high correlation between mother and infant behavior occurring synchronously (in the same $1/24$ of a second) is striking. This may result from mother and infant having sufficient daily experience with the timing, rhythm, and sequencing of each other's motions so that short runs of synchronous behavior could occur—when there is not sufficient reaction time for a stimulus-response explanation. In between synchronous runs, movements are initiated by one and responded to by the other. A waltz serves as an analogy. Certain steps and turns will be cued by one partner—in between those cues both know the program well enough to move synchronously for short periods.

(c) *Differences between the twins in motor responsiveness to maternal motion.* Do the two different dyads show the same mutual approach-withdrawal pattern? Does it occur to the same extent in each dyad? Does it occur

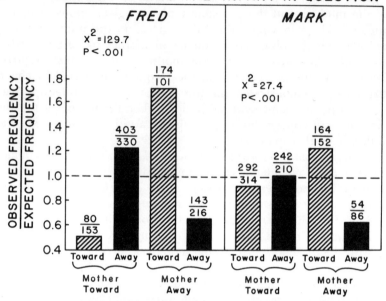

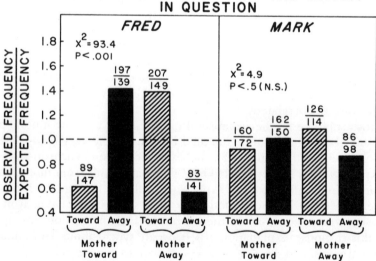

Figure 2
Effect of the direction of maternal motion on the direction of infant head motion, when mother is facing or facing away from the infant: comparison between the twins (expressed as the ratio between the number of observed occurrences and occurrences expected by chance)

under the same conditions for each dyad? Figure 2 compares the effect of the direction of maternal motion on the direction of Fred's and Mark's movements when mother is facing and when she is faced away from the twin in question. The twins show divergent patterns: (1) when the mother is facing them, the direction of head turning of both twins is highly correlated with her behavior in a pattern of mutual approach-withdrawal. The correlation is greater for Fred. (2) When mother is facing away, Fred's head turning continues to correlate highly with the mother's behavior, whereas Mark's head turning becomes random relative to her behavior. By this measure, Mark's behavior is no longer related to hers. Fred's continuation of the approach-withdrawal pattern

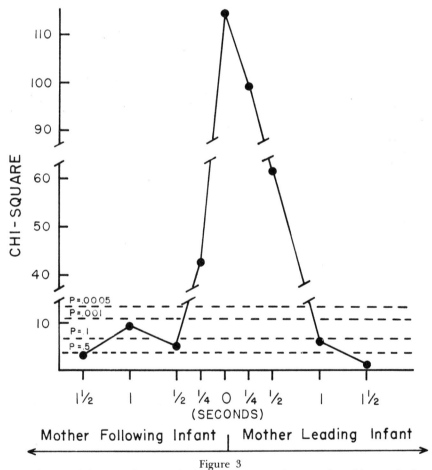

Figure 3
Significance of the mutual approach-withdrawal pattern (expressed as chi-square) when the direction of infant motion in a given frame is correlated with the direction of maternal motion occurring in the same frame and $1/4$, $1/2$, 1, and $1\frac{1}{2}$ seconds earlier and later than the infant motion

when mother is faced away is another indication (along with the duration of his facing positions) that he does not discriminate as well as Mark the mother's facing position.

The presence of maternal speech slightly influences the approach-withdrawal pattern, but is not the crucial variable. The difference between the two dyads under the two conditions obtains when analyzed for periods when the mother is speaking as well as for periods when she is not.

Discussion

This interaction in which the maternal behavior appears "controlling" and "overstimulating" is not solely directed by the mother. It is (at this point in its formation) a mutual interactive event—an event in which specific infant and maternal behaviors together produce repetitive sequences. A characteristic repeating sequence between mother and Fred goes as follows:

(1) If mother and Fred are facing one another, Fred will avert his face after a very short period of mutual facing (in anticipation of an unwanted approach?). (2) Mother responds with an approach toward Fred. It was earlier stated that the mother turns away when Mark averts his face slightly, but approaches if Fred does. This may not reflect simply a differential responsivity on her part to their face positions. When Fred is turned partly away, the direction of his small head motions remains highly dependent on her behavior and she receives the impression that he is still in contact with her. This may act as a discriminative stimulus for her. She then tries to establish further contact at the level she wants. (3) Her approach then forces him to a more exaggerated face aversion to turn her away. (4) She turns away, and (5) relatively quickly (compared to Mark), Fred turns back to face her. While he is facing her and she is turned away, he continues to execute approach and withdrawal movements dependent on her motions, even though those motions are not directed at him. His movements, plus his rapid resumption of the facing position, may recapture her attention. (6) She then turns to him, he quickly turns away, and the sequence is reinitiated.

A vicious cycle, cued by specific behaviors of both mother and infant, is repeatedly instituted. The cycle is also time-consuming so that mother and Fred generally spend more time interacting together. It is, however, mutually unsatisfying. In this sense each of them is "controlling" of the other.

The specific infant behaviors involved in a repetitive interactive sequence are of developmental interest because they constitute an important part of the infants' executive or adaptive experience of being "in" that particular relationship. We were thus interested in the fate of

Fred's use of face aversion in later social interactions. A second question to be answered by later development concerned the issue of independence and dependence. One of the striking differences between the dyads at $3^{1}/_{2}$ months was Mark's ability and Fred's inability to terminate contact with mother successfully. Fred could not remain turned away from mother, nor could he cease responding to her motions. However, he was also unable to maintain face-to-face contact, as Mark could. For some infants, establishing mother-infant contact may prove less of a developmental issue than acquiring the ability to terminate successfully that contact. This may be especially true with controlling and overstimulating mothers. From this point of view, Fred may be expected to have more difficulty with individuation and independence than Mark.

With these findings and speculations in mind (they were completed when the infants were 7 months old), it was of considerable interest that observation of the twins at age 12 to 15 months revealed Fred to be a more fearful and dependent child. He greets people with a fearful expression, refuses to make prolonged eye contact, and regularly executes extreme face aversions in social situations (usually to the side and down). An example of this face aversion, which has become a persistent social behavior, is drawn in figure 4. His stranger reaction was more intense and lasted longer than Mark's. He has had transient pho-

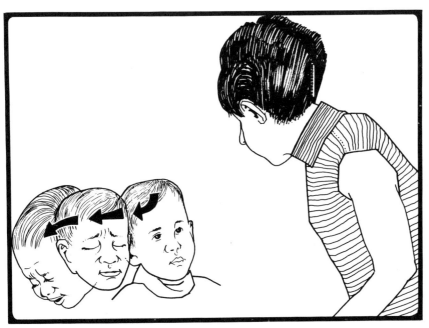

Figure 4
Fred's characteristic head aversion, drawn from film taken at age 14 months

bias, and he will not freely wander far from mother or get deeply involved in play without frequently checking back to her with a fleeting
glance, or running back to her but without looking directly at her.
Mark greets people well, he makes prolonged eye contact, and when
averting his face from a stranger, does so with a combination of behaviors that maintain the contact: his face averts only slightly so that good
peripheral regard remains; he turns his head up, not down, and characteristically smiles as he averts. He wanders off more freely and gets
deeply engrossed in play without any regard for mother's whereabouts.
The performance of more complex behaviors at 12 to 15 months is
consistent with the interpersonal patterns and behaviors developed at
$3^{1}/_{2}$ months with visual motor behaviors.

In subsequent studies we have further examined the nature of the
social interaction between mother and infant, in particular: how they
gaze at one another (Stern, 1974a); how they vocalize to one another
(Stern et al., 1975); the quality and nature of infant-elicited maternal
behaviors that constitute the social world of the infant (Stern, 1974a,
1974b); a conceptual framework for understanding the goal and structure of the mother-infant play activity (Stern, 1974b); and the temporal
patterning and rhythm of maternal social behaviors (Stern, 1975). In
each of these studies we have focused primarily on the nature of the interaction, but also indicated the implications of these findings for the
development of early coping and defensive ego operations.

Summary

An example of "controlling" maternal behavior with $3^{1}/_{2}$-month-old
twins is studied by a method of frame-by-frame film analysis. Characteristic infant behaviors regulating social contact with the mother are
identified and followed through 15 months.

A method for identifying and examining early social interactive patterns is described and may prove useful in further exploring the influence of the mother-infant relationship on the development of specific
infant behaviors and mental operations.

11

ISSUES IN EARLY MOTHER-CHILD INTERACTION

Louis W. Sander, M.D.

One of the principal aims of our longitudinal study of early personality development, begun at the Boston University School of Medicine-Massachusetts Memorial Hospital's Medical Center in 1954, was the investigation of the mother-child relationship. The study was of a naturalistic exploratory type, planned to provide frequent opportunities to observe mother and child together in a variety of situations over a period of the first 6 years of life. Most of these observational situations were structured quite consistently from contact to contact. Only primiparous mothers were selected to keep the factor of mothering experience comparable in the groups. Detailed descriptions were made at each contact of the behavior of the mother, of the child, and of the interaction between them. Thus, for each mother-child pair a longitudinal descriptive account was obtained of the progression of the outstanding characteristics which their interaction demonstrated in these well-defined situations over the years of the study. Comparable observations have been gathered on 22 of the mother-child pairs from birth through age 3 years. We have begun to analyze this extensive interactional material, and present here one of the avenues of approach. This approach consists of dividing the interactional data gathered for each pair into a sequence of time segments and making evaluations of interactions prominent in each segment. We are using these evaluations to study the proposal that in this early period there are a series of issues that are being negotiated in the interaction between mother and child. I present the theoretical considerations and the observational material which have suggested such a possibility.

In investigating the early mother-child relationship, we wished especially to study the way a particular maternal personality exerted its influence on the child and on the course of his development. In the origi-

Reprinted from the *Journal,* 1 : 141–166, 1962.

nal research design, primiparous mothers were chosen whose personalities showed the widest contrasts we could find along a range
of emotional maturity and immaturity, in order that we might observe
clear-cut contrasts in their behavior with their infants. We felt that this
would make interactional behavior more readily assessed in relation to
the developmental course taken. Such obvious interactional contrasts
were encountered in the sample of mother-child pairs. We were faced
with the task of weighing their importance in relation to the course of
development that followed and of comparing similar interactions across
the sample of mother-child pairs.

Ernst Kris (1950b) discussed the difficult problem of investigating
the mother's personality "in order to establish a link between her behavior and the symptomatology of the child." He stated: "The situation
in a specific crucial period can no longer be described only in terms of
psychosexual development; equal consideration has to be given to that
of the aggressive impulses, to the development of the ego, and to that
of object relations" (p. 36). He suggested as an example that the particular balance existing in parental relationship in respect to "the alternatives between indulgence and deprivation (discipline)" might have a
phase-specific appropriateness, requiring more of one at one point and
more of the other at another to improve the infant's chances for successful conflict solution.

In *A Genetic Field Theory of Ego Formation* (1959), Spitz presents in detail his concept of the part played by the adequacy or inadequacy of object relations in the epigenesis of early ego development. He asks (p.
84): "Will disturbances in infantile object relations result in deficient
ego formation according to the critical period at which they occur?"
After describing the relationship between "synchronicity" and integration, he proposes that a "developmental imbalance" results when
asynchrony exists between a maturational period of early ego development and particular features of object relations appropriate to it. The
question that at once arises is: which features of object relations are appropriate to which periods of early ego development?

This question has been extensively dealt with by Erikson (1950a,
1950b) in his presentation of stages of development and the interactions that are associated with each. He discusses the influence on later
developmental outcome of cultural variations in these interactions, as
well as variations stemming from individual personality characteristics
of caretaking figures. In the first two stages of his schema, covering the
first 3 years of life (which is the span we are studying in our interactional analysis), he describes in considerable detail the interactional
elements we have selected for evaluation in our mother-child pairs.
Furthermore, he describes these features as alternatives with a
considerable range of possible variation between the extremes. He im-

plies that, in the individual's object relations, some point of equilibrium will be struck in this range between alternatives which will be characteristic for that individual. For example, in regard to the alternative of supply vs. frustration experienced in the establishing of the particular ratio of trust vs. mistrust that will be characteristic for a given child, Erikson writes (1950b, p. 57): "Now, while it is quite clear what *must* happen to keep a baby alive (the minimum supply necessary) and what *must not* happen, lest he be physically damaged or chronically upset (the maximum early frustration tolerable), there is a certain leeway in regard to what *may* happen; and different cultures make extensive use of their prerogatives to decide what they consider workable and insist upon calling necessary." Each individual mother also possesses the same prerogative. She exercises it in accord with the consistencies that characterize her particular personality makeup. This factor touches upon certain considerations which underlie our approach to the evaluation of interactions in the various periods of early ego development, and which I shall discuss briefly before turning to the specific interactional elements of early object relations I have selected for study.

If the behavioral consistencies that characterize a mother's particular personality makeup could be viewed from the position of the infant's experiences with them, they could be conceived as coming to be represented by certain expectancies or anticipations that he would develop in respect to these features of his relationship with the mother. It might take a certain period of time for a trend to become established and for the expectancy to be an accurate estimate. The simple repetitive situations that are a part of the daily life of mother and child in this early time of life should lend themselves admirably to a solid set of reliable anticipations about many dimensions of the mother's behavior. A longer span of time for the same degree of certainty to be established would be required in the face of maternal inconsistency or marked expressions of ambivalence in her activities. The estimate should finally approach the point on the range between alternative possibilities for each element of early mother-child interaction that would be characteristic for the pair.

We have tried to capture these relationships in our evaluation of interactions by representing the reaching of such a point as the negotiation of an issue of interaction. The *New Century Dictionary* gives several definitions for the word "issue." It cam mean "a point in question," or it can mean "an outcome." A third definition puts these two together as "a point, the decision of which determines the matter." The issue would be negotiated when the child's expectancy for the element of maternal behavior became crystallized. In this respect, "an average expectable environment" (Hartmann, 1939) would be one in which such expectancies would be reached in an average chronology and for average points on the range. This concept of developmental relationships has been delineated by Erikson (1950a, 1950b) in his formulation of a series of epigenetic stages determined by the points at which certain precursors of personality function come to their ascendancy, meet their crises, and find their lasting solution through decisive encounters with the environment. Deviations in timing and range of behavior in these encounters lead to the "asynchrony" referred to by Spitz (1959). In our evaluation of interactional material, for each time period of early ego development, we have worded an issue that concerns one especially prominent feature of interaction during that span of months. Rather than define the issues in terms of whether or not a given feature of interaction will appear, we have framed them in respect to the degree or extent to which the feature will appear.

Our observational material of the first 18 months of life seemed to fall into five large time segments, each with a prominent feature which was encountered extensively in our data for that period.[1] The first period corresponds to the "undifferentiated phase" of early ego development (Hartmann et al., 1946), namely, the first $2^1/_2$ months of life. Characteristics of the mother-child relationship at this time have been discussed by many students of early development (e.g., Spitz, 1954, 1956; Escalona, 1952; A. Freud, 1936; Hartmann et al., 1946). A central issue in these months concerns the degree of specific appropriateness that the mother can maintain in her response to the cues the baby gives of his state and needs. The second period, from $2^1/_2$ to 5 months, is the segment most thoroughly described by Spitz and Wolf (1946), in which smiling behavior is developing and coming to play a central role in the relationship. The degree to which truly reciprocal interchanges are established between infant and mother has been selected for evaluation. The third period, 5 and 9 months, has interested us especially in regard to the way in which the baby's expression of initiative for social exchange and for various preferences is responded to by the mother. This formulation was suggested by Bowlby's conceptualization of the nature of the child's tie to his mother (1958a). The fourth period, between 9 and 12 or 13 months, has been delimited somewhat more arbitrarily. The feature of interaction which impressed us most forcibly during this phase concerned the intensity and insistence with which the child made demands on the mother and the manner in which she dealt with them. Descriptions of this focalization of demands on the mother have been made by E. Kris (1950b), A. Freud and D. Burlingham (1944), and Mahler (1968). The fifth period, extending from 12 to 18 months, has been described in detail by Erikson

1. It is obvious that a number of other interactions and issues might have been selected for a study. The prominence of these in our material may relate to the sample of subjects chosen and to our methods of observation and recording.

(1950a) in relation to the establishing of early autonomy. We have been especially interested in evaluating for each mother-child pair precisely how the self-assertion of the child is dealt with, particularly when it is in opposition to the mother's wishes.

By arranging the data according to these time segments, descriptive features of the observations can be compared in different subjects at roughly the same point in the life of the child. Individual variations in the chronology of significant interactions then become apparent.

DESCRIPTIVE CLINICAL MATERIAL

I shall describe in detail the characteristics of mother-child interaction in each of the first five periods, illustrating the range of behaviors we have observed in our sample, and indicate the issues that have been extracted relating to these elements of the emerging relationship.

Period of Initial Adaptation (0–2¹/₂ months)

There seems general agreement that in the initial period of adaptation [2] the primary adaptive task consists of a suitable meshing of mothering activities with the cues the baby gives of his state, necessary for him to live and thrive. This primary adaptation is usually achieved by the end of this period and is reflected in the child's adoption of some reasonably predictable rhythms of feeding, elimination, sleep, and wakefulness. If the environment is an "average expectable" one, there also emerges a capacity for discrimination, shown by the child in his responsivity to handling by the mother. He usually becomes more responsive, and quiets more readily for her than for others. A measure of the successful negotiation of the adaptive requirement may be seen as early as the third or fourth week in the mother's spontaneous comment that she now feels she "knows" her baby, which may be accompanied by a perceptible moderation of her anxieties about the baby's care.

This period is one which reveals a great many of the mother's insecurities and anxieties, and puts to test many of her attributes. The dimensions of the child's organization can remain unknown to her for a considerable time if she is not perceptive of the cues supplied in his behavioral feedback to her. Although variations of interaction in this earliest time have been extensively described, we found it a noteworthy experience to observe the striking contrasts revealed in our sample of a "normal" population: the range of adaptation achieved lies truly on a broad spectrum. The extent of adaptation ranged from the barest semblance of a behavioral synchrony between mother and child that was

2. The time span ascribed to each period is that being used in the cross-case comparisons. It represents an approximation only, inasmuch as individuals may show considerable variation.

consistent with life [3] to a varied and harmonious interaction, specific in its accuracy of matching stimulus and response, infant need and maternal care. Such synchrony might occur in only one or in many sensorimotor channels. There is quite clearly a quantitative and a qualitative dimension to the *specific* appropriateness of maternal ministrations in respect to the baby's state. A measure of appropriate social stimulus initiated by the mother is included here as one of the infant's needs, and is observed, for example, in her efforts to produce a smiling response in her baby.

The degree to which mutuality will be established seems to depend, in part at least, on the balance the mother can maintain between her empathy with what she feels are the child's needs and her objectivity in viewing him as an individual apart from her own projections and displacements. A measure of objectivity is essential if the mother is to pick up the unique functional qualities an infant can show from birth. The balance a given mother can maintain between empathy and objectivity is characteristic for her and stems from her particular personality structure. This balance determines the unique combination of areas in which infant need may be met by appropriate response or further intensified by inappropriate stimulation or lack of response.

Thus the evaluation we make in this first period concerns the quantitative and qualitative aspects in the dimension of "specific appropriateness." The issue has been worded thus: *"To what degree in the adaptation established between mother and child will the mother's behavior be specifically appropriate to the baby's state and to the cues he gives of it?"*

For each pair, a rating on a 5-point scale was given, and the particular areas of inappropriate behavior were noted. In ensuing development the fate of these areas is watched and kept in mind in evaluating later unique aspects of behavioral style.[4] The range of mother-child interaction that was encountered in our sample is illustrated in the following two examples.[5]

1. The interview with a Mrs. C. was held in the hospital after she had been shown her baby for the first time.

3. In one mother-child pair the mother was so preoccupied with the fear of her otherwise normal infant choking to death with feedings that she fed only a minimum amount. The baby had gained but 1½ pounds over the birth weight by 3 months of life. We had real fears for the baby's survival.

4. In one instance, the only outstandingly inappropriate maneuver of the mother in the first period was an extraordinary amount of tactile stimulation which she gave the child. A hair-clutching gesture of the infant's, which had already been observed in the neonatal period, came to be used by the infant at 7 months in response to excessive tactile stimulation. A few weeks later she began intense scratching of her own skin, and in the second year of life, the hair-clutching came to be recognized by the observers as a signal of distress.

5. All the descriptions presented in this paper have been taken directly from the records of the original observation.

She was very pleased and enormously proud of her son. She said that the baby was crying intensely when he was brought to her, but when he was laid beside her, he immediately quieted and was quiet the whole time he was with her. She said she felt that her baby knew her because when the nurse came to take him again, he began crying again. She said she had stroked his cheek and he had smiled. When she had tried to feed him the water, he had known it was water as soon as it had touched his lips and he spit it out because he wanted milk.

Objectivity was at a minimum here. Her empathy with her newborn child hinged on the meanings she gave to his behavior. She viewed him to a great extent in a framework consisting chiefly of her projected feelings. The limitations of such a framework become evident when these feelings are highly ambivalent. The problem is compounded when the mother cannot decide when they match reality and when they do not.

The following report of a home visit with the same mother at 4 weeks is given below. The baby was asleep in an adjacent room.

After about a half hour there was a slight whimpering sound from the other room. Mrs. C. immediately alerted to this, although it was only the faintest sound and then said that she had better wait until he really cried as she half got out of her seat, then sat down again, and then immediately got up and went to the baby. I followed her into the bedroom to look at him. The infant was lying in prone, head to the right, with some slight frown which did not seem like crying to me particularly. Mrs. C. turned him over and he lay quiet again. Again Mrs. C. said, looking at me questioningly, "I'd better wait until he really wakes up" and came back into the kitchen and sat down again. At another slight sound she got up again almost immediately, picked the baby up and brought him out, holding him first against her arm. He looked very sleepy and as though discomforted at being moved and he closed his eyes again. Mrs. C. then put him back in the bassinet; soon after this he began to cry, and she picked him up again. The whole sequence had a quality of a kind of disorganized indecision about it, as though Mrs. C. never once settled on any kind of action for more than a minute. Almost before she decided on one move, she was already reversing it.

Once it was definitely ascertained that the baby was awake, Mrs. C. took him into the kitchen and held him against her arm in a sitting position. As he quieted, she tapped his nose and chin; this seemed to be an irritant that set him off crying, and Mrs. C. now shifted him against her shoulder. He looked very cozy in this position, his legs drawn up under him so that he was curled up in a kind of little ball, and cuddled against his mother's shoulder, very quiet now.

As Mrs. C. had not given the baby his bath yet, she now decided to do this, taking him to a shelf by the sink and laying him down in supine. Actually there were a few moments of indecision again as she thought that she would give him his bath, then looked at me questioningly, and then continued to hold him, and finally got up and made the actual decision to bathe him. The baby began to cry as she laid him down, and Mrs. C. shifted him about, tapped his chin and nose—all of this with a kind of uncertainty. It seemed to me that she made a great many small movements that gave me the sense of acute discomfort in watching and seemed to have a similar effect on the baby.

As the baby activated his arms, he seemed to try to get his hand to his mouth. He seemed not able to do this and cried briefly and then quieted. Mrs. C. spoke to him, tapped his nose, and he again began to cry and Mrs. C., looking very distressed, pushed a pacifier into his mouth. She said that he was hungry and that he didn't like the pacifier, but the baby quieted again. As he yawned and stretched his arms a bit, the pacifier dropped out and Mrs. C. immediately put it back in. It would drop out again soon and the baby would seem to be yawning and stretching. But Mrs. C. seemed to take this as the beginning of a cry, although the baby looked quite content to me, and pushed the pacifier in his mouth again. This was repeated several times. Mrs. C. said to me, "I'll let you watch him and go finish my cigarette," and indicated that she would like me to stand by him as she went toward the table. The pacifier very soon dropped out of the baby's mouth and I picked it up ready to put it in again; but, as he seemed to be yawning and not discomforted, I held it in my hand. Mrs. C. returned again very quickly and asked, "Doesn't he want it?" watched for a moment, and then decided that she would get the bath ready.

2. The second illustration provides a contrasting description of a mother child interaction during a home visit. Nancy was 3 weeks of age.[6] Her mother was, in contrast to Mrs. C., at the other extreme of our personality grouping. Earlier in the visit, the mother had described how Nancy had indicated her preference for the prone position; she had told of a characteristic posture that the baby adopted before going to sleep. The mother also had been quick to pick up that her infant's wakening process was very slow. It took her daughter some time between her first whimpers of arousal until she was ready for her bottle; the mother had already learned to pace her feeding accordingly. During the visit, the baby had been sleeping until this time.

After Nancy had been sleeping for some time, she began to move about, though still asleep. She pulled her knees up under her and seemed to be stretching her arms and turning her head about on the pillow, her skin taking on a reddish tinge with the effort. Finally she made slight squealing sounds. Mrs. D. now turned Nancy over on her face, accomplishing this again with a quite easy but gentle movement. Nancy, as before, remained quiet for a few minutes, her eyes open, her mouth moving minimally; then she began moving her arms and legs about, finally putting her fingers to her mouth and then beginning to cry. As Nancy lay on her back, Mrs. D. stood beside Nancy chatting with us and holding Nancy's feet very lightly, touching rather than restraining, lifting the baby's nightgown to show how chubby Nancy was getting, and occasionally feeling the diaper to see if Nancy was wet.

Mrs. D. finally picked Nancy up, not letting her cry very long, and cradled her very comfortably and gently in her arms, looking down at her in a very warm, half-humorous, accepting expression. She held Nancy in this way for a

6. The deliveries of both these babies were observed as part of our routine. Resuscitation was uneventful in both. Lusty crying was established in the first minute and good color and muscle tone within the next three minutes.

while, pinching the infant's cheeks between her thumb and forefinger in a quick, repetitive gesture, then tapping her on the chin a few times playfully; and then, after a while, Mrs. D. put Nancy back on the couch on her stomach. At one point, while Mrs. D. was holding Nancy and the infant's fingers were going to her mouth, Mrs. D. commented, "I'd bet she'd suck my finger if I put it in her mouth." This time, as Mrs. D. placed the baby in prone on the couch, Nancy's face came into contact with the pillow, and she lifted her head slightly, twisting about and kicking her legs, and seeming a little discomforted. Mrs. D. reached out her hand and patted Nancy with gentle rhythm on her back, and the baby quieted very quickly. Mrs. D. said, "That has always worked." The infant began moving again after Mrs. D. stopped patting, and then the mother took the baby's feet in her hand, holding them very lightly as before, seeming to be establishing contact rather than restraining in any way.

We see here the mother's respect of the infant's gradual awakening and her reporting of her observations of the various idiosyncratic preferences of her child, her reaching out to contact the child, and the specific quieting effect of this behavior. In spite of her wish to demonstrate the baby to the visitor and to participate in Nancy's performance, she did not seem to carry this activity too far. She put the baby down. We also see the quality of her attention: she divided it between the visitor and the baby, and she maintained tactile contact with the baby after placing her in a prone position.

It is likely that the impact on these two infants of the experiences illustrated will be profoundly different. In our cases in which a mother failed to achieve appropriateness sufficiently specific for her child, the father often could establish it. He then became the one who could more successfully quiet the baby and the one who first elicited the smile.

Inasmuch as observations were recorded every 2 to 3 weeks, evaluations of the outcome of the issues were based on a review of a series of contacts. This check, which is one of the strengths of longitudinal data, served to modify extreme impressions which a single contact might elicit. In general, mothers showed a high degree of consistency within any given period.

Period of Reciprocal Exchange (approx. 2^1/$_2$-5 months)

By the time of this second period, the mother had usually surmounted the anxieties of providing an environment adequate to sustain the life of her infant. One usually saw her now involved in the increasingly delightful experience of stimulating and responding to the emerging smiling behavior of her infant. It is one of the most pleasurable (and obvious) of the early interactional phases. We have attached importance to the crescendo quality occurring in the well-developed smiling play, in the way it spreads from the facial area to bring the whole body,

including the voice, into a primitive organized effort. This extension of
the response to its limits occurs as the smiling behavior of the infant is
elicited in a series of repeated reciprocal activities on the part of the
stimulator and the baby. A brief pause allows the infant his first response, then the mother's smiling face is brought closer, another pause
for the infant to react again, another presentation of mother's face,
each time with some new stimulus added—perhaps now an open
mouth, or the touch of a finger, or a vocalization. The infant's initial
localized facial response extends to involve arms, legs, trunk, and voice
in an exuberant, wriggling, infectious, joyful display.

Again, however, we discovered somewhat to our amazement that
there were some mothers in our group who never reported, and were
never observed entering into, this kind of interaction with their infants.
There were others who engaged in it so intensely and over such a
prolonged period that the child would break into crying, a response
which would bring the mother to her senses and lead her to stop the
stimulation. There is, therefore, a wide range in the experiences which
an infant can have in respect to this element of interaction, one which
is so often taken completely for granted. Other variations include the
age at which a mother will attempt first to elicit a smile from her baby,
as well as the amount of effort and attention she devotes to getting the
smiling response started. There is a considerable variation in the age at
which smiling behavior reaches its peak.

We have operationally defined "reciprocal" interaction as that showing the quality of stimulus-response alternation, back and forth, between mother and child in the fashion just described above. (Some
mothers will stimulate their infants to smile, but the interaction is intended only to produce a reaction in the child, and not truly to begin a
reciprocation with him. In others, the interaction may consist of reciprocity of vocal exchange rather than in the general area of smiling
play.) The issue for this period has been worded then as follows: *"To
what extent will the interaction between mother and child include reciprocal
sequences of interchange between them, that is, back and forth, active-passive al-
ternations of stimulus and response?"*

The following extract is taken from an observation during a home
visit, which was made when the infant Helen S. was 3 months, 17 days
old. If the mother's interaction with the child is compared in this example with the father's, the subtle differences in reciprocal quality of
interaction became apparent. The observer writes:

> Helen lay on her back in the bassinet, appearing pleased with the activity
> around. Her arms and legs moved about quite actively, and she smiled read-
> ily as Mrs. S. leaned over and spoke to her. Mrs. S. talked to Helen in a very
> animated, stimulating fashion, chucking her under the chin, calling her "Lit-
> tle Fatty." She moved her head toward Helen and back in rapid succession as

she did this. Helen responded, looking at her mother with an expression of pleasure and moving arms and legs in excitement. As Mrs. S. discontinued this, the baby continued her excited movement for a bit, looking at her mother as though anticipating a return engagement. As it was not forthcoming, she quieted her movement and began to fuss minimally. She soon turned her attention to me, looking at me, breaking into a spontaneous smile as I spoke to her. Mrs. S. leaned forward and kissed Helen on the cheek in quick pleasure as she did this, seeming very delighted at the baby's display of responsiveness to me.

Mother and visitor became involved in conversation and Helen began to fuss as no attention was paid to her, making a series of separate little cries, her arms spread wide and up as though wanting to be picked up. After a while, Mrs. S. said, "I'll hold you for a while," picked Helen up and held Helen on her lap against her left arm. The baby quieted immediately and sat looking at me for a moment, seeming very contented having reached her objective. She soon leaned well forward from her mother against the table and became interested in looking at something on the table; Mrs. S. talked to her, asking, "What are you looking at? You looking at this?" She spoke in a very animated way, with Helen paying no attention, simply continuing to focus her gaze completely absorbed on something on the table. Mrs. S. said one could not distract Helen when she was interested in something. She had a mind of her own. Mrs. S. said the baby was very sensitive to know who would pick her up and who would not, implying that Helen differentiated between her father and mother in this respect. She spoke in a very definite way of her own imperviousness to the baby's "winding" (whining), implying that the infant knew who was the boss and of the uselessness of fussing.

Mr. S. came in after the mother had again placed Helen in the bassinet. He stood looking down at the infant, and she now turned to look up at her father, spreading her arms wide and a little upward as though appealing to him to pick her up, and she now began to fuss a bit again. Mr. S. made no move to pick her up, but after a while he leaned over and patted her on the stomach, moving her body back and forth very gently in a kind of quick awkward movement as though pulled to make some response to the infant's appeal. The baby made no response to this; she neither activated nor quieted, but waved her arms and legs as he spoke to her. Mr. S. made no other approach to Helen, simply standing looking down at her as he made small conversation with me.

It is difficult to illustrate a mother-child pair in which the reverse situation is exemplified, inasmuch as the judgment of a relative lack of social reciprocity can be obtained only on a review of all our material. However, we have found that in those pairs in which the mother did not take advantage of the easy opportunity for this reciprocal exchange, the delightful readiness for response in the child nevertheless might be observed. The mother might be pleased and gratified as she watched her baby interact with others, or at the pleasure the baby showed at her approach, but she was not observed entering into the interchange herself. The following example is an illustration of this. It was taken from a home-visit observation of a mother whose personality showed strong obsessive-compulsive trends. She was restrained,

gloomy, overanxious, and complaining. She had had an extremely anxious time in her initial period of adaptation. This observation was in
the fourth month, and the observer noted immediately that there was a
lightening of the dark cloud of grave concern that had previously hung
over them. The beginnings of interchange were evident, but no reciprocal play was noted.

> There seemed to be some quality of closeness between the mother and child
> which had been completely missing before. For example, at some point the
> baby lay staring at me and then turned to his mother to look at her as though
> for assurance, and Mrs. K. commented, "He's asking, is it all right, Mommy,"
> in a quite pleased tone of voice. (She was not induced to play here with the
> child.) At other times the baby would smile at her and was very responsive
> when she picked him up or touched him, quieting almost immediately. Mrs.
> K. seemed to enjoy his responsiveness and to be pleased at his smiling at her
> or at her being able to quiet him. She even talked to him spontaneously *in
> response* to his smiling or looking at her, but her behavior was still limited
> pretty much to asking "What's the matter?" though in a much more conver-
> sational tone, and at one point she even ventured a "Goo."

We note here that it was the mother who was responding to her baby
and not the baby who was being stimulated by the mother. We observed later that this child was of unusually serious demeanor and
showed relatively little spontaneity. One could sense here a separateness between child and mother. She talked to the baby without spontaneous *exchange* with him.

We are interested in studying the extent to which a lack of specific
appropriateness in the first period can be made up for by a satisfactory
experience during this second phase. We are also interested in following the later outcome in children who do not experience an easy reciprocity with their mothers at this time or until some later age. We have
examples in which this reciprocal feature did not really begin until
speech was well enough developed to permit simple conversation. The
mother-child relationship then seemed to take on a new meaning and
liveliness for both of them, and especially acquired a positive affective
tone that had previously been missing. In other pairs we observed that
reciprocal interaction almost disappeared by the time speech was developing. When this quality of interaction disappears from the relationship, the child appears unhappy and distressed; mother and child
give the impression of having "lost" each other. It has been of interest
to watch, as time moves on, the point at which reciprocal interchanges
of smiling play begin to disappear from our observations; in many instances, this occurred by the eighth or ninth month.

We suspect that much of importance for the child's development
hinges on the continuance of reciprocal exchanges in some other area
of interaction. Whether it persists or not seems to depend a good deal
upon the mother's lead in continuing this quality of interaction in a
new area such as vocalization and speech, or upon her ability to play

spontaneously on the level at which the baby may be in his development. This is illustrated in the following example during a home visit
to Mrs. Q., whose child was 10 months old.

> Although there was virtually no direct physical contact between Mrs. Q. and
> Ellen during my visit, Mrs. Q. did a lot of direct talking to Ellen, offering her
> a glass of milk and leaning over and whispering, in a somewhat tender and
> feeling way, various little unimportant statements. Ellen responded very
> nicely to these, paid close attention to her mother, and seemed to be very in-
> volved in their relationship.

Period of Early Directed Activity of the Infant (5–9 months)

The social interchange between mother and child has been presented
largely in relation to the mother's initiative in eliciting and sustaining it.
However, the baby's initiative in establishing social exchange with the
mother begins to come into play as the smiling response reaches its
height. The child attempts to reach out to the mother and stimulate
her to respond to him. The manner in which the mother responds to
the baby's initiative forms the basis for the third issue, which has been
worded as follows: *"To what degree will the initiative of the infant be successful in establishing areas of reciprocity in the interchange with the mother?"*
When this effort is successful in bringing the mother into smiling play,
the infant learns to anticipate her response to him and can reproduce
some of the joyful excitement of the experience by actions associated
with this anticipation. The mother's ability to respond to the infant's
initiative for social interchange is related to her general affective spontaneity, the gratification her child's pleasurable reaching out gives her,
and the general level of interchange she shows in interpersonal relations. It also seems to be related to the priority given her child in the
organization of her perceptual awareness.

Subtly and easily obscured are the tender beginnings of the child's
directed activities in this period, as shown in the following example of
Mrs. G. C. whose baby was 7 ½ months old:

> I remained a while longer as Mrs. G.C. began the feeding. She held the baby
> on her lap with his head resting against her arm as she spooned the food to
> him and although she had expected that he might refuse it since he had not
> been eating well the past few days, Douggie took the food quite readily, and
> the feeding went very smoothly. Once or twice during the feeding, Douggie
> would seem to want a brief respite from taking the mouthfuls of food and
> Mrs. G.C. would wait until he was ready. A couple of times when this oc-
> curred, he put his head back and looked directly up at his mother, com-
> pletely engaging her in visual contact, and Mrs. G.C. seemed extremely de-
> lighted and, I thought, quite excited by this contact, returning his gaze and
> then seeming a bit embarrassed and pulling herself away and offering him
> the next spoonful.

We first paid attention to the baby's initiative in regard to its influence in starting social exchanges with the mother. However, it seemed

obvious that the mother's response to the baby's initiative in general must be a large part of the issue at stake in this period. The baby is beginning to show preferences of all sorts, and is attempting actively to control the stimulations reaching him as well as those disappearing from him. Some of his efforts in the direction of his mother encounter a response in kind from the mother, a back and forthness, or a feedback of reciprocal quality, whereas some of his other efforts do not. We have assumed that those activities which the infant initiates and which lead to a reciprocal exchange with the mother must be clearly distinct in the infant's perception from those which do not. A dimension of anticipation must therefore be set up in the child's expectancies which reflects the balance of success or failure the child has experienced in establishing new areas of reciprocity with his mother. In our contrasting groups of maternal personalities, there was a wide variation in the respect the mother showed for early preferences stemming from the initiative of the baby, just as there was a wide variation in the mother's availability for reciprocal interactions.

The period from 6 to 9 months is a time which demands of the mother a certain keenness in reading and appreciating the cues of her child; it further demands that she respond as appropriately as in the initial period of adaptation. However, it has the flavor of a more passive response in adaptation on her part than the more active role she took in the first period. This difference is frequently observed as the mother begins the feeding of solids. The average mother who has negotiated the two earlier issues adapts so readily to the new pressures of the child's budding initiative that it is usually not readily apparent that an important issue is being settled. However, when we see an infant, who has progressed solidly through the first 4 or 5 months, meeting then an implacable barrier to his initiative, the picture is different.

The following example is taken from a tape-recorded interview with the mother whose son, Ned, was 9 months old. Mother and child had experienced a satisfactory initial adaptation and a delightful early period of social smiling play. However, the battle of initiative had shown its first beginnings in the area of motor activity when Ned was $4^{1}/_{2}$ months old. At that time, he was able to pull himself to the edge of his carriage and was promptly harnessed because the mother feared he would fall out. The struggle extended in the following months until we felt entitled to label this period for this mother-child pair as "the battle of the high chair." Some weeks before the interview, the pediatrician had suggested that the mother could try again to introduce solid foods. The interviewer reported:

> I.: Well, to get back to Ned again. How is the feeding situation going?
> M.: It's picked up very good. He's got the idea that he's gonna gag. You know, he's always gagging on his vegetables. And that's why he won't take

it—and—or he didn't like the taste. If he didn't like the taste, he'd gag like. I'm disgusted. So last Friday, he was mad. He took a fit, he was mad. My husband was sitting there, and he was crying for my husband to pick him up, and I was feeding him and he was cross. I don't think he knows what I'm giving him—the mixed vegetables and the soup and his bottle.

I.: Well, what was he—spitting it out?

M.: He just quit taking them. I don't know what's wrong.

I.: What do you mean?

M.: He'll be happy and all. If you pick him up in the morning, he'll be so quiet and never say a word—up in his high chair. He'll just sit there and play. And we used to give him tea, a cup of tea or something. He'd be quiet, and then I'd feed him, and maybe he'd get cranky and be tired. But when I pick him up *now* and walk to the high chair [to feed him], he don't want that [makes crying sounds]. Sit down, sit down—he don't want that. He wants to go.

I.: But when you do sit him down, then he—.

M.: Then he goes, then he runs all—he pushes and he kicks and he bangs his head, and he'll just sit there. And look at him, he's crazy. I says I don't know. If he bumps his head enough times, he'll stop. Then he'll stop and he gets mad. Mm—mm—he'll start crying, and there's nothing to do but just let him cry.

I.: Uh-huh.

M.: If you keep on picking him up, you'll get nothing done and you won't accomplish anything. So, we leave him there. Then we give him a toy to shut up.

This baby, who had been one of our most attractive infants in his fourth and fifth months, lost all signs of spontaneous, pleasurable affect in the early part of his second year of life. He was completely defeated by his mother in this early struggle. This mother-child pair provided an instance in which the usual sequence of issues had not followed in order. The threat which the initiative of her infant posed for this mother was revealed by the fact that she suddenly went to work for 4 months, leaving the 7-month-old baby in the care of her husband. She gave up this solution and returned to resume her control in the household because the husband was now yielding to the baby's demands to be picked up. She said, "That was the last straw." The outcome of the next two issues for this mother and child could have been easily predicted at this point. The self-assertion usually seen in the early part of the second year of life submerged. In a recent follow-up at the age of 5 ½ years he showed a striking passivity and almost an avoidance of investment in the few activities he could begin himself.

Period of Focalization on Mother (9–15 months)

The issue has been worded as: *"To what degree will the child succeed in his demands that the mother alone fulfill his needs?"* One of the roots of autonomy in the first year of life stems from the outcome the child experiences from the activities that he initiates. There are a series of steps by which this primordial autonomy widens its foothold vis-à-vis the outer world. Once Issue 3 is satisfactorily negotiated, the way is immediately opened in the relationship between child and mother for the next issue to come to the fore. This concerns the extension of initiative in the child to achieve something of a manipulation of the mother, especially a focalization on her as the person who meets his needs. During this period, there is a further discrimination of mother from other caretaking people. Whereas previously the child might have accepted a feeding as easily from father as from mother, it is now only the mother who is clearly preferred for this activity. It is only the mother's lap that is sought for comfort or security. Such a process of focalizing interaction on the mother has been termed "monotropy" by John Bowlby (1958a). He considered it an innate characteristic of developmental behavior in the animal kingdom that the specific stimulus-response patterns become focalized in one parent animal.

Although from the beginning the mother has been responding to her child's demands, these have gradually become more and more specific. Whereas the first demands of the child are diffuse expressions of discomfort, they now become directed efforts to possess and manipulate. It is one thing for a mother to come to the aid of the helpless infant, and quite another for her to yield to a clearly intended demand of her year-old baby. The demands of this period on the mother are intense and unremitting and involve the mother in the deepest threats to her integrity. One could say that this period separates the women from the girls, those with flexibility from those without, those whose sense of identity as mothers is secure from those who are only partially committed. The smooth and satisfactory negotiation seems to depend upon the mother's ability to yield or to compromise by keeping the baby in her awareness while she pursues her own interests. Her freedom to do so depends partly on her freedom to limit. Fear of strangers, strong at this time, is an additional factor serving to push the child toward the mother. The dangers from which a child in his beginning motor explorations must be protected are another factor binding the mother's attention to the child. On the other hand, the mother who is secure enough in herself and has confidence in the ultimate separateness and integrity of her child can enjoy and yield to this possession by him. When she does so, preserving areas of reciprocity with her child, she acts as a stable base of operations for him as his growing motility and inevitable curiosity carry him away from her.

The range of interactions that can be seen here was illustrated by one of our mothers whose principal preoccupation was to maintain her child's involvement with her. She welcomed any turn of the child toward her, and kept herself always available. The period was passed with little sign of the child's demand on her mother. On the contrary, notable efforts were made by .the child to move away from the mother.

We have observed that by 9 months, the focus of the mother's attention is a percept which the child clearly has come to appreciate. The child struggles for her attentive involvement. One of the consequences of the perception of attentive focus of the mother and its employment in the interaction is that such a simple signal can come to represent actual exchanges of considerable duration and complexity.

The capacity to find gratification in the outside world apart from the mother, to transfer the experience of gratification from interaction with her to interaction with the world is, we feel, related in part to a certain degree of success in negotiating this fourth period. Unless a satisfactory level of certainty of the mother's availability is established before the self-assertion which follows in the early months of the second year, the child is faced with an important asynchrony in respect to his mother: he is still seeking to assure himself of her while he already must begin to assert himself against her.

A single illustration will show the way the child exerts his possessive pressure in this fourth period. It is an excerpt from a tape-recorded interview with a mother whose child was 12 months old.

> M.: But she gets into everything. She won't play by herself and she wants me to play with—and she won't stay out on the porch by herself. She likes to go out there, but she won't stay by herself.
> I.: She won't play by herself?
> M.: No, for a while she will, and then she always comes in to me, and she's either in the pantry or in the cabinet, or in the closet—and now she pushes the car bed away and gets into my closet.

This behavior continued as illustrated in the following example taken from a tape-recorded interview with the same mother when the child was 14 months:

> I.: Does she ever let you get away from her or—.
> M.: She bothers me all day. I can't do anything. I can't sit down to read a paper or do anything because she always tries to get up on me, and when I'm in the pantry, she's in the pantry; when I'm in the kitchen—if I'm sweeping, she's gotta sweep. No matter where I am she's gotta be. And she won't stay out on the porch, although she has been for the last couple of days playing at the door, but when the screen door closes, she doesn't like it. It's only a little porch. But when the door closes, she doesn't like it and she cries. And you know the bathroom has to be closed at all times.

Period of Self-Assertion (12–18 months)

The clarity of this fifth issue and the timing of its onset follow on the outcome of Issue 4. The fifth issue we have stated as: *"To what extent will the child establish self-assertion in the interaction with the mother?"* We might add *"In what areas?"* and *"At what cost?"* This period extends over the early part of the second year of life and corresponds to the well-known phase of negativism. This is the time of appearance of autonomy (Erikson, 1950b; Spitz, 1957), which emerges *pari passu* with the restriction of volition that is occurring. For example, Spitz (1957) writes: "The jurisdiction of the fifteen-months-old eventually is limited practically to his own body." This factor has been described in relation to the struggle over toilet training in which the child may be pressed to retreat to a last fortress of assertion of volitional control, i.e., in control of his body functions. In these present times, however, where the least well-educated of our mothers may have read when to begin toilet training and may not begin it until the close of the second year, toilet training itself may not enter so clearly into the picture. Yet, just as surely, the problem of self-assertion, the attempt to possess the initiative, results in conflict.

However, except in unusual instances in our material, we found, instead of a complete defeat of the child, that there are different areas in which self-assertion is achieved. Possible conflicts had been in evidence since the beginnings of self-assertion in the third phase, but now these reach an outspoken struggle. This represents the time of "decisive encounter" as Erikson (1950b) has described it in his discussion of the emergence of autonomy. The areas of self-assertion achieved are of a wide variety, unique for the mother-child pair, and again reflect the particular character of the mother and her household. The following example is extreme for our population, but not an unfamiliar picture to those acquainted with mothers who find it difficult to set limits. The description is taken from a home visit with Dora I. at 17 months:

> Dora runs the apartment and the family. Mrs. I. is unable to study for her examinations because she can't open a book when Dora is up. It has gotten to the point where Mrs. I. can hardly go down to the laundry in the basement with Dora because Dora runs around and gets into so much mischief, like opening the other washers and taking out the laundry, and so on. Dora's things are all over the apartment and the whole bedroom (only one bedroom in the apartment) belongs to Dora. Mrs. I. is constantly trying to anticipate Dora in the nicest possible way, but it is difficult for Mrs. I. and difficult for Dora. This home is almost too child-oriented. The walks outside are talked about as though it is Dora who determines where they should go. Mrs. I. is constantly at Dora's beck and call, although Dora does have trouble settling down to anything and really being satisfied with it.

The more usual state of affairs is better illustrated by the two following excerpts which are taken from observations of Mrs. D. and her child Nancy. The first is from a home visit when Nancy was 15 months, 23 days, about which the observer wrote:

> Mrs. D.'s handling of Nancy was warm and permissive. She was supporting, approving, and seemed to enjoy her very much. She wanted Nancy to "perform"—fold her arms, tap her nose, play peek-a-boo. She was not the least insistent or annoyed when Nancy wouldn't comply; said rather philo-

sophically, "She never does things when you ask her to," quite accepting of Nancy's own will to comply or not. She relates that Nancy wants to do everything herself now; she refuses to be fed; she insists on holding her own spoon. Mother lets her, is not concerned with lower food intake when Nancy feeds herself. Lets her do as many things for herself as possible. Mrs. D. did not seem threatened by Nancy's quest for independence, but accepting of it and supportive. She made no mention of any troubles or mess resulting from this self-feeding; she only spoke of it in terms of what Nancy wanted and needed to do. Her eating habits are changing. She no longer wants baby food, but wants to (and does) try all adult food. Mrs. D. still tries to give her baby food for lunch, sometimes opens four to five cans to give her a choice, but Nancy turns them all down. "She really likes roast beef and steak," said Mrs. D. with a chuckle. She drinks very well from a cup. She rarely wants her bottle now, except for going to sleep. She is fed a little before the parents eat, then nibbles at their food during their dinner as well. Nancy no longer naps as long as she used to. She used to sleep for two hours in a blanket on the floor; now naps one hour at the most.

The second illustration at 16 months, 12 days shows how the degree of self-assertion possible becomes ascertained by the child. The observations were recorded while the mother was conversing with the pediatrician prior to the examination of the child:

> Then Nancy looks up at camera, walks to mother's pocketbook on small table, pulls it off, vocalizing, takes it to mother. Sits on floor with it and proceeds to empty it. Takes out diaper first, then keys, at which point mother bends down and takes pocketbook. Nancy gets up and cries out in an angry squeal. Keeps crying while mother shakes keys in front of her to divert her, while continuing to talk to pediatrician. Nancy's cries become more urgent. Finally, mother gives her back the pocketbook. Nancy lets out a frustrated squeal. Mother bends down, I believe to open the pocketbook for her (here mother yields), Nancy quiets, proceeds as before. Takes out diaper, keeps rummaging inside the pocketbook. Real pleasure evident in this activity as it had been in moving screws on the table previously. Takes out box of Chiclet chewing gum, looks at it, holds it high in one hand, gives mother back pocketbook, keys, diaper. Holds chewing gum box, shakes it, and is just about to open box when mother takes it and puts it back into her pocketbook. Nancy screams loudly, inconsolably. Mother picks her up. Nancy holds arms into air, as if pulling on something, touches her hair, her ear. Angry, piercing screams as mother sets her on table. She quiets somewhat when the pediatrician hands her a roll of adhesive and scissors to play with. [This mother had always been quite concerned about the child's choking on small items, i.e., the gum, that she might put in her mouth.]

Such illustrations show the push and pull of forces between mother and child. The child wins the pocketbook and its entire contents except for the one item. Such equilibrium regarding limits is reached at a particular point on the range of possibilities for limits by each mother-child pair in an individual way. The process appears more complicated when the previous issue 4 has been unsatisfactorily negotiated. The asynchrony can be observed in the frantic efforts of such children to reestablish themselves with the mother after such a rupture, and the implications of frustration seem more total. The child is struggling for an adequate assurance of the availability of the mother, while at the same time he is struggling to assert himself against her. The possible relationship of developmental phases to levels of equilibria between infant and environment was suggested in Piaget's (1956) discussion of the part played by equilibration processes in the psychobiological development of the child. Assessment of the issues we have delineated will provide a means of exploring this concept.

The second 18 months have been divided more arbitrarily into three 6-month periods, from 18 to 24 months, 24 to 30 months, and 30 to 36 months. There are four issues being studied in reference to these periods. The first two are concerned with the destructive aspects of the child's aggression and the manner in which he directly challenges the mother's will and convictions. The other two involve the way the interaction with the mother includes the emerging secondary process activities of the child and the preoccupations he develops with his body functions.

SUMMARY

I have presented our modes of organizing the complex longitudinal descriptive data of early development in respect to one of its facets, namely, that of the mother-child interaction. The approach we are utilizing was conceived in response to the necessity of making cross-case comparisons of this detailed observational material in a sizable number of cases. It also stemmed from the challenge to examine new (i.e., behavioral or observational level) elements of the child's early object relations and to look for new relationships between those elements which appeared prominently in the material. We have developed a hypothetical schema in which these elements can be studied in a phase-specific, epigenetic context. It provides a set of dimensions in respect to object relations which occupies an intermediate position between the levels of phenomenology and of the dynamic constructs by which meaningful information about object relationships is usually communicated. This intermediate position provides a bridge between prenatal appraisals of maternal character, observations in chronological sequence of maternal and infant behavior, and outcome in evaluations of later ego organization in the child. Exploration into the manner in which maternal character might exert influence on the early personality development of the child was one of the original interests in launching a naturalistic study of this type.

A method of analysis based on a hypothetical schema must, of course, itself be exploratory. A rough scaling of interaction has been devised on the basis of the concept that the adaptation between mother and child in a given period involves the settling of an issue. This assumption determines for the period the point of equilibrium that will be characteristic for a mother-child pair in respect to a particular element or dimension of interaction. Marked variations in the range of behaviors encountered in a "normal" population of mothers, such as ours, can be quite clearly delineated by this means and thus communicated more easily. These phase-related variations can then be correlated with evaluation of variables in later ego organization in the children. We hope that the effort to represent events occurring between mother and child in terms of the anticipatory function of the developing ego will open further avenues of study, as should our attempt to relate the epigenetic phase relationships of early development to a sequence of equilibrial positions of interaction between child and environment (mother in this case).

12

CONCEPTS RELATED TO CHILD DEVELOPMENT

Irene M. Josselyn, M.D.

THE ORAL STAGE

The question of the significance of the impact of a culture upon the development of the personality during the psychological maturation of the individual has challenged writers in many disciplines. As the theoretical concepts of psychoanalysis have become a part of the basic formulations of those disciplines, the scope as well as the clarity of microscopic details have greatly increased. This development has in turn enriched psychoanalysis. The tendency, however, has been to explore distant horizons rather than to examine the immediate environment as closely as would seem indicated in view of the changes in our cultural patterns since Freud first formulated a dynamic concept of personality development.

The present interest in direct observation of infants and in the longitudinal studies of child development will undoubtedly provide an opportunity for reevaluation of many of our formulations. The scrutiny of the infant and child who is exposed to our particular cultural patterns of child rearing will probably confirm many of the basic tenets which seem valid in the reconstruction of the childhood of adult patients and in the therapy of disturbed children. Such scrutiny may in the next several years add a great deal that is new to the basic theoretical concepts of psychological development. The demonstrable applicability of certain psychological formulations, no matter what culture is studied, would imply that these represent basic factors that are universal in the human species and probably are, in the human species, a refinement of what is characteristic of all complex living organisms. However, it is possible that certain psychological configurations now considered universal will be found to be largely culturally determined phenomena. It is therefore important continually to review our evi-

Reprinted from the *Journal,* 1 : 209–224, 1962; 2 : 357–369, 1963.

dence indicating the nucleus of the psychological structure, its inherent maturational patterns, and the nature of the effect of the culture upon these patterns.

The content of this chapter, for the most part, is not original. Many points are to be found, better stated, in the child psychoanalytic and psychiatric literature. I shall not quote the literature since a valid review of it would constitute a chapter in itself, and a brief sentence out of context would be an injustice to the author of the original article. My comments are based upon my own clinical observations; from these, I can only raise questions and suggest hypotheses. One conclusion to me seems clear. Our professional language and theories have not kept up with our knowledge of infant behavior or with cultural changes. Without question, our application of the theory to clinical practice is not to the same degree the victim of semantics.

A striking example of the inaccurate use of words to conceptualize infant behavior is the description, so often found in the literature, of the neonate as "passively receptive." [1] This terminology results in a theory based upon an inaccuracy of perception. Other students, especially those experienced in observing infants, point out that this picture is incorrect. No nursing mother would comprehend any description of her sucking infant that implied passivity on his part.

The earliest period of life is not completely accessible to exploration. To a certain extent an understanding of its significance is dependent upon reconstruction from extremely fragmentary material, upon creative interpretation of later personality constellations, and upon extrapolations from observed phenomena at a time when the infant is too undeveloped to manifest psychologically determined, goal-directed behavior. However, observations of neonatal behavior would suggest that the extrapolations have been affected by wish-fulfilling fantasies of what a return to infancy would provide. The wish-determined conclusions have become a part of our theoretical psychology and have been utilized in the diagnostic appraisal of certain patterns of regression.

At no time during the sucking period is an infant passive. The nursing sequence is characterized by an active sucking, active seeking for an object to suck, and active participation in deriving nourishment from that object. The infant is not cognitively aware of the goal of his act in seeking the breast and sucking, but lack of knowledge is not to be equated with passivity. Only if this activity proves futile and the infant experiences unrelieved distress does he cry. The infant's exhaustion ending in sleep, occurring when adequate nutrition is not obtained, is

---

1. This terminology apparently originated in the concept that the aim of an instinct is to attain a state of absence of stimulus tension, and, in the neonate, to take in through sucking. This formulation of the aim of the instinct was then utilized to describe the behavior of the infant in the process of achieving that goal.

the measure of the actual expenditure of energy. The sleep following adequate relief of hunger may be due not only to the state of satiation and thus the absence of stimulus tension, but may in part be due to fatigue. When such a level does not result, the infant's postnursing state may be different. Many studies indicate that a state of sleep is not the only alternative to discomfort-wakefulness in the neonate. There are also periods of nonsleep in which it appears probable that the stimuli to which the infant is responding are not producing intolerable tension but rather are compatible with a state of equalization between stimulation and response. This state may follow appetite satiation in the neonate.

Sucking appears to be an inherent discharge mechanism irrespective of the nutritional benefit derived from it.[2] Perhaps the most successful therapeutic result I ever had was in the case of a 6-week-old infant who was a persistent fist sucker, not only when awake but also when asleep. My therapeutic tool was to suggest to the mother that she buy new nipples for the infant's bottle so that the milk would not flow so freely. The infant stopped sucking his fist, once an urge for active sucking could be gratified by a stiffer nipple.

That the child is, because of the limitations his immature state imposes upon him, dependent upon an outside source for succor is obvious. He is an infantile version of the early tiller of the soil who was considered self-sufficient as the result of his own labors. He worked hard to suck out of mother earth the nutrition essential for survival. He was not a passive, receptive person but rather found in mother earth the passive giver upon whom he was dependent. So with the infant!

It is in reality the nursed mother, not the nursing infant, who experiences passive gratification when the infant is at the breast. It is true that physiologically she actively produces and stores the milk. In response to certain psychological as well as physiological stimuli the glands will discharge the milk. But in the nursing process itself the infant *takes* from the storehouse. The mother's willingness to have the milk taken prevents this act from being larceny. The physical response of the breast to the stimulus does not disrupt the mother's psychological state of relaxation and contentment. It is in part through the mutuality of the mother's willingness to give passively and the infant's willingness to take actively that the infant-mother oneness is maintained in spite of the physical severing of the umbilical cord. From many case histories it is apparent that when the mother actively gives, as illustrated in pressuring the infant to eat, or when the infant makes little or no effort to

2. Studies have indicated that if an infant is fed from birth from a cup, the sucking response is not present and the object sucking one would theoretically expect does not occur. There are many possible explanations for this; some will be discussed in section 2.

obtain food, the unit, infant and mother, may prematurely disintegrate, with later serious repercussions.

The language of mothers seems to confirm this meaning of the infant's nursing to them. When breast-fed babies are weighed before and after nursing to determine the amount of milk that was consumed, the mother most typically will say, "He took so many ounces," or, "I had so many ounces." It is unusual for a nursing mother to say, "I gave him," or, "He held" so many ounces. The typical mother apparently does not see her infant as a hollow cylinder to be filled, but rather as an active organism, taking from her that which she gladly allows to be taken.

A more unfortunate use of a term to indicate the taking rather than receiving role of the infant is the categorization of the less regimented feeding schedule presently popular as "demand feeding." In choosing this term rather than one such as "need feeding" the pediatricians indicated, probably quite unconsciously, the active seeking of the infant and the desired passive compliance of the mother.

From whence then comes this fantasy of a relationship with the mother symbol in which the mother is not the passive but is the active giver? While the nursing period is part of the amnesia of later life, a memory trace apparently becomes the thread that is woven into a fantasy. It finds expression in our concept of the passive-receptive oral stage; we fantasy with nostalgic longing that in infancy manna flowed from heaven.

The more deeply buried experience of neonatal life is that of the degree of active behavior involved in obtaining gratification of nutritional needs. This experience is so deeply buried, it does not find expression even in fantasy. In the semantics of our psychological theory, we deny what we actually know from observation and we believe our fantasy of passive receptiveness to be a fact. If the living organism is ever so passively receptive as such a fantasy indicates, it would be during intrauterine life. If it is experienced at that time, the state of passivity is abruptly interrupted by birth.

There is perhaps a clinical aspect to this theoretical concept. Are there not two types of patients in whom regression to or fixation at an early infantile state is observed? One type is not passive in seeking immature gratification but will spend a great deal of energy in attempting to please so as to be rewarded in the framework of an immature, dependently gratifying relationship with another. The regressive nature of this behavior is obvious. The individual attempts to please as a small child attempts to please the mother. Just as a small child, wishing to be secure in the mother's love, does not passively wish for it but actively attempts to hold the parental love, so likewise does this type of regressed patient. The patient's psychological investment of energy as well as that of the small child may have an anlage in the infant's investment of physical energy to obtain food. The adult patient has regressed to, or is fixated at, an early phase of development, utilizing previously effective but immature ways to earn a psychological living.

In contrast, another clinical picture of regression to, or seeming fixation at, the early period of life is that of the individual who is frustrated if gratification of a desire to receive without effort on his part is not forthcoming; here we see the psychological phenomenon of the true, passively dependent personality. The wish inherent in this behavior cannot be explained by the simple formulation of regression to, or fixation at, the oral level of development. It must either be a regression to an earlier period in which the organism was truly passive, which, if true, would mean a return to intrauterine life, or it is a withdrawal into a fantasy as to what life was during the neonatal period, but which in actuality it was not. Within the limits of our present knowledge, the patient's response seems to be indicative of an attempt to make a fantasy real.

The latter type of patient raises an interesting point for speculation. Is the clinical phenomenon of this type of regression related to the time when self and object were not differentiated? In this case the manifestation of the regression actually indicates a new attempt to attain a self-identity, an attempt which now is in the service of avoiding rather than reestablishing the true infant-mother interaction. This would imply that the patient is saying in effect, "If I were the mother, I would not make the infant struggle for nutrients. I would be a good mother and would actively give. Thus, as a baby I should be given to, not have to work to attain." The identification sought is with the passivity of the mother which will then be gratified through a fantasied state of passive receptiveness in a freely giving world.

The first group of patients, in my experience, is much more responsive to therapy than is the second. Those of the first type, no matter how immaturely they woo one to be a rewarding mother, eventually can gain sufficient insight and possibly realize enough gratification from a corrective emotional experience in therapy that they can find satisfaction on a more mature level. They attain some capacity for interpersonal relationships of a nature which is a component of the psychologically adult personality; dependency upon others is no longer a direct or disguised manifestation of infantile dependency.

This shift to a more mature form of dependency is the result of a maturational process in the patient. In theoretical, diagnostic, and therapeutic work a great deal of emphasis is placed upon the dependent needs of small children and the immature nature of dependent longings of certain adult patients. For semantic economy the word "dependence" has come to be used as the equivalent of immature dependence.

This has resulted in some lexical confusion. Psychological maturation from early infancy to adulthood is not characterized by a gradual relinquishment of dependent relationships. One of the significant components of any civilization is the capacity of its adult members to be maturely interdependent. The so-called "dependent" adult patient is characteristically an *immaturely* dependent person.

The behavior of the second type of patient described above is not only an indication of a desire for gratification for immaturely dependent needs but has an additional significance. They are expressing an unwillingness to tolerate the abandonment of their fantasy of what the mother should be. They are like the child who told me to instruct his mother to love him because, as a mother, she *had* to love him. She was bad if she did not. In discussing with a colleague an alcoholic patient of his, I commented on this differentiation I had hypothesized. He responded that this second group is composed of those people who bite the psychological breast that feeds them. It will be interesting to see, as a result of the current longitudinal studies, if the latter type of regressive syndrome is statistically more frequent in those individuals whose early feeding history was one of minimal zest during the nursing period, in contrast to those neonates who sucked with vim.

Current patterns of infant feeding have not been fully incorporated into the present conceptualization of the significance of the neonatal period. While there are outstanding examples in which it is not true, many references to the breast in current literature refer to the oral gratification derived from the breast and thus its significance as a primary object. But many of our patients were never breast-fed, during neonatal life probably never saw a breast, yet the breast appears in their material as it does in that of people who suckled at the breast for their early nutrition. I have not treated an adult who, having been bottle-fed during infancy, used the bottle as symbolic of mother love. Even the alcoholic craves what is in the bottle, but does not value the bottle per se. I would be interested in anyone's experience with an adult patient who did utilize the bottle as a representation of the primary object and of mother love.

A patient of mine, an adult, when dealing with the roots of his intense jealousy of his younger sister developed a milk "addiction." He could not seem to get enough milk to satisfy his craving for it. Prior to that time he had not cared for milk. I knew he had been breast-fed and this craving for milk, developing as it did as he probed deeper and deeper into the etiology of his jealousy, seemed to be related to his jealousy of his sister at the mother's breast. Further inquiry established the following facts. He was born in Germany immediately after the First World War. There was no food for him except that which his mother's breasts could provide, and this was very little. During the first year of his life he was in a chronic state of near starvation. His sister was born after the Hoover Commission provided milk for infants. His sister was *bottle*-fed. With this information it became apparent that the jealousy of my patient was not rooted in envy of the nursing sibling, but in envy of nutrition itself.

Cathexis of a nursing bottle is seen in small children who have been bottle-fed. Mothers are encouraged to follow a "demand" (*sic*) feeding schedule, and many mothers offer a bottle to the infant whenever and for whatever reason an infant is seeking comfort. Thus the bottle has a great deal of meaning other than that of nutrition to the small infant. It becomes a substitute for many other gratifications that are sought but not forthcoming.

As a result we see infants who have cathected the bottle and value it after the need for sucking gratification has normally receded. Occasionally one sees an infant carry a bottle around whether it is full or empty. This suggests that the bottle might become of lasting symbolic value. However, except in extremely disturbed children, this prolongation of attachment to the bottle is relatively short-lived and usually disappears in the second or third year of life when other activities become more available and enjoyable.

During therapy, an older child will at times suck a real or toy bottle. This is often done somewhat humorously. The humor hides the regressive type of gratification the behavior provides. However, regression to an infantile level in therapy of children more often is shown by lap sitting, clinging, and other direct bodily contacts, rather than by undisguised orality. In my experience, the prognosis of the case is better if the child, sucking a bottle during a therapy session, wishes that experience to be coupled with body contact or other sensory stimulation. The prognostic significance of this can be explained by interpreting such behavior as evidence of the existence or absence of object relatedness. However, that alone does not encompass the total meaning of the behavior. The relatedness to the human object, when it is present, is expressed by patterns that are a part of, not by a symbolic representation of, infancy.

In a nonclinical setting, I observed an infant's response which would be hard to explain on any basis other than an unusually early awareness of the gratification derived from being held. The infant was just 4 months old. Her mother and her 2-year-old sister had been away from the infant for approximately three hours; they returned accompanied by the children's grandmother. During that time interlude her father had given her a bottle, holding her during the feeding period. The infant knew her grandmother well, and on her arrival readily accepted being held by her. She relaxed comfortably in her arms, and watched her sister's choreography as the latter danced in front of her, sucking orange juice from a bottle. The infant smiled and cooed. The older child then leaped into her father's arms and, lying in a nursing position, continued to suck the bottle. Immediately the infant became tense and cried. She could not be comforted. But as soon as her father dislodged the older child and took the infant in his arms, she quieted down and became her characteristic good-natured self. The nursing bottle did not enter the picture at all.

Curious about this behavior, I questioned the pediatrician about the infant's usual care. I anticipated that she was frequently held at times other than during the feeding periods. He indicated that the actual situation was quite different; in fact, he had planned to discuss it with the mother. Because the older child was a rather demanding child, and the younger very placid, the infant was getting little attention. She spent most of her time, when physical needs did not require attention, lying in her crib in a room alone. He felt she was being seriously deprived.

This youngster is now 3 years old. It is interesting to observe her response at this time. She has continued to be a rather placid child, but quickly woos people. When she is held she is "cuddly," not, however, in a way suggesting a regressive pattern, but rather with a warmth of responsiveness typical of a 3-year-old who likes and feels secure with people. Undoubtedly the physician's advice led to the infant's receiving more attention and thus the potential dangers from her early life experiences were obliterated. But it also appears that any holding was a source of real gratification to her. A very early form of jealousy was aroused when another was offered, by a primary person in her life, an experience she enjoyed. Undoubtedly this response was reinforced by the fact that her father had just recently fed her. But to me the significant fact was that this response did not come when she saw her sister sucking the bottle, but only when her sister lay in her father's arms. Yet her experience with this type of gratification had been limited so that one cannot assume it was an acquired taste on her part resulting from an unusual amount of physical attention. It also suggests that this youngster probably should be classified with a group of infants whose early response to the stimulation inherent in being held is strong.

Thumb sucking is interesting to consider at this point. Thumb sucking is recognized generally as having two possible roots. Early in neonatal life some infants apparently do not have sufficient gratification of their sucking urge after their nutritional needs are met and they augment their gratification by nonnutritional sucking. This is undoubtedly why my therapy with the 6-week-old fist-sucker was so successful. Later thumb sucking is considered to have a different significance. Then it appears to be characteristically related to a vague sense of insecurity or comfort deprivation. It may develop when a child, exposed chronically to an intensity of stimulation he cannot handle by a direct response, is not adequately supported by others. In that event, he is frequently a habitual thumb-sucker. When a child who is only an occasional thumb-

sucker faces an atypical situation which is overstimulating and therefore cannot be mastered, he will suck his thumb. At this age thumb
sucking has become a psychological phenomenon on a level higher
than that of an inherent pattern of response.

Early thumb sucking or fist sucking can be modified if a pacifier is
substituted for the fist or thumb. Such a substitute is not so easily accepted later unless there is a continuity between the early and later patterns of sucking. It is true that in the later period the self and object
have become differentiated, but this is a fact, not an explanation of the
refusal to shift the suckable object. It would seem that on the basis simply of a wish for oral gratification from an object as a substitute for the
breast, an object separate from the self rather than a part of the self
would be chosen, once self and object have been differentiated. In
some cases blankets, for example, are habitually sucked. People suck
pens, pencils, and cigarettes. But the habitually sucking infant more
often persistently sucks his thumb rather than another object. Many
times a blanket or other object is used for *cutaneous sensory gratification*
while the thumb is sucked.

Is it possible that this choice of the thumb to suck in preference to an
object has another facet of significance? When the thumb is sucked, two
experiences are provided, that of sucking and that of being sucked.
The gratification of the oral component may be coupled with a pleasurable sensory experience in the thumb. A suggestion of the value of this
component to some children is the observation occasionally reported by
mothers that the child gave up thumb sucking when the thumb became
chapped and sore as a result of the almost continuous wetness caused
by the sucking; no substitute object was chosen. Furthermore, when the
barbaric custom of splints and the like are utilized to break the child of
thumb sucking, he often develops other symptoms. In most instances
(there are exceptions), the new symptom is not that of sucking other
objects. Something enjoyed, for which there is no substitute, is absent
when the thumb is no longer available. Is it possible that it is the sensory experience in the thumb that is missing?

It is important to consider other sensory experience the infant has
during nursing or at other times, in addition to those related to the oral
mucosa. Whether an infant is breast-fed or not, the natural position of
the infant in the mother's arms is for the head to be pillowed against
the mother's breast. If the infant is fortunate enough to have a mother
who, in spite of refusal or inability to nurse the infant, at least provides
the nonoral, cutaneous experience of pillowing the infant's head
against the breast, the infant has sensory gratification from the breast.
That gratification has no oral component. It may be this sensory experience that explains in part the acceptance by some infants of a substitute object such as a blanket rather than a bottle when under stress.

The warmth and softness of the blanket is equated with the warmth and softness of the mother's body. Actually, some infants experience cutaneous pleasure only from blankets and in those cases the blanket is the real object rather than a substitute for or symbol of the real object.

Infants who are attached to a blanket will lie down, pillowing the head on the blanket instead of using the blanket for a cover, or, if sucking the thumb, will hold the blanket close to the cheek. This latter is the counterpart of the breast-fed baby's experience, and suggests that the thumb is the substitute for the nipple of the breast or bottle. The bottle-fed baby is repeating an experience, either with cutaneous sensations created by the soft breast or the softness of other parts of the mother's body. Recently "Peanuts," the pen child of the cartoonist Schulz, clarified the value of his ever-present blanket. He explained that his blanket "absorbs all my fears and frustrations." What theoretician could describe as succinctly the meaning of an object that provides security not by giving but, as Peanuts' friend responded, by being a "spiritual blotter?"

It is interesting that the bottle-fed baby does not perpetuate into later life a cathexis of the bottle, as we assume the breast is cathected by the breast-fed baby; rather, he will shift to use of the breast as a symbol of mothering as he develops capacity for symbolic thought. The use of the breast as a symbol of mother love and of infantile gratification is possibly a sociological heritage, carried down from its origin through our art, literature, and language. At one time, in the not-too-distant past, the mother's breast was the only source of nutrition to the neonate. It was thus a priceless object to the individual and to the race, being a symbol of the contribution by the mother to basic survival. It has been retained through our social heritage. It symbolizes, as the individual develops an ability to utilize symbols, all the multiple facets of the vaguely remembered comforts the infant experienced from the mother figure. Probably this heritage is reinforced by a memory trace of the gratification other than nutritional that many individuals as infants had as they were held. It is this experience of the past that requires no activity on the infant's part. This is perhaps the nirvana of infancy.

The infant experiences many pleasure-providing sensations during neonatal life. If certain of these become excessively erotized, they may become a part of the foundation for neurodermatitis, possibly arthritis, and perhaps other psychosomatic or neurotic symptoms. However, every relatively psychologically healthy adult has retained a capacity for pleasure derived not only from orality but from the other erogenous zones dominant in neonatal life. Unless they are considered as a part of forepleasure in heterosexuality, they are often described as a displacement of orality and as substitutes, by a very circuitous route, for that primary source of pleasure. It is less confusing to consider the possibility that multiple sources of infantile pleasure remain through life, retaining their original value, whether or not they also come into the service of the psychological economy of symbolic representation. Those erogenous zones are manifested in an exaggerated form and often used symbolically if early patterns were overly accentuated, or have been contaminated by a reinforcement through displacement from another erogeneous area. The achievement of a heterosexual level of libidinal discharge, via the vicissitudes of the developmental steps of orifice erotization, is not challenged by this concept; it only questions whether the concepts of psychological distortions and health have not been too narrowed by a study of only one component of that roadway. The neonate has been seen as a sucking mouth, rather than a whole organism of which one part is the mouth.

Freud pointed out that he had emphasized one aspect of the total psychological gestalt because that was his area of interest, but indicated that other areas should also be explored! As a result of the present study of infancy, it has seemed sounder to attempt to understand the important infant-mother entity in the earliest phase of life, its vicissitudes and its development, through consideration of the totality of the interflow between mother and child. This includes not only the feeding experience and cutaneous sensory stimulation but also mutual experiences of all types, those, for example, resulting from visual and auditory stimulation, the multiple aspects of rhythmic movements, and the subtle communication that is based upon the muscle tone of both mother and infant.

An adult patient, whom I had unsuccessfully attempted to treat as a child of 7, came to see me at the age of 19 for analysis. During the earlier attempt at therapy she had been very resistant to coming in and often had to be forcibly dragged to the door. During the hour she showed very little interest in the play equipment, talked only to complain of how mean her mother and friends were, and became very hostile and sullen when I made any friendly verbal or physical gesture toward her. Her mother withdrew her from therapy because she felt it would be fruitless to continue. I apparently agreed, for I did not urge her to stay in therapy. A colleague had made a similar attempt to treat her earlier, with the same discouraged response, both on the part of the mother and the therapist herself.

There were many developments in this case, interesting in the light of the picture that was presented at the age of 7, but I would like to describe only one aspect, unsatisfactory as it is to present it separate from the complete case. I knew from the earlier history that the patient had been breast-fed until she was 5 months old. Frequently, associative material brought a recall of her early contact with me, which in reality extended over about ten therapy hours. Gradually, during her analysis she recalled more and more concerning my waiting room and therapy room, recalling some details that I had difficulty at times confirming by my own hazy recollections of 12 years ago. One object was always a part of her recall, a bowl of artificial oranges. These oranges became, in the analysis, a symbol of what she wanted from me. She often said if only I still had the oranges and would give them to her, she would be well. The oral implications and the breast symbolization seemed clear. This wish to receive from me orally became the focus of that phase of the analysis. But both to her and to me as she reacted to the material, there was a hollow ring.

She recalled that I always offered her candy and cookies during the hour. Sometimes I had the kind she liked. She remembered how angry she felt when I made this offering and that, even though she was a compulsive eater, she always refused. She wondered speculatively whether she had really wanted something else but did not, either then or now, know what she wanted. Characteristically, she did not respond to the concept of longing for the breast as a symbol, but as a realistic object. She had little capacity through much of her analysis to utilize symbols. As much as this was a complication in the analysis, it did serve to bring forth the subsequent material.

After a time, her behavior on the couch and her associations changed. For several hours she seemed to nestle on the couch, and in a dreamlike state she would talk of wanting to sink into the couch and remain a part of it, to be a part of my room, and to be constantly with me. She wanted to curl up in my lap, not to talk, to do nothing but just experience the sensation of lying there. Finally, during one of these dreamlike periods, she suddenly said, "That's what I wanted. I wanted to live with you, to always be with you—for you to be my mother. I knew I couldn't, and it would have hurt too much to know that was what I wanted. All I felt was anger." She was referring to her earlier therapy experience. This patient was subject to a neurodermatitic type of skin lesion during her adult life. The lesions occurred whenever she felt that people were not giving to her but rather were making demands upon her.

This material, as it was worked through over several weeks, heralded the beginning of reintegration in the analysis. There were two very interesting external indications of this change. One was in her response to my absence. Previously, any trip of mine brought about panic, a need to eat excessively, acting out, or a fantasy of acting out her previous characterological symptoms, and an inability to handle any frustrations. The next and subsequent trips on my part she handled very adequately. Secondly, she no longer accused me of treating her only because I wanted her father's money. Quite unexpectedly to herself as well as to me, she said one day, "You like me," expressing both in her tone of voice and her ruminations about her remark her wonderment at knowing her statement was true.

From the sequence of the material in this analysis it seemed to me that the symptomatology, which was classical for those of fixation at an early oral level, was related not primarily to specific oral deprivation, but rather to the lack of oneness with the mother, experienced through the unsatisfactory bodily contact with the mother. The mother was a narcissistic woman, who, it was apparent in the history obtained when the child was 7, emotionally abandoned the child whenever she failed to serve as a narcissistically rewarding extension of herself. The breast feeding per se was adequate, it was over-all mothering that was absent; this lack resulted in a significant deprivation. This patient's obsessive eating during the periods of emotional turmoil appeared to be the result of offering herself the one satisfaction her mother had given her in infancy. She was not sexually aroused by intercourse, but enjoyed the physical closeness it provided. (Intercourse had other meanings also, not so directly related to this phase of her analysis.) After working through her wish to be physically one with the couch, my room, and myself, and the sensory longings involved in this, she was able for the first time to experience an orgasm, although she had much to work through before she finally became maturely sexual. She handled a period of emotional disturbance through a new psychological closeness with her current boyfriend and without any urge for excessive eating. Since this woman had not developed the severe pathology attributed to the failure of the symbiotic relationship between infant and mother, she provided an opportunity to observe the nonoral aspects of fixation at a very early developmental level.

Clinically the broader aspects of the infant-mother relationship during neonatal life are a part of our therapeutic conceptualization. Many writers have stressed other important experiences. However, when we attempt to define the symptoms of regression to early infancy as an attempt at oral incorporation, or as an attempt to return to the state of passive receptiveness when manna seemed to flow from heaven, we are crippling our therapeutic selves by too narrow a formulation of the infant's experience. Unless we carefully define our use of the term *oral stage* we invite serious misunderstanding among those for whom *oral* means *mouth*. As wounding to our sensitive souls as Freud's expression (1905) was, his definition of the infantile instincts as "polymorphous perverse" was a significant concept.

WEANING

The significance of weaning to the infant has been stressed in theoretical discussions of early infancy and in descriptions of the impact of early experiences upon the development of the adult psychological configuration. Weaning is frequently referred to as one of the earliest traumas in the normal maturational experience of the infant; it deprives the infant of a primary object. According to certain theoreticians, this loss of a primary object often occurs when the infant's response to the breast changes from that of "passive receptiveness," more accurately from "sucking," to "oral aggressiveness"; in other words, when the infant bites the breast, the biting is being attributed in part to the infant's hostile aggressive impulses or to his wish to cannibalistically ingest the breast. Furthermore, it is implied that weaning is imposed upon the infant by an outside agent, with the infant seeing that act as motivated by hostility on the part of the one who deprives him. It is assumed that this hostility is interpreted by the infant as an indication of the withdrawal or absence of love, or as retaliation for his own hostile aggressive or cannibalistic impulses.

During this period the infant will hit an object with another object; he will break objects if they have a fragility that is in proper ratio to his strength; he will squeeze live or toy animals; he will bite any solid form available. The intensity with which he carries this out suggests that he enjoys the activity. This behavior also has been interpreted by some as evidence of an inherent destructive pattern related to hostile aggression.

I would question whether this shift from sucking to biting and the behavior that results in injury to or destruction of an object is as psychologically determined as this concept of aggression implies. It is possible that it is more related to neurophysiological development which results in coordinated movement and, as far as biting is concerned, a more effective utilization of the muscles involved in mastication. Furthermore, the tenderness of the gums related to beginning dentition, in many instances, may encourage the biting response. The sensory experience of biting down on tender gums and the response of the individual whose breasts are bitten may lead later to the use of biting as a direct or symbolic expression of hostile aggression and finally, being found pleasurable, become identifiable as an expression of either masochistic or sadistic impulses. It seems somewhat questionable, however, to assume that in infancy this response is either masochistic or sadistic.

Abraham (1924) in his original formulation of the oral character indicated that neuromuscular development enables the infant to bite, that this act is pleasurable, and that the later character traits reflecting oral sadism are "built upon the ruins of an oral erotism whose development has miscarried." It was in the enlargement of this concept that the psychologically goal-directed behavior of the infant as sadistic in nature became a part of the theory of personality development. But a wish to hurt another cannot take form until the infant not only conceptualizes himself as separate from the object but can also identify with the object to the extent that he can conceive that another feels pain that he himself does nc: experience. When the infant is weaned at an early age before such differentiation, it most often has a deleterious effect. That would suggest that some other factor than mutual hostility may be involved.

If a breast-fed infant is suddenly weaned, his behavior often indicates that the experience is a stressful or traumatic one for him. This can be observed directly at the time of precipitous weaning. It is frequently clearly described in the history obtained from parents concerning their child's infancy. The effect can be observed whether weaning was due to the mother's attitude toward nursing or because of some reality need. Probably the mother's unwillingness to continue nursing the infant has negative repercussions more often than when reality, not her attitude, determines the cessation of breast feeding. This would suggest, as so many other observations in other areas have, that preverbal communication through multiple channels of physical contact and physically defined experiences, and characterized by a two-way flow, exists between the infant and the mother. The observation that some infants accept the shift from breast to bottle without manifest disturbance does not invalidate the conclusion that for many infants it is a traumatic experience. It does not invalidate the observation that if the infant does bite the breast and the mother reacts by angry withdrawal, such a sequence of events can have future significance. It only suggests that although such reactions to a traumatic stress do occur, they are not necessarily universal.

Many children of today are not weaned from the breast because they have not nursed the breast. They are weaned from a bottle. More significantly, they are not weaned suddenly. They are gradually weaned and complete the weaning process themselves. There are two phases in the weaning experience of the present-day infant. On the one hand, he is partially weaned from the breast or bottle very early as a result of the introduction of semisolid food in his diet. This typically occurs when he is about 3 months of age. At first the infant sucks the food from the spoon; later he develops the more mature skill of shoving the food off the spoon into his mouth and biting down upon it. When the infant shifts from sucking the food off the spoon to utilizing his lips and teeth to push the food into his mouth, he has begun to wean himself. During this phase of development the typical infant feeding regime of the present does not deprive him of continued sucking experience. Frequently he is given a bottle during or after solid food is ingested and after liquids have been taken successfully from a cup, particularly at bedtime, until well into the second year of life. Many mothers allow the infant to continue to derive some of his nutrition from a bottle until the infant on his own initiative forsakes the bottle.

A pediatrician pointed out to me a common observation he has made in watching the development of his young patients. He noticed that an infant will react positively to being given milk from a cup and will refuse a bottle before he would anticipate that the infant was ready to relinquish the latter. He assumed that this was either in imitation of the mother or in response to her teaching him the skill. This response typically lasts for a few meals. Then the infant rejects the cup and the wise mother returns to offering milk in a bottle. Later the infant again accepts milk from the cup, will strive to handle the cup himself, and will show progressively less interest in the bottle as a source of supply irrespective of the mother's stress on either the bottle or the cup.

The histories of infants whose mothers did not insist that the bottle be given up often indicate that the infant himself discarded it eventually. This suggests that if weaning from the bottle is not imposed from without, it will be self-imposed. From a physiological standpoint it appears that this shift would be related to neurophysiological development. As indicated above, this development facilitates the use of muscles involving mastication. The shift to mastication occurs frequently before the eruption of teeth. Any new neurophysiological development stimulates utilization of the activity related to it with a concomitant increase in the rate of the neurophysiological maturation process. Paralleling this neurophysiological maturation, which results in the infant utilizing other mechanisms in addition to sucking to derive his nutrition, I would hypothesize that there is a psychological maturation process. The core of this maturational process is the urge to wean the self.

A mother who is concerned over work created by an infant feeding himself with fingers and spoon is well aware of self-weaning that extends beyond weaning from the bottle or breast. Not only does the infant show interest in obtaining food in a manner other than sucking, he protests against being fed by the mother; he attempts to grab the spoon or to fill his buccal orifice with a food-smeared fist. While the attempt to use the spoon may be imitation of the mother, a response to her teaching, and awareness of her pleasure in observing his developing skill, the use of his fist can scarcely be so explained. It resembles more a prehistoric pattern by which, in a practical way, to obtain nutrition. When the infant develops a coordination that enables him to put things into his mouth, a talent that he indulges in to the point of putting any available object into his mouth; when the utilization of that ability leads to the availability of tasty food and relief of hunger; and when he is ready to shift from sucking to biting—he follows the table manners of his forefathers. The infant's attempt to feed himself suggests not only that if weaning from the bottle is not imposed, it is instituted by the infant himself, but also that even though he cannot provide the nutritional substance, he weans himself from direct dependency upon another for its intake. His fortuitous experience of using his skill and being rewarded with good food enhances the value of the skill and also provides a way to wean himself.

That breast-fed babies are more reluctant to wean themselves is dramatically indicated in observations concerning children in those cultures in which the lactating mother's breast is available for three or four years. These observations do not necessarily invalidate the preceding concept. One would have to know what else of mothering is available to the child before assuming that an infant will cling to an adequately flowing breast until it is withdrawn. It would also be important to consider what the nutritional alternatives are, and how adequate both in quantity and quality they are. It is, however, possible that with the tendency to bottle-feed babies and the encouragement of early intake of solid foods, infants are being precipitated into self-weaning somewhat prematurely.

Material obtained from older children and adults supports the concept that frequently the weaning process did create conflicts that, overtly or in a more disguised form, are manifested in the presenting character structure or in neurotic or psychotic behavior. The psychological configurations that have been understood as the effect of stressful weaning experiences and the observation of infant behavior when weaning is not imposed by another indicate the desirability of further study of the weaning process itself, the object from which the infant is weaned, and the nature of the weaning conflict, if present, particularly when the weaning was not demanded by others.

Self-imposed weaning, I would tentatively hypothesize, is a manifestation of the infant's growing awareness of himself. It is thus a step in the evolvement of narcissism, a shift from a pattern essential for survival to investment in the psychological self. It is the beginning crystallization of the "I." The "I" is defined in part by doing *for* the self as well as being aware of what is being done *to* the self. When the infant discovers that fingers smeared by food through his own act provide the pleasure the mother-managed spoon provided, he has found an important way of establishing his own separateness.

Mahler and Gosliner (1955) have referred to the time of the establishment of the self-object relationship in contrast to the symbiotic relationship of the infant and the mother as a second birth phenomenon. This concept is very important. They indicate that this occurs during "the period from twelve-eighteen to thirty-six months" (p. 196). It is probable that at least the inception of it is earlier, at that point in development when the infant begins to minister to the self, not only in the terms of food but also in other activities. The exact time of this occurrence cannot be determined because it is a gradually evolving phenomenon. Prodromal factors are the infant's gradual awareness of objects in the environment, his ocular ability to follow moving objects and to focus on objects, his observation of movements of his hands and feet as well as those objects not a part of himself, the awareness that touching himself results in a dual sensation, touching an object in only one sensation, and the acquiring of ability to perform certain movements such as reaching which appear to be goal-directed. He gradually becomes aware that objects are separate from himself and thus that the self and the object are different entities. This step is related to the neurological growth that is occurring, probably primarily in the development of subcortical-cortical connections and the association fibers in the cortex itself. This growing awareness of the self as differentiated from objects is an essential initiation of the self-weaning process. It is my impression that the actual self-weaning is recognizable as a psychological pattern at an age that corresponds to Spitz's (1957) 8-month anxiety.

If self-imposed weaning begins with the differentiation of the self and the object and parallels the development of 8-month anxiety, it suggests another dimension in the interpretation of the latter phenomenon. Spitz has stressed the significance of the presence of strangers in arousing the anxious response of the infant. When the stranger, in the absence of the mother, appears within the infant's visual range, it is easy to follow Spitz's concept. "The child produces first a scanning behavior, namely, the seeking for the lost love object, the mother. A decision is now made by the function of judgment 'whether something which is present in the ego as an image, can also be re-discovered in perception' (Freud, 1925). The realization that it cannot be rediscovered in the given instance provokes a response of unpleasure. In terms of the eight-months anxiety, what we observe can be understood as follows: the stranger's face is compared to the memory traces of the mother's face and found wanting. This is not mother, she is lost. Unpleasure is experienced and manifested" (p. 54).

However, if the mother and stranger appear together or if the stranger appears when the mother is already holding the infant, the scanning, seeking ocular behavior of the infant must result in the infant alternately seeing the mother and the stranger and at times seeing both. The infant under such circumstances may appear uneasy, cry and will often turn away to burrow his face into the mother's body.

It is obvious that any evaluation of an infant's behavior has potentiality for many errors. We do not know factually that to which the infant is responding; we can only conjecture. If the infant's comprehension of external reality is such that he can recognize that his perception of the stranger is not compatible with the image he has of the mother, he must equally recognize that the mother is like that image. Is it not possible that the presence of the stranger is sharpened evidence of self-object separateness, and the turning away and the intensifying of physical contact with the mother are actually not only reconfirming the mother image but also trying transiently to reestablish the oneness with the mother, a return to the unity of the symbiotic relationship?

There is another common pattern of behavior in infants at approximately this same maturational level. If awake he objects to his mother leaving him, he appears to wish the mother to remain within his field of vision. He will lie quietly in his crib watching his mother straightening up the nursery or will play with his toys only to cry lustily as soon as she leaves. However, observations of infants in their normal home environment suggest that visual contact with the mother is not the sole source of contentment. Often if the mother is not visible, the sound of her voice or even of her activities will quiet him. Is he able under these circumstances to tolerate separation because the visual or auditory experience stimulates the fantasy image of the mother and also provides a channel for returning to a state of nondifferentiation? If so, that would indicate that the infant is beginning to fantasy an image under the stimulation of other sensory experiences associated with the object and from this gains a sense of security. The capacity for simple fantasies increases the tolerance for separation and also may enable the oneness to be reestablished. If so, this would suggest that possibly fantasy always offers an opportunity to be one with the person imagined, a component of certain highly meaningful relationships that does not disappear with weaning. It would become a significant part of certain more mature facets of interpersonal relationships, such as the capacity for empathy.

Undoubtedly the infant does not mature from nondifferentiation to differentiation of the self and the object in one brief moment. There is an appreciable span of time in which this perception of the self and the nonself as separate entities gradually evolves. Under ordinary circumstances it is likely that the infant passes through a psychological phase of several weeks' or possibly months' duration in which there is a pendular swing between nondifferentiation and differentiation, the infant vacillating between noncognitive fusion with the mother and self-object awareness. The maturational force and cognitive development lead toward the establishment of the self as an identity, but the earlier phase cannot, with ease, be relinquished.

If weaning is considered as encompassing a broader experience than being weaned from the breast, and is considered in this more comprehensive definition as self-initiated weaning from the symbiotic relationship with the mother, a conflict different from the conflict created by the growing recognition of the frustrations imposed by the external world may be present. This alternate conflict would be between two internal urges, only secondarily related to external impositions. The narcissistic urge to establish the self as an object separate from other objects undermines the security provided by the sense of being one with the object; thus the narcissistic need to establish the self as an object separate from other objects is in conflict with the more primitively narcissistic need to retain the secure oneness of the earlier symbiotic relationship. When the mother leaves the infant, the urge for separateness is fulfilled, but not at the will of the infant or tempered to the infant's own capacity to tolerate separation. The security which oneness provided is destroyed. Equally so, strangers recognized as such accentuate the separateness of the individual. In that situation there is no preestablished pathway that a pendular swing can follow. These precipitous or transient weaning experiences are beyond the ego capacity of the child to handle and anxiety is manifested. This concept would possibly explain why sudden weaning or too early weaning proves traumatic in many instances. It not only deprives the child of sucking gratification prematurely, but, particularly when the weaning is from the breast, it prematurely precipitates the infant into being either a separate entity or only a partial one. Furthermore, the security an infant experiences during the normal phase of differentiation is rooted in confidence that he will be cared for and in the awareness that the pendular swing to self-identity can be reversed and the symbiotic relationship can be reestablished. If the symbiotic relationship is prematurely weakened, this confidence is lacking.

Aside from the recognizable picture of the infant seeking to feed himself, his self-initiated abandonment of the bottle, and the phenomenon of stranger anxiety, there is another behavioral characteristic of this maturational stage that suggests further that self-weaning from the symbiotic relationship creates conflict. Just before the infant achieves the neurological maturity that enables him to walk, he is frequently fussier than he has been previously. Mothers will, in a nonscientific way, describe their impressions; the infant to them appears frustrated. This state they may attribute to the infant's "wish to walk" and inability to do so. They may describe its etiology more broadly, saying that the infant wants to do many things he is unable to do. Also at the same time he demands more attention. He wants to be played with, to be held. He is discriminating in seeking that attention, wanting it primarily from his mother or others with whom he has had frequent, rewarding contacts. He is, it appears, struggling to establish his separateness, struggling to achieve new independence from his partner in the earlier symbiotic relationship. To protect himself from being overwhelmed by his own strivings he seeks the presence and services of the mother or an adequate substitute in order to deny that separateness. The fussiness is a manifestation of a conflict—but not one originally between the external world and his internal impulses but rather one between two internally rooted, incompatible impulses; the wish for oneness and the urge to establish the "self" as an entity.

If this interpretation of self-weaning is valid, the adult's material related to weaning can be understood not solely by knowing how the mother weaned the child but also from clues as to how the infant weaned himself and what in the latter process might have been traumatic. This concept may have significance in understanding those patients who present material suggesting a weaning trauma. The meaning of this material may not always have been determined by an early conflict between an internal need and a reality demand. It may in some instances be rooted in a conflict between two incompatible internal urges, a conflict intensified in some instances by too rapid weaning imposed by others.

During the terminal phase of psychoanalytic therapy this conflict may be reactivated. The wish to be on one's own and the wish to remain in a dependent relationship with the therapist are often interpreted as the final struggle between the adult and the infantile self. I have been impressed by material in some cases in which the struggle appears to be at an earlier level, particularly in those cases in which pregenital problems were prominent in the analysis. For example, a patient during a period of marked resistance wished to terminate his analysis because consciously he thought he was ready to do so since his symptoms had disappeared. He stated he really wanted to stop because he would not know who he was as a person until he was functioning independently of analytic sessions. Analysis of this revealed the nature of the resistance. It was structured by his feeling that he could not be sure where I ended and he began. His wish to wean himself in order to establish his own identity as sharply demarcated from me was in conflict with a wish to perpetuate a state of being one with me.

In less neurotic attempts at termination an effective working through of the termination may in part be the process of reestablishing the self-object status, not just becoming reconciled to the fact that one must be weaned from a breast from which nutrition flows. In a discussion of this point a colleague pointed out to me that if this hypothesis is correct, material concerning weaning from the breast brought out during psychoanalytic therapy may have the same significance as primal scene and early seduction associations do. In the latter example, what was once considered to be a memory of actual events has now been recognized as frequently a recall of an infantile fantasy.

I have been particularly interested in what appears to be a reactivation of the self-nonself conflict, the sense of oneness with another in conflict with the need to be an individual, as manifested in the response of certain adolescents in therapy. An adolescent girl sought therapy with me on her own initiative. She complained of her inability to love others. She was able to reconstruct her early life with surprising clarity and to pinpoint the time at which she became aware of many characteristics of her own personality. This occurred when a younger cousin who had been a very conforming, warmly responsive child died. The patient was aware that she had both loved this cousin with whom she had been very congenial and also had been very jealous of her. She believed, a concept which also came out very clearly in her projective material, that the good, like her cousin, died, the bad, like herself, survived. She was aware that she valued herself as a hostile, unloving, and unlovable person. She also wanted to be loved; if she did not love others, they would not love her.

The case was baffling. In spite of her recall of many episodes of childhood which he had interpreted as evidence she was not loved but which she could now reevaluate, in spite of a conviction early in therapy that she was very much loved by her parents, later a certainty that she was completely rejected by them, and finally a realistic recognition of her parents' attitude toward her, an ambivalent one with the negative aspects intensified by the girl's own behavior, there were no changes in her overall behavior, her emotional responses, or the contents of therapy hours. I then did what proved to be catastrophic; I made an extremely premature interpretation. I told her in effect that while she consciously wanted to be loved by others, she actually feared it. To be loved she would have to respond to others in a fashion they found pleasant. Then she would be like everyone else instead of different and an individual separate from others; this would mean to her a loss of her own self-identity. This interpretation, given much less directly than this summary implies, created acute panic in her. She described a feeling that something terrible was about to happen to her and she would cease to exist. She returned for a few more hours, always recalling this comment of mine, how ridiculous it was, and denying the panic she had experienced. Finally she withdrew from treatment, stating I could not help her. She insisted that she did not want to change; she just wanted to find some people who liked her as she was. She confided to her parents that she was afraid of me because I understood her too well.

In retrospect it is my belief that at the time I made this remark she was actually fending off a wish to be close to me. My "understanding" of her increased the temptation to fuse with me; this threatened her with a loss of her own identity. Sometime later she consulted me for recommendations for a therapist in another city. At that time she confirmed my formulation to the extent that she could recall wishing that I would tell her, step by step, how to act like I did so that she would be loved. This type of interpretation I have made with wiser timing to other adolescents, and it has frequently resulted in rich material and important therapeutic gains shown both in clinically manifest behavior and also in the substance of the therapy hours.

Another adolescent early in therapy always moved her lips as I talked. This mannerism gradually disappeared without any explanation of its meaning. After several weeks of supportive therapy, she suggested that she would like to use the couch. For a few hours the sessions were relatively uneventful even though I rather abruptly shifted my role, offering little direct support and remaining relatively silent. Finally some new material came to light, and she immediately sat up. I made some comment in regard to her last association and her lips moved in unison with mine. After this continued for several minutes I commented upon it. She disclaimed being aware of it, but described her anxiety before sitting up and a sense of being one with me as soon as she saw me. "I guess," she commented, "that I am talking to myself as if we were one." That this was a true description of her psychological state at that point seems probable since I had not considered this possible explanation and had not been aware in the therapy how much she experienced our contact as one of fusion. Later as she was able to tolerate more typical analytic sessions, this feeling that we were one became clear.

It is my opinion that in adolescence the young person struggles again with the conflict between being one with the loved parent, evidenced by dependency, and the establishment of what Erikson (1956) describes so clearly as *identity*. The adolescent institutes a self-weaning process which creates for him many of the psychological crises characteristic of that age group. It is a recapitulation of the self-weaning struggle of infancy. Its manifestation is colored, as is true of any of the earlier conflicts reactivated during adolescence, by the effect of maturation, by the capacity for richer fantasy, by the impact of superego demands, and by the patterns of the culture.

In summary, the psychological trauma of weaning and the scars that have often resulted from that trauma may be in some instances the result of unwise weaning from the breast, imposed prematurely or precipitously by an outside agent, the mother. On the other hand, in view of the present patterns of child rearing in which the infant is not breast-fed and often is not deprived of the bottle until he himself abandons it, it is likely that if weaning is not imposed from without, it will be self-imposed. This self-weaning involves not only weaning from a suckable object but also weaning of the self from the symbiotic relationship. Initiated by a growing capacity to observe and recall experiences, it is indicative of a maturational step toward psychological differentiation of the self from the object. This maturational experience creates an internally determined conflict; an urge toward self-identity which is incompatible with the longing to maintain the undifferentiated, secure oneness with the mother. The conflict is intensified because the differentiation is still so hazily defined and not continuous. It is experienced in recurrent short intervals and can be erased or interrupted if stimuli exceed the infant's integrative capacity. During the latter half of the first year of life this conflict is revealed in the infant's behavior; it is often recapitulated during the terminal phase in psychoanalytic therapy and during adolescence. The "weaning trauma" is, broadly speaking, a consequence of the ego's inability to deal with the stress created by the recognition that the self and the source of primary security are separate entities.

CONCLUSION

It seems to me essential that conceptualizations concerning psychological development and the conditions that distort or inhibit that development be constantly reviewed. Two sources of new material of great value are becoming available from those who are observing groups of infants, both under controlled circumstances and also in their home surroundings, and from those who are following infant development over the years considered critical in the evolvement of the personality. From these studies should come a wealth of information concerning "typical" as well as "atypical" patterns of maturation. I have suggested that certain concepts that have been considered nuclear in the theoretical formulations of the significance of very early infancy may require some modification as a result of such studies.

13

DEVELOPMENTAL AND MOTIVATIONAL CONCEPTS IN PIAGET'S SENSORIMOTOR THEORY OF INTELLIGENCE

Peter H. Wolff, M.D.

In the introduction to his Edinburgh lectures on natural religion, William James (1902) wrote:

> Medical materialism seems indeed a good appellation for the too simple-minded system of thought which we are considering. Medical materialism finishes up Saint Paul by calling his vision on the road to Damascus a discharging lesion of the occipital cortex, he being an epileptic. It snuffs out Saint Theresa as an hysteric, Saint Francis of Assisi as an hereditary degenerate. . . . Carlyle's organ-tones of misery it accounts for by a gastro-duodenal catarrh [p. 14]. A more fully developed example of the same kind of reasoning is the fashion, quite common nowadays among certain writers, of criticizing the religious emotions by showing a connection between them and the sexual life. Conversion is a crisis of puberty and adolescence. The macerations of saints, and the devotion of missionaries, are only instances of the parental instinct of self-sacrifice gone astray. For the hysterical nun, starving for natural life, Christ is but an imaginary substitute for a more earthly subject of affection [p. 11f.].

In this manner James prepared his audience for the psychological exploration of religious experience that was to follow in subsequent lectures, by indicating that he would not attempt to reduce complex human experiences to neural excitations or to neurotic instability and other disorders of the mind; in later passages he proposed that such explanations might yield necessary, but could not yield sufficient, explanations of the phenomena in question.

What was fashionable among certain writers in James's time has become an established Weltanschauung among some schools of clinical psychiatry, which look to a unitary causal explanation of behavior. Regardless of our particular theoretical persuasion, as clinical psychiatrists many of us are sometimes inclined to view behavior as if it were deter-

Reprinted from the *Journal*, 2 : 225–243, 1963.

mined only by motivational causes and completely reducible to genetic sources.

My primary assignment today is an exposition of Piaget's sensorimotor theory of development, but I shall also use the opportunity to focus attention on his causal conception of behavior, to show how a comprehensive psychological system which does not postulate inherent internal forces or motives accounts for behavior and development in an internally consistent manner. To highlight those features of Piaget's causal conception that distinguish it from our clinical mode of thinking, I have chosen David Rapaport's definition of motivation because it transcends parochial arguments among schools of motivational psychology, and abstracts the formal characteristics that are apposite to all motivation concepts. His definition states: *"motives are appetitive internal forces.* The defining characteristics of the concept of appetitiveness as I am using it here are the following: (a) peremptoriness, (b) cyclic character, (c) selectiveness, and (d) displaceability" (1960b, p. 187). Within the context of Piaget's theory I shall try to show that under some conditions of internal equilibrium, and with respect to particular kinds of action, Piaget's conception may broaden our general understanding of the causes of behavior and development.

By intention Piaget is a philosopher of science and not a psychologist. His empirical writings culminate in the formulation of a genetic epistemology and a demonstration that the perennial philosophical question, *how man knows the world,* may be fruitfully studied by the empirical methods of developmental psychology.

The fundamental assumptions which Piaget (1936, 1937, 1945) set out to demonstrate are:

1. Intelligence is only one aspect of a general biological adaptation to the environment.

2. Intellectual adaptation is the progressive differentiation and integration of inborn reflex mechanisms under the impact of experience.

3. From the simplest symbolic play to the most complex logical thought, *mental* functions are derived from *motor* actions on concrete objects; the growth of intelligence may be viewed as the progressive transformation of motor patterns into thought patterns, the latter transcending the concrete circumstances out of which they arise.

4. The differentiation of reflex structures and of their function gives rise to the mental operations by which man conceives of object, space, time, and causality, and of the logical relationships which constitute the basis of scientific thought.

Piaget sought to answer, for example, how the newborn infant, equipped with stereotyped reflex behaviors, grows into an 18-month-old child capable of searching for an object after it has disappeared from vision, of inferring unobserved causes from observed results, of constructing spatial relations in thought, and of arranging sequences of action into means-ends relations. He sought to answer how the 18-month-old child, equipped for the first time with representational thought patterns, develops into an adolescent who can formulate abstract problems in the absence of concrete objects, and can solve these by reversible mental functions that approximate the logical operations of algebra.

To outline the model of behavior that is implicit to Piaget's theory, I shall first consider the normal newborn infant who is capable of sucking, grasping, auditory and visual pursuit, and other stereotype behavior patterns. The patterns are primed so that they will be activated by nonspecific stimuli in the average expectable environment. After a reflex behavior has been activated by accidental encounters a sufficient number of times, it is repeated spontaneously, or without additional external stimulation. In the case of reflexes, the act itself serves as a sufficient stimulus to propagate the behavior. In the case of acquired behavior patterns, the infant seeks to renew contact with novelties after he has encountered them; apparently he seeks to repeat newly discovered actions. Action patterns conserved by self-repetition are called *circular reactions;* as each of the reflexes is repeated through circular reaction, behavior corresponding to it is executed with increasing efficiency. Although at birth the child is able to suck at the breast, practice improves his facility and gradually coordinates the ensemble of components making up the sucking act into a stable action adapted to its goal of taking nourishment; but without such practice the component parts present at birth would not be integrated.

At a later stage in development the hand, while moving at random by reflex circular reaction, contacts the mouth and initiates sucking movements. The mouth, already adapted to the breast and to nonnutritive empty sucking, now sucks the hand, and the infant makes repeated efforts to suck his hand. Although the initial efforts are clumsy, the new object (the hand) is not so foreign as to disrupt sucking activity, yet it is sufficiently novel to create a relation of *disadaptation* between the infant's behavior and his environment. After the hand has been brought to the mouth repeatedly by chance, the arm is directed to the mouth, the mouth shapes itself to "receive" the hand before actual contact, and the hand prepares itself to fit the mouth aperture. Gradually a new circular reaction of thumb sucking emerges and persists until the infant sucks his thumb skillfully. After thumb sucking becomes an established form of behavior, the child retains the capacity for empty, nonnutritive sucking and nutritive sucking at the breast. Thus, when two or more behavior patterns coordinate to give rise to a new unit of behavior, the component parts are retained and may still be applied under appropriate circumstances.

From examples like these we can infer the basic model of Piaget's theory of sensorimotor development. The observations show that at least some of neonatal behavior is *organized* as distinct and repeatable action patterns. From this we infer the existence of psychological structures which insure that behavior will be repeated in relatively stable form. The psychological structures existing at birth we call the *reflex schemata*. For each newly acquired motor pattern, such as hand sucking, and for each later thought pattern, we postulate comparable acquired structures or *schemata proper*. In each case the schema is conceptualized as the central guarantee that behavior will be stable and repeatable.

With each repetition behavior changes by an imperceptible increment in the direction of greater adaptation. From this we infer that each activation of a circular reaction alters the behavior to some degree, and that the change is cumulative rather than abrupt. Since the new motor patterns that emerge with practice are also repeatable in stable form, we deduce that the reflex schema itself undergoes change through experience, and that some actual properties of the encounter must also accrue to the schema to change it in the direction of greater adaptation. The function by which each encounter between infant and environment accrues to the schema is defined as *assimilation*. It represents the incorporation of novel encounters into the assembly of all past experiences of the same kind. The function by which the schema changes as the result of assimilation is defined as *accommodation*. It represents the active reorganization of past experiences of one kind which brings the past into closer correspondence with the assimilated novelty. Development is therefore a constant interplay of assimilatory and accommodative functions. Only when the assimilation of a novelty no longer forces a further modification in behavior will we consider that the behavior is adapted or that a balance between assimilation and accommodation has been struck.

Sensorimotor theory postulates assimilation as the universal function that characterizes all living organisms, the function that selectively incorporates specific material substances into organ systems at the organic level, and at the psychological level incorporates sensorimotor data and ideas into already existing mental structures. Assimilation thus broadens the organism's contact with its environment by differentiating the existing internal structure and producing a more accurate inner representation of the relation between individual and environment. It is the intrinsic developmental factor of Piaget's theory.

Fundamental to the concept of assimilation is the notion that new structures are built *because* the organism actively renews contact with specific stimulus situations and integrates these into the already existing structures, and not because the world of stimuli impinges upon a passive organism. The external stimulus plays a vital role since it determines the direction of adaptation, but assimilation is not identical with the reflex response to stimulation. Only those stimuli are assimilated for which an approximating internal structure already exists, and the organism imposes an order on its surroundings in terms of the structures at its disposal. Nor is accommodation identical with response; rather it refers to the organism's constant restructuring of past experiences in keeping with present circumstances. The schema that is generated by assimilatory activity is therefore in no sense an association chain of discrete sensory stimuli and motor responses.

Sir Frederick Bartlett, among the first to introduce the concept of schema to psychology, defined it as "an active organization of past reactions, or of past experiences which must always be supposed to be operating in any well-adapted, organic response. Whenever there is any order or regularity of behaviour, a particular response is possible only because it is related to other similar responses which have been serially organized, yet which operate not simply as individual members coming one after another, but as a unitary mass" (1932, p. 201).

Whatever the schema assimilates is defined as *aliment;* the nature and complexity of aliment that can be assimilated at a given stage is always determined simultaneously by the child's developing structures and by the "action potentialities" of the object encountered—whether the action is concrete behavior or mental activity, whether the object is a concrete thing or an idea.

Aliment does not mean the same as stimulus, which by definition remains identical to itself at successive developmental levels and is defined independent of the organism, while aliment can only be defined in terms of the relation between organisms and object at a particular stage in development. The newborn infant, for example, assimilates the breast, the bottle, or the finger, as something to suck or to see or to grasp, because he is endowed only with reflex schemata which can encompass such global action properties of objects; and his corresponding accommodation consists simply of sucking or looking or grasping all those objects which suit the action. By 3 months, when grasping and looking are coordinated, the appropriate object (e.g., the bottle) also offers aliment for looking and grasping, although the stimulus object has not changed from the "objective" point of view. At 8 months the child assimilates not only the action properties of objects but also their spatial and causal characteristics; then his accommodations will include the effort to see what is on the other side of the bottle, and what happens when he drops it. Thus the meaning which the child attributes to objects and to their interrelations constantly changes as he develops, and is determined neither exclusively by the object's stimulus properties nor exclusively by his apperceptions.

So far I have considered only the mechanisms of action but not the causation of behavior in Piaget's sensorimotor theory. We have seen that as long as an action is not adapted to the stimulus object, each repetition slightly alters the behavior pattern; from this we inferred that assimilation and accommodation had not completed their adaptive work. Until the repetition of an act no longer changes behavior, the corresponding schema is said to be in a state of *disequilibrium,* or the action pattern is said to be in a state of *disadaptation.* The theory assumes that disequilibrium (at the level of mental constructs) or disadaptation (at the level of behavioral descriptions) gives rise to a *need to function,* or a need to repeat action to the point of adaptation.

The need to function is the exclusive concept of causation in sensorimotor theory. It refers to all occasions when assimilation of an aliment and accommodation of the schema to it are not in balance. The term does not imply an *a priori* need of the organism to adapt ubiquitously and without specification to any and all objects, as do terms like the instinct for mastery, need achievement, and competence motivation; need to function is a generic term that acquires specific definition only in each particular context of action. For example, when the child who is able to suck at the breast encounters a new object with his mouth which he can suck, the cause of action is the need to suck, but now in the new way already experienced; when two or more action patterns are coordinated into a new circular reaction, the need is created by the fact that the two separate action patterns have intersected while using the same object and it consists, for example, of the "need to see what is grasped and to grasp what is seen." When the child discovers for the first time that a ball will roll down an inclined plane all by itself, he repeats this experiment out of the need to explore the causal properties of objects that he now experiences as being independent of himself. In each case the need arises within a context of action and persists until a full assimilation of the specific datum encountered and a corresponding accommodation are achieved. Since every circular reaction on one object exposes the child to a variety of new circumstances, each of which he can partially assimilate and to which he is not fully adapted, the state of adaptation always remains an ideal goal which gives direction to development, but a goal which is never achieved.

Having now considered Piaget's concept of the causation of behavior, we can contrast it with the concept of motivation as defined by Rapaport.

1. Unlike motives, which are conceptualized as *internal* forces, the need to function is neither generated within the organism nor imposed on the organism as an external force (that is, as a stimulus of academic and Pavlovian learning theory). Both the goal and the aim of action are determined by the context of the encounter, and the cause is located simultaneously in the environment—the novelty, and in the organism—

the tendency to assimilate all possible aliment. The child is "caused" to act, or has a need to repeat his contact with specific objects, because he has already acted on them. Encounter with novelty motivates repetition or circular reaction, and it is the *action* which engenders the *need* for further contact rather than the internal *need* which prompts the *action*.

2. Unlike the motivation, need to function is not cyclical; functional need for activity is not terminated by consummatory action. It arises in the course of action and abates after the appropriate modification within the psychic structure has taken place.

3. The need to function is not peremptory. If circular reaction is disrupted before adaptation is completed, the behavior remains in a state of disadaptation until appropriate environmental conditions allow for the necessary practice. Disruption or interference with action, therefore, does not result in increasing internal tension, as is the case with motivational forces.

4. The need to function, unlike motivation, cannot be displaced from one goal to another. Therefore it does not give rise to substitute action on substitute objects when the intended object is not available. Although the child may alternatively perfect his global sucking schema by acting on his lips, his thumb, or the breast, each object serves as aliment for the stabilization of the global schema of sucking to the extent that the different objects are suckable and for the child identical at this stage of development. Later, distinct objects will generate their own specific action schemata, thereby differentiating the global schema. The concept of object permanence will be assimilated equally from action on disappearing dolls, disappearing faces, or disappearing fingers, since object permanence is a property universal to and therefore abstractable from all of them. But the child will also elaborate differentiated schemata for recovering the doll, the fingers, or the face of another person, since the recovery of these different objects requires distinct means of action.

According to Rapaport's definition (1960b), as he has pointed out, Piaget's *need to function* is not a motivation in the true sense, but rather another psychological causation of behavior. I shall now consider the role of this cause in intellectual development in relation to Piaget's observations and experiments.

I have already referred briefly to the data of the first stage. The child simply repeats and strengthens the reflex patterns given at birth. By repetition the reflexes are stabilized. Slight degrees of differentiation in sucking patterns do occur, and as a result the child can for the first time make practical judgments about various related objects in terms of the differentiated actions which he applies to them. During this first stage the need to function is, however, primarily the need to repeat inborn behavior patterns as such. As long as the child does not distinguish between action and object he has no knowledge of objects except while he acts on them, and they exist for him only as something to suck, or something to see, or something to grasp, but not as something to grasp *and* to see at the same time. Since action is hardly differentiated from object, and since action is both the adaptive action and the source for further aliment at the same time, the need to repeat is identical with the act itself.

During the second stage reflex patterns are coordinated into new actions or *primary circular reactions*. Until now the hand has moved independent of visual control; grasping movements developed in a sequence which was similar to that of sucking, while the eyes practiced visual pursuit and began to accommodate to near and far objects. While the hand is repeatedly brought to the mouth, it will sooner or later pass before the eyes, and then it becomes an object for the eyes to follow as well as for the mouth to suck. As the chance encounters between sucking, visual, and grasping activities are coordinated, the hand begins to linger in the visual field before going to the mouth, while the eyes adapt themselves by keeping the hand in the visual range in order to observe the different movements of the fingers. Eventually a new behavior pattern emerges in which everything that the child grasps is brought to the eyes, and everything he sees evokes an effort to grasp. This intersection of two behavior patterns creates a new need and an anticipation of looking whenever the hand grasps something, and of directed grasping whenever the eyes see something. The child becomes aware that the object is something distinct from action in progress when he learns to anticipate those other actions which experience and coordination have linked to the action in progress. Thereafter, when he sucks on something, the object exists for him not only by virtue of its "suckability" but also by its visual and graspable properties, although he "knows" of the latter two properties only by an anticipation or a readiness for appropriate sequences of action to follow. In subsequent stages as he acquires more diverse ways of acting on objects, and as these actions are linked into complex anticipation patterns, he will eventually regard the object as something that is entirely independent of action and therefore external to him.

Between the fifth and eighth months (the third stage of sensorimotor development), the child directs his action to the novelties as if they were somewhat separate from, although still dependent on, his action but he does not yet adapt his action to the spatial, objective, and causal properties of the events. While kicking for the sake of repetition, for example, the child happens to kick a toy suspended from his crib. He stops kicking, looks at the toy as long as it moves, and when it stops he kicks again while looking intently at the toy. His attitude of expectancy clearly suggests that he anticipates seeing the toy move again after he kicks. He appears to act in order to repeat events which are independent of his action, and for this end uses *procedures* or motor anticipation patterns. However, as *procedures to make interesting spectacles last* are stabilized, the child generalizes them indiscriminately to all other novelties he perceives, and thereby betrays the extent to which for him object permanence still depends on action. He kicks his feet to make a noise recur, or to repeat the movement of a distant window curtain that is causally unrelated to his action, and expects that it will recur. Such observations show that procedures, although they have become ready-made action pattern or a "practical concept" which can be generalized to various circumstances, still have a *"magical"* quality, and that the child still considers his action to be sufficient cause for all external events, or that the object is still at the disposal of his action ("magical" conception of causality).

During the eighth through the twelfth month, the child actually accommodates his action pattern to real circumstances. He abandons "magical omnipotence" (that is the subordination of all causes to his action) for the intention to achieve actual results by intelligent action. For example, when he wants to reach a doll but the path to it is blocked by a pillow, he discovers in the course of his groping that he can displace the obstacle and reach the doll by striking at the pillow. Unlike in previous stages, he is no longer distracted by the spectacle of displacing the pillow, nor does he rely on magical procedures which will not yield the desired result in "reality." He uses the removal of the pillow as a mediation between his wish and his final goal. In time, means such as displacing one object to obtain another can be linked to various goal actions in sequences appropriate to the causal-temporal-spatial context of the total situation. Then the motor anticipation pattern of striking becomes a stable tool of behavior independent of the specific context in which it was learned and capable of unlimited adaptive generalization as a *mobile schema.*

When the child executes one movement as the intermediary to achieving a goal by a distinctly different movement, we infer that during the delay the child remains aware of both the goal and the goal-directed action, even though he is not acting directly on the goal; and that he must literally "keep the goal in mind" while engaged in detour behavior. Piaget considers such awareness of the goal independent of action as the hallmark of all intelligent action, and calls it *intentional* or *purposive* behavior. As the schemata themselves have differentiated during the first four stages of sensorimotor development, so the simple need to repeat inborn reflex patterns has evolved into a complex, psychological causation that is identical with purpose.

As in earlier stages, the source of a complex cause such as intention resides simultaneously in the novel situation and in the child's tendency to assimilate. But now as the child is able to assimilate the goal, the obstacle, and the relation between them at the same time, his functional need encompasses the goal object as well as its spatial-causal context.

Throughout the first four stages the need to function has been directed by the past, and it resulted simply in the repetition of action discovered by chance. Even during the fourth stage, although the situation was novel, the child used only familiar behavior patterns in new sequences. During the fifth stage when the child encounters a novelty, he acts as if his purpose, instead of repeating what he has already seen, were to explore possible variations which he has not yet perceived. For example, when he pushes with his finger on the matchbox and discovers that it tilts, he systematically pushes the box from various angles at various points, and causes it to tilt in different ways, each novelty leading him to discover a new way of pushing. He may not know what the result will be, but in some primitive sense he must be aware that there are unrealized possibilities of tilting the matchbox, otherwise he would be engaged in repetitive movements or random behavior.

What *causes* the child to invent new variations by trial and error rather than repeating old ones? The need to repeat can no longer provide a sufficient explanation since the child actively creates novelties. Nor can concepts like the instinct for mastery, need achievement, or competence motivation do more than describe the behavior in general terms, since they tell us nothing about the direction which a particular action will take once a novelty is encountered, and therefore nothing about the purpose which directs this action. Piaget argues that the child now explores what the object can do by itself precisely because he has acquired a partial concept of object permanence which is independent of his action; because he has acquired a partial concept of physical causality which is independent of his participation; and because he has acquired a concept of physical space in which he can anticipate the placement of objects independent of his action. The child assimilates the novelty to a whole array of internalized action patterns (mobile schemata) and subordinates these in means-end relationship to the discovery that a matchbox can be tilted by pushing. Each latent action pattern subordinated to the controlling schema of tilting the box then suggests to the child a new way of tilting. Because ready-made anticipation patterns through generalization were freed from their initial context of origin, they are applied freely in entirely new circumstances, but are now applied so as to fit into the spatial-causal context of the present and therefore no longer as magical procedures. The functional need is still generated by the encounter with novelty, but the greater differentiation between self and outside allows the child to explore the properties of objects rather than repeating actions on them.

During the sixth stage the child invents new procedures and discovers new combinations in almost the same way as in the fifth stage, although inventions now take place in thought and by spontaneous rearrangement, rather than by concrete action and by trial and error. Slowly, during the preceding five stages, motor actions have become internalized as thought patterns; at the second stage actions became motor anticipation patterns, at the third stage novel spectacles activated ready-made anticipation patterns or procedures; and during the fourth stage these internalized anticipation patterns became the tools for means-end behavior. During the fifth stage the internal anticipation patterns are sufficiently liberated from their context of origin to engender a systematic creation of novelties.

The complementary roles of assimilation and accommodation remain the same, although in the sixth stage the intermediate steps between the initial desire and the final goal are no longer directly observable. For example, when the child loses sight of a ball as it rolls under a couch, he walks around the couch to retrieve the ball on the other side rather than crawling under it. From such directed behavior we infer that the child invents a new spatial displacement which he relates to the ball's projected displacement so as to bring himself and the ball to the same end point, in thought prior to action. From this it follows that the child is able to represent the ball to himself although he no longer sees it; and that he has acquired the concept of object permanence. It follows that he can represent to himself a space in which various objects, including himself, can be displaced in relation to each other, and that he has acquired a mental representation of space. Finally, it follows that he attributes independent motion to the ball, and that he has differentiated psychological from physical causality.

The end of sensorimotor intelligence marks only the first step in the total sequence of intellectual growth. What was achieved within a context of immediate action on concrete objects must now be repeated at the level of mental representations. When the child acquires language, and as linguistic symbols replace motor anticipation patterns, he must distinguish all over again between himself—in this case his mental representations or *signifiers*—and the things and relations that are represented—or the *significations*. The differentiation between symbolic signifier and signification, and the socialization of differentiated signifiers into a system of communicable signs, are the work of intellectual growth still before the child. At the level of mental representations we can again measure the progress of intelligence in terms of the differentiation between assimilation and accommodation. Now, however, this process is reflected in thought rather than in concrete action. Although we still infer the work of intelligence from its end product in adaptive action, action is no longer the direct expression of intelligence, but simply the observable index of representational thought; in subsequent stages motor action will further be replaced by verbal behavior as the index of intelligent adaptations.

1. To the extent that the two functions are undifferentiated and accommodation has primacy over assimilation, the child responds to novelty without integrating his action fully into the totality of past experiences. He acts in the present without relating his action to his (inner) past, and as a result imitates the models in his environment without comprehending their veridical implications. Like intelligence in general, imitation has its roots in sensorimotor behavior of the first 2 years. At 1 year, for example, the child watches his father open and close a matchbox. Then he opens and closes his fist while keeping his eyes on the box; he makes a sound which resembles the scratching of the matchbox, and at the same time opens and closes his mouth. The strange matchbox has created in the child a functional need to encompass in some way what he saw but did not yet understand. In contrast to intellectual adaptation proper, the child does not assimilate the spatial properties of the object to his thought schemata of space and causality, in order to understand them, but imitates the model as he has perceived it. His primary aim appears to be to reconstitute the novelty to himself, to conserve it without seeking to comprehend it. At this stage imitation is still motor action related to objects in his presence, and there is nothing in his behavior to suggest that he has an internal image of the model. One year later, after the symbol has been fully divested of its action context, the child imitates the action of a servant he has observed scrubbing the floor several days before, or he pretends to sew with a thread and needle as he observed his mother do on a previous day. Such *deferred* imitations imply that the child has at his disposal an image of the model to project it as an independent representation which has an inner and therefore an external constancy; and that he can reproduce it at will when the model itself is no longer present. It is imitation rather than intelligent adaptation insofar as the child does not understand the significance of the model he imitates.

2. To the extent that the two functions remain undifferentiated and assimilation has primacy over accommodation, the child incorporates novelties into his private world without modifying that inner world in correspondence to the real properties of the novelty. Thus, the present acquires meaning for him only as he relates it to his inner past; he relates the outside world to himself but does not relate himself to the outside. Thereby he engages in *play*. Like imitation, play has its roots in early sensorimotor behavior, and becomes symbolic after thought schemata replace motor anticipations. At 14 months the child engages in practical make-believe games that utilize the sensorimotor actions at his disposal. He pretends to drink or eat, although there is nothing in his hands. The nature of his play suggests the child's dawning awareness

of "pretending" and suggests the concomitant first realization of the difference between the object as idea and the object as thing. He uses pebbles at one time as if they were candy, at another time as if they were building blocks. He disregards the physical properties of objects to make them fit into his play of the moment, and does not change the action to adapt it to the real properties of the thing with which he is playing. By 4 years the child makes up stories by organizing fragments of conversations he has heard on previous days into coherent accounts. Although the story may have no basis in reality and is constructed to fit the child's need of the moment, it employs freely interchangeable linguistic symbols. Such use of symbols is "ludic" or playful rather than intelligent adaptation insofar as the child manipulates ideas in disregard of the veridical world that he is capable of perceiving. Only after the child can clearly differentiate between the idea as subjective reality and the thing or phenomenon as objective reality, will intellectual thought become capable of the unlimited combinations and generalizations that characterize abstract logic. In all its developmental manifestations, play therefore serves a crucial function in intellectual growth because it allows for new combinations and inventions that are not bound by the concrete realities of the present.

3. To the extent that assimilation and accommodation are differentiated and integrated, the child assimilates novelties to his representational schemata, and at the same time alters these to make them correspond with the veridical world and its social conventions. Not only does he assimilate the present to symbolic representations of his experiences (as in play), but now he accommodates his inner world to coordinate it with the realistic aspects he has perceived. Thus, at $2^1/_2$, the child adapts his reasoning process to observed events. When he calls his father who does not answer, he concludes that his father did not hear. When he sees his father preparing hot water, he infers that the father is going to shave. By 4 years, adaptive intelligence allows him to classify objects into categories, although such categorizations still often lead to incorrect solutions. When he acquires a concept of classes, he identifies an animal as a horse because it has a mane, on the proposition that all four-legged animals with manes are horses; but because he cannot differentiate logically between horses and mules, he is confused by the fact that mules also have manes. Later as he acquires the mental operations of class inclusion and class multiplication, his class concepts acquire an objective permanence. Then he can decide that the universal class of four-legged animals with manes includes both horses and mules, each constituting a subclass with special attributes (by class multiplication) and both subordinated under the universal class (by class inclusion).

Imitation, symbolic play, and cognitive representation are only three aspects of a general process of intellectual adaptation. Since imitation always combines assimilatory with accommodative functions and can never be pure accommodation, it always increases the child's understanding of real circumstances, although the focus of action is on the reproduction of models rather than on the assimilation of their meanings. Since symbolic play always combines accommodative with assimilatory functions and can never be pure assimilation, it always increases the child's understanding of the real world by altering his mental representation of it, although the focus of action and thought is to subordinate new experiences to already acquired private meanings.

At every new phase in development, the causation of intellectual function remains the same as during the sensorimotor stage. The need to function arises when the child encounters a novelty which he is able to integrate in part but to which his actions or thoughts are not fully adapted. Whether the result is imitation, symbolic play, or cognitive representation, the child is caused to assimilate and to accommodate all novelties he encounters, and the cause resides simultaneously in his fundamental tendency to assimilate, and in the world of objects to which his intellectual structures are partially adapted.

I have devoted so much time to discussing a limited segment of Piaget's general theory of intelligence to show how it accounts for the causation of behavior without invoking the concept of motivation. As a ubiquitous explanation of all behavior, *functional need* is surely as insufficient as other unitary concepts of causation, whether these invoke a classical stimulus-response sequence or one of various motivational forces. From clinical experience we have learned that a concept like the need to function cannot account for all observable behavior, and that motivational factors which antedate experience (that is, causal forces which do not arise in the course of action) are significant and powerful determinants of behavior and organizers of experience. Clinical experience also suggests that without dynamic and economic considerations we cannot adquately account for the peremptory quality of some behavior and for the phenomena subsumed under concepts like directed attention and altered levels of consciousness, for which Piaget's theory provides only *ad hoc* explanations. Clinical data suggest that contrary to Piaget's assertion, affects *are* structure-building forces which give rise to semipermanent emotional predispositions (e.g., moods, character traits, etc.), and that when so structured, affects may also serve as defenses to ward off other affective experiences. The clinical investigations of individual life histories have shown that specific variations of early social experience individualize the person's social, intellectual, and affective adaptive pattern and style. The need to function as the exclusive concept of causation cannot easily account for the fact of individual differences. Finally, clinical experience teaches us that the need to function and the intellectual structures that such a causation generates are always indissociably linked to motivational factors, to defensive organizations, and to the derivative discharge modes arising from defense formations; and that adaptive mechanisms are always only *relatively* but never *absolutely* autonomous from motivation and conflict. The indissociability of affective and cognitive-perceptual development is a truism postulated both by comprehensive motivational theories of development and by Piaget, although neither theory has studied this interaction systematically. For developmental psychology, the significant question regarding the relative autonomy of structures is not so much whether affects speed up or slow down the *rate* of cognitive development, as it is whether affective forces (and more generally motivational forces) *change* the sequence of developmental steps, *modify* the nature and content of cognitive structures elaborated in the course of adaptation, and thereby *alter* the direction of the need to function.

Piaget did not intend to study the relation between affective and intellectual development. It might be argued that a study of cognitive development which does not pay systematic attention to emotional influence cannot yield valid results. Such an extreme view does not seem justified in view of the complexity of developmental phenomena. It would be equally just or unjust to assert that a study of emotional development, which does not at the same time systematically study cognitive mechanisms, will not yield valid results. To arrive at first approximations of personality development, it is apparently necessary to make an arbitrary division of its affective-motivational and cognitive-perceptual aspects, and then to integrate the partial results. The task remains for us to study *how* motivated behavior, which has been the primary concern of clinical psychiatry, and nonmotivated behavior, which has been the primary concern of some cognitive theories, exercise their mutual influence. Far from achieving such an integration, I have only tried to show how Piaget's data suggest that at least under conditions of relative internal equilibrium, and at least with respect to certain sequences of total development, the psychological causation of behavior resides in the encounter between the individual and the real circumstances on which he acts.

In conclusion, I would like to remind you of Freud's admonition to his circle of students, which states in seven simple words the point for which I took an hour—namely, that sometimes a cigar is also a cigar.

14

PRIMARY PREVENTION AND SOME ASPECTS OF TEMPORAL ORGANIZATION IN EARLY INFANT-CARETAKER INTERACTION

Louis W. Sander, M.D., Gerald Stechler, Ph.D., Harry Julia, Ph.D., and Padraic Burns, M.D.

The work described in this paper was carried out with infants who were selected to meet rather stringent criteria for normality, and it was limited to observations within the first 2 months of life. These two considerations introduce at once the question of the usefulness of this material in a discussion of primary prevention and the high-risk infant. The relevance of further normal developmental data to a discussion of primary prevention can be challenged in the face of the appalling scale on which existing infant-rearing conditions close at home reveal obvious and often abysmal deficiency. There seems little doubt that "intervention" by a wide assortment of individuals in the early developmental situation will be rapidly increasing in the years to come. Whatever action is carried out by these individuals in the name of "primary prevention" will be based on the conceptualizations they happen to have of the process of development going on at that earliest time of life. The long-term effectiveness of their actions will depend on the adequacy of their point of view. It is the contribution which the study of normal development can make to our understanding of the process into which we step in intervening that makes it relevant to an Academy symposium on primary prevention.

CONSIDERATION OF ORGANIZATION OF BEHAVIOR IN EARLY INFANCY

Recent infancy research, especially in the areas of early perception and learning, is giving us a new picture of the sensitivities and capabilities

Presented at the 1971 symposium in Boston, and based on a study "Adaptation and Perception in Early Infancy," 1965–1969, USPHS Grant #HDO-1766.

of the neonate, and an appreciation of new levels in the early interaction between genomic and experiential factors. Just what these recent findings imply for the subsequent development of the individual or for our comprehension of the early developmental process is not at all clear, however, and reflects a huge gap in our present understanding. The gap in large measure concerns ignorance of the lawful principles which govern postnatal organization of infant functions and the characteristics of the organizing process over ensuing months. The meagerness of substantive empirical data in early infancy has made it well-nigh impossible to consider an attack on the problem of early organization as a suitable or proper research aim. However, the accumulation of empirical research will in time inevitably demand precisely such an approach.

An illustration of the relationship between empirical findings and the problem of organization may be found in the monograph of Bell et al. (1971). The authors report on the findings of an NIMH project in which 75 infants were studied both as newborns and at the 27-33-month level. Bell et al. were impressed with the relatively few links which could be established by significant positive correlations between variables measured at one age point and those measured at the other. On the other hand, they were impressed by the finding that variables (e.g., measures of respiratory rate, tactile threshold, reaction to interruption of sucking) which measure overly intense behavior in the newborn period (in terms of frequency, speed, and amplitude) showed significant correction with variables measuring *low* intensity at the 27-33-month point. (Variables here were interest, participation, assertiveness, gregariousness, and communicativeness.) They conclude, "In other words, there was a longitudinal inversion of intensity." How should we understand or account for such an inversion? The answer lies somewhere in the, as yet dimly conceived, machinery of "organization."

It is the lack of correlation between variables measured in early infancy and those measured later which has made the construction of developmental scales in early infancy so difficult, and their usefulness in assessing early development so limited. It is this issue with which Hebb (1949) was concerned when he emphasized that there is something different about the effects of the first learning experiences of the infant organism on his development, in contrast to effects of later experience and later learning. He proposed that the difference was that the initial phase concerned the organization of certain autonomous central processes related to perceptual experience which would then underlie later, more complex learning and problem-solving behavior. However, the effects of first learning or first experience may not be limited to a primary perceptual or sensorimotor development, but may be related to the establishing of overall regulatory mechanisms involving the infant as a whole in relation to his environment and basic to any subsequent adaptive functioning. Mechanisms of regulation on the level of "the infant as a whole" appear as highly complex integrations involving many subsystems.

In emphasizing the need for a field of "integrative physiology," Mason (1968) stated that "the distinction between analytic and integrative approaches seems clearly of bedrock fundamental importance" (p. 804). He made clear that he regarded the analytic and integrative approaches as complementary rather than antithetical: the study of the relationship between parts is obviously dependent upon prior study and characterization of individual parts. Mason reviewed the enthusiasm during the first third of this century in the study of integrative processes and biological organization and pointed out the difficulty of finding any clear historical continuity of this interest in the past three decades. "While there has been some movement in the direction of more emphasis on regulatory mechanisms, the single system model has usually been employed and there has been very little work on coordinative or integrative mechanisms" (p. 801f.).

In proposing his conceptualization of "overall hormonal balance as a key to endocrine organization," Mason restated an old issue in biology, namely, that comprehension of organization of the organism cannot be grasped at the level of analysis of individual variables alone. He proposed that before the role of a single endocrine system could be defined, its contribution to the balance maintained in the complex interaction of the entire array of endocrine systems must be determined. The role of the single endocrine system might be in one direction (anabolic) in one context, and in another context it might be in an opposite direction (catabolic), synergistic and antagonistic combinations with the other endocrines shifting with the shift in total context. The context in which a variable is measured is thus as important as the measurement itself, if one aims to understand lawful relationships between variables. The identification itself of salient contextual parameters represents a major step in this understanding. We hope that the material presented in this report will evoke discussion of the implications of the issue of "organization" for primary prevention, a concern distinct from the implications of data related to single variables or systems. We shall describe a study of temporal organization in early infant care interaction and discuss its relevance to primary prevention.

RESEARCH STRATEGY

Our point of departure is the notion that a conceptualization of organizing mechanisms cannot be pursued suitably at the level of the individual infant alone, but requires consideration of a next level, namely, the infant plus the caretaking environment—that part of the surround with which he is in exchange. We have assumed that infant-caretaker dyads should be compared, rather than babies; furthermore, that the study of relationships between variables requires repeated measurement of more than one variable over an adequate span of time.

Since organism-environment exchange depends at the biological level on mechanics of regulation, conceptualization of infant and caretaking environment as a regulatory system seemed to promise a good starting point. Infant and caretaker could be visualized as becoming joined in a regulatory system as the behavior of each, through recurrent encounters, is modified toward the establishment of stable (expectable) configurations in the exchanges between the partners. One of the outstanding features of postnatal exchange between infant and caretaker is that the recurrent encounters themselves take place at intervals which begin irregularly, and gradually take place with greater regularity. In the usual instance, postnatal caretaking is a matter of two individuals, disparately organized at many levels, but especially in the temporal distribution of their states of readiness for activity, having to live together around-the-clock day after day. It is precisely this continuous 24-hour-a-day feature of encounter which makes the time of occurrence of events and their duration all-important issues to both partners. Under such conditions, organization of events into a daytime and a nighttime of occurrence becomes a feature of real concern, as does the emergence of a pattern of recurrence of sufficient stability to constitute a comfortably predictable 24-hour frame of reference.

Attention to the time distribution and the various temporal relationships between events became, then, our second point of departure in this study of organization of an infant-caretaker regulatory system. The method of continuous monitoring of infant and caretaker which was developed in this investigation led directly to the finding of the periodicity characterizing recurrent infant states. This finding required a consideration of the contribution of biological rhythms to the mechanics of organization of exchanges between infant and caretaking environment.

METHODOLOGY

The infants, 9 in each group, were taken into the study one at a time, after meeting rather stringent pre- and perinatal criteria of normality based on a detailed newborn examination. The three caretaking conditions, the methods of observation, and some of the variables have been described in previous publications (Sander and Julia, 1966; Sander et al., 1969, 1970, 1972), and need be reviewed only briefly.

The first of the three caretaking conditions was lying-in nursery care with 4-hourly scheduled feedings; infants experiencing this caretaking were designated as group A. This caretaking was limited to the first 10 days of life. The second caretaking condition was foster care with infant-demand feeding provided around-the-clock by one individual acting as surrogate mother, rooming in with the baby on the hospital maternity floor; infants experiencing this caretaking in the first 10 days of life were designated as group B. The third caretaking condition was natural mother care provided around-the-clock by the infants' own mothers, first in a hospital rooming-in facility and then in the home (again infant-demand feeding); these infants were designated as group C.

Infants for groups A and B were drawn from a population of infants for whom adoption was being planned, and their availability for the study during the first 2 months of life depended on the time taken for the completion of agency arrangements. (In the interval since the study took place, these agencies have now reduced this time span.) Groups A and B were matched for prenatal and background factors. Group C consisted of infants of selected multiparous mothers of stable family situations and was not intended as a matched group, although the babies came from similar socioeconomic levels. We wanted a group which represented relatively optimal rearing circumstances, inasmuch as the 24-hour data we were collecting were unique, and there was no way to guess on which side of more optimal caretaking conditions the data collected for groups A and B might lie. Findings will be reported chiefly for groups A and B.

There were three time periods in the study, illustrated in figure 1. The design of time periods was intended to provide examination of, first, the effect of first 10-day caretaking on behavior over the remaining days of the month, since, after day 10, both groups A and B re-

Group	N		CARETAKING PERIOD I (0–10 days)	CARETAKING PERIOD II (11–28 days)	CARETAKING PERIOD III (29–56 days)
A	9		Nursery	Single Care-taker (X or Y) Rooming-in	Foster Home
B	9		Single Care-taker X or Y Rooming-in	Single Care-taker Y or X Rooming-in	Foster Home
		0–5 days	6–10 days		
C	9	Natural Mother Rooming-in	Natural Mother At home	Natural Mother At home	Natural Mother At home

Figure 1
Design of infant and caretaking groups over the first 56 days of postnatal life

ceived similar caretaking, i.e., between days 11–29. What is the effect of the infant's experience, for even this brief 10-day period, of an environment (lying-in nursery) in which there is no respect for the temporal organization of his recurring states of awake or sleep, and no mutuality of modification in arriving gradually at a stable regularity of daily events?[1] The second aim of the design was to study the effect of substituting one experienced caretaker for another at the end of the first 10 days of life (carried out for group B only). Does the initial adaptation between infant and caretaker depend on nonspecific factors related to the furnishing of adequate feeding, holding, quieting, or does a stable coordination between infant and caretaker depend upon some quite idiosyncratic pattern of exchange related to individual differences in characteristics of regulation in the partners and reached by mutual but specific modifications?

There were five major observational methods employed: (1) a 24-hour-per-day recording bassinet which monitored, automatically and continuously and in real time, infant crying, motility, caretaker approach, caretaker removal of infant from the bassinet and return of infant to the bassinet; (2) a 24-hour record of clock time of observed onset of major sleep and wake periods; (3) daily event-recorded feeding interactions; (4) systematic observations of infant behavior when confronted by visual stimuli, such as the human face; (5) pediatric neurological examination, adapted from an early format of Brazelton's newborn examination method (1973).

FINDINGS

The first finding dealt with the activity of the newborn, that is, a greater *duration* of relatively more active states during the initial postnatal days. This finding became evident only because around-the-clock records could be obtained day after day over the first month of life. The total daily *duration* of more active states of the infant (ones characterized by crying, increased motility, and/or removal of infant from bassinet) was greater over the first days of life than it was again until the end of the first month of life. This held whether the infant was in group A or B. Until this study, we had supposed that the newborn baby in the first few days of life was recovering from the exhaustion of the delivery and the depressing effects of medication and, that as he recovered and grew older, he steadily grew stronger, gradually day-by-day remaining active for longer periods; in other words, a linear increase in duration

1. The temporal asynchrony between infant activity and that of the nursery caretaking environment has been described (Sander et al., 1969; see also Aldrich et al., 1945); the variable of "delay time," the time elapsing between onset of infant crying and the initiation of an intervention, has been used to study this asynchrony in the nursery situation.

of active states over the first month of life. But the picture is more like that shown in figure 2.

We emphasize that we are here talking about the *duration* of more active states, not about intensity or quantity of activity. The group B infant whose caretaking was relatively unchanged over the first 10 days of life spent less time crying in the second 5 days of life; but the group A baby also showed reduced crying over the second 5 days of life, even though he was receiving significantly less caretaking time in the second 5 days than in the first 5 days of life. What might be the adaptive significance of the longer time each day in states of relatively greater arousal during the first few days of life? Is there a reason for a relatively greater readiness for interaction with the caretaking environment at the outset?

If each awakening provides an opportunity to experience repetition in specific contingencies between a sequence of infant states and a sequence of particular caretaking activities, the first days of life might be providing an opportunity for establishing certain stable patterns in the infant-caretaker interaction. There are great infant differences in the sequence and in the time course of state changes over an awakening from the end of one sleep phase to the onset of the next sleep phase. The behaviors which an infant characteristically displays with his changing states, especially in the transitional segments, become clues for the experienced caretaker to guide her decisions. They constitute

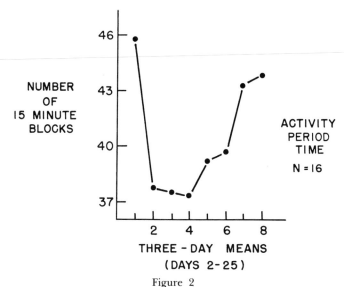

Figure 2

Activity segment time per 24 hours. Each point represents a mean for 3 days for which the totals for 8 group A and 8 group B infants are combined. Quadratic $F = 27.84$ df $= 1/84$, cubic $F = 7.36$ df $= 1/84$, linear $F = 1.46$ df $= 1/84$ (Sander et. al. 1972)

the configurations which identify the unique individual qualities of a particular infant. It is just these individual differences which are being learned by the caretaker and are being modified by the infant as they establish adaptation through mutual coordinations.

A second finding was that the emergence of day-night differences in distribution of relatively more active states was under some environmental control. As long as group A infants were in the lying-in nursery on the 4-hourly scheduled feedings, they continued to cry more at night (6 P.M.-6 A.M.) than in the daytime (6 A.M.-6 P.M.) and to be in these more active states longer at night than in the daytime. As soon as they were transferred to the care of the surrogate mother on day 11, in the first 24 hours in fact, this distribution reversed. As soon as caretaking became contingent to change in infant state, the infant slept for longer periods.

With demand-feeding caretaking by the infant's own mother, the longest sleep period per 24 hours migrates to the night 12 hours within the first 10 days of life. In the group B situation, day-night differences in 24-hour distribution of variables, highly correlated with awake states, appeared already in the first 3-day block and became highly significant

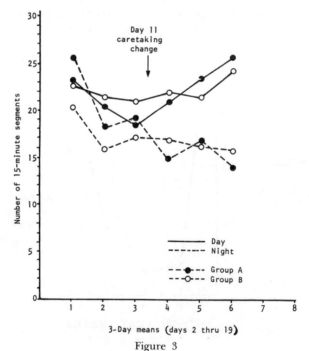

Figure 3

Activity segments days 2–19. Equal number of days before and after change of caretaker on day 11. Anova, days 2–19 (DN × group × period) F = 2.80 df = 5/60 p<.025. Infants experiencing nursery caretaking do not show day-night differentiation in activity segment time until after removal to surrogate mother situation on day 11 (Sander et al., 1972).

within the first 10 days of life (see fig. 3). Obviously, once the longest sleep span becomes stabilized in the night segment, the day segment can be occupied only by the briefer sleep periods and the awakenings. This raises the question whether extrinsic environmental factors may, in part, determine the linking of subphases of sleep—the REM and NREM periods—into one longest sleep period per 24 hours and, in part, determine its stabilization in the nighttime hours.

Day-night differentiation in distributions of sleep and wake states is one of the earliest indicators to the mother of the progress which her infant is making in settling down and becoming predictable. Our data show wide individual differences in the rate of advance of day-night differences for normal infants who have been cared for by the same individual as surrogate mother. One *abnormal* infant we observed showed no significant D-N difference over the entire first 2 months of life. Work which has come from the laboratories of Prechtl (1968), Aschoff (1967, 1969), and Stroebel (1969) has caused us to wonder if there is a connection between the way an infant becomes organized in respect to the 24 hours of the day and the temporal organization or phase synchrony which exists or can become established intrinsically between his various physiological subsystems. Such intrinsic coordination is usually considered a matter of genomic determination, as are rates of change for the most part. The data we have obtained have suggested the possibility that *extrinsic* determinants may have a significant role in modifying both rates of change and the temporal organization of *intrinsic* infant subsystems, that is, the relationship of the phasic characteristics of one function in respect to another.

A third finding which also surprised us was the persistence of effect of the first 10 days of caretaking. We found that these same group A infants, who suddenly began sleeping more at night when transferred to the single caretaker on day 11, also after day 11 now suddenly began to show a significantly *greater* day-night difference in sleep distribution than did the group B infants. During days 11–29, both group A and group B infants were receiving similar care on a one-to-one basis in the rooming-in situation. The group B infants had shown a gradually increasing day-night difference from the first days of life. There was therefore not only an abrupt change at 11 days for group A infants in their around-the-clock behavior, but then an overcompensation, a precocious advance with greater time awake during the day hours and less sleeping.

Was there a possibility that the individual who provided the care between days 11–29 was producing this effect? Fortunately, only two women had provided the care, so it was possible by analysis of variance to determine that there was no significant effect on day-night difference being contributed by the individual currently caring for the

baby. The only factor which made the difference was whether or not
the first 10 days had been spent in the lying-in nursery. How could
something or some things that had happened in the first 10 days of life
be exerting such a continuing effect on the time in the day of sleeping
and waking over the rest of the first month? And possibly some unknown effect on the timing of the fluctuations in the infant's other
physiological subsystems with respect to each other?

Some may see a relevance here of reports from animal research concerning the effect of "stress," in the form of early handling, on regulatory characteristics of the adult animal or on appearance of day-night
differences in activity. Preweaning handling or electric shock in rat
pups appears to produce an adult that shows relatively more exploratory behavior and less emotionality (Ader, 1969; Ader and Deitchman, 1970). It has been proposed that in the adult, this represents a
regulatory system that is cabable of more graded responses in contrast
to all-or-nothing responses.

Ader and his coworkers (1969, 1970), however, also showed that
shock or early handling advances the time of appearance of a 24-hour

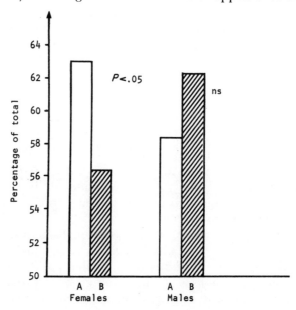

Group A   Nursery caretaking first 10 days of life
Group B   Single caretaker first 10 days of life

Figure 4

Activity segment time occurring in daytime days 11–25. Anova for days 11–25
(DN × group × sex) F = 5.99 df = 1/12 p = .05. Females having had nursery caretaking
in first 10 days show greater day-night differentiation in days 11–25 than do females who
have had rooming-in caretaking in first 10 days. Males show the opposite tendency (Sander et al., 1972).

rhythm in output of adrenal cortical steroids, and that handling of the pregnant mother advances the time of appearance in the pups of a 24-hour activity rhythm. Thus, in this animal and under these conditions, rates of development in certain functions or subsystems may be sensitive to environmental inputs.

Obviously, in the human we have no idea as yet what the early or later effects of neonatal "stress" are, or of early stability or instability, or of shifting the developmental rate of change in one function relative to another, on the kind of basic regulatory organization the individual will have, or on the intrinsic coordination between his various physiological subsystems. What may be gained adaptively by the adult for one kind of a later environment may be lost by the same adult for another kind of later environment.

Returning to our data, we found *a difference between male and female infants in the effect of first 10-day caretaking experience,* which gives further impetus to the task of specifying the interaction of intrinsic and extrinsic factors in rates of advance in 24-hour organization. We found that the precocious advance of group A babies in day-night difference during days 11-29 was contributed chiefly by the *female* infants. Girls experiencing the less stressful individual caretaking of the group B condition, by contrast, advanced only in the slowest and most gradual manner. The males, on the other hand, showed their most rapid advance in days 11-29 when they had received the individual care of the surrogate mother during the first 10 days of life. They were retarded or slowed down by a first 10 days lying-in nursery experience (see fig. 4).

This finding seems to add further evidence to the suggestion, already proposed, that we are possibly dealing with a different set of rules from the outset for the organization of little girls and of little boys. Findings of sex differences appear to be ubiquitous in current research reports in early infancy. A further example: in our study, total sleep per 24 hours was significantly greater for girls than for boys. At this point in infancy research, the implications of these findings for "preventive intervention" do not seem nearly as exciting as the implications that by further detailed examination of male-female differences, we may stumble on a better grasp of basic mechanisms of organization of the infant-caretaker system.

A further interesting finding relevant to the temporal characteristics of sleeping and waking emerged from around-the-clock observations of sleep-wake onset, during days 11-29 of life, which were made by the two nurses who carried out the surrogate mothering on most of the infants. The infants care for by *one* of the two surrogate mothers developed significantly longer first- and second-longest sleep, and first- and second-longest awake periods per day than did infants cared for by the other. This was a finding of which we became aware only with data analysis. Both women were under our daily observations, both were adhering to the rule of not waking the baby for a feeding, both were recording sleep and wake onsets reliably. In contrast to the effect of the group A or group B experience on day-night distribution, this time statistical analysis revealed *no* effect of first 10-day caretaking experience on the length of sleep or wake periods during days 11-29. The key determinant appeared to be which of the two women did the caretaking.

There were many differences between the two women. We are unable to specify causative factors, since mechanisms of phase control are too little understood. The babies having the longer epochs showed more total crying and more often cried after being put down in the crib; those with the shorter epochs were more often asleep or nearly so when returned to the bassinet. The mean difference between infants, grouped according to surrogate mother caretaker, in duration of longest sleep epoch was 45.6 minutes, and in duration of longest awake epoch, 26.4 minutes. These durations, together approximating the duration of a basic rest-activity cycle, suggest the possibility that we are encountering here some mechanism by which temporal adaptation is being effected between infant and caretaker, perhaps by determining the phase relations between the basic rest-activity cycle and the major sleep or wake periods.

When examined day-by-day in detail at the level of the variables we have utilized, groups A, B, and C appear to be clearly following different courses over the first two months. Other variables and the way the three groups differ in respect to them will merely be listed. The response to twice-weekly presentations of visual stimuli over the first 2 months of life indicates that the infants of the three groups may be developing their styles of handling visual information quite differently. Burns et al. (1972) presented evidence based on their study of the feeding behavior of group A and B infants, before and after the change at 11 days, that regulation of feeing behavior may, already in the first 10 days of life, become dependent upon specific adaptation to the one individual caretaker who regularly feeds. The impression gained from group C indicates that regulation in the natural mother situation is idiosyncratic to a greater degree than in groups A and B, reflecting rather than modifying unique individual differences. Group A is distinguished from B and C over the first 2 months of life in terms of the greater instability week-to-week in the rank order of infants within each of the three samples when ranked on the basis of values obtained for the variables we have studied. One thing which this greater week-to-week rank-order instability indicates is that individual infant differences are not becoming established as consistent individual characteristics of group A babies. What does this greater instability at the outset of life imply for the coordination between subsystems within the individual, or for eventual characteristics of self-regulation in the adult? This may indicate further that initial variability [2] is as important in the description of the dyadic system as of the individual infant.

Not only, then, is the temporal pattern of exchange between infant and caretaker different for groups A, B, and C, but the course of development of various infant functions shows important differences between the groups as well.

DISCUSSION

The task remains to find some way to bring these findings together as a coherent picture and to focus the question of their relevance to the subject of primary prevention. The points reviewed above suggest that it may be possible to establish systematic empirical connections between part and whole; namely, connections linking characteristics of early temporal organization of exchanges between partners in the dyad, and the early course of differentiation of certain of the infants' functions (e.g., feeding or perception). Distribution over the 24 hours of the day of the infant's behavioral states along a sleep-wake continuum is one major determinant of the pattern of exchange in the dyad. This cyclic recurrence of states not only constitutes a category of individual infant differences which affect the pattern of exchange in the dyad in a major way, but also provide an avenue by which the characteristics and role of certain cyclic or periodic phenomena in the early developmental picture can be investigated. What is it about infant state that requires our central attention?

The manifest state of the infant, governed by interplay of activating and inhibiting systems, represents a confluence of at least (1) an intrinsically generated time course of phases in a basic rest-activity cycle (Kleitman, 1939); (2) a summation of *intrinsic* inputs arriving from a variety of infant subsystems, e.g., nutritional, respiratory, excretory, sleep-wake (possibly at the outset of postnatal life, each with a semiau-

2. Our recent work with 24-hour monitoring of infant state indicates that variability may have quite a different meaning when regarded from the standpoint of the individual than when regarded from the perspective of the system. Furthermore, just as within-day variability in the values of variables can be distinguished from across-day variability, so also can within-subject variability be distinguished from between-subject within-sample variability. Within-day within-subject variability appears related to the fluctuations of circadian rhythmicity and is greater in the normal than in the at-risk infant. On the other hand, the stability over time, i.e., week to week, of the rank-order position an infant holds in relation to his peers appears to be more a characteristic of regulation in the dyadic system. When individual infant differences are playing a significant role in the establishing of interactive regulation in the postnatal dyadic system, regulation becomes based on these unique individual characteristics so that their consistent expression becomes established as well.

tonomous temporal organization); and (3) *extrinsic* inputs representing recurrences of periodic events in the infant's caretaking environment. We realize that it is precisely those infant behaviors generated over the course of the periodic fluctuations of infant state which provide the behavioral clues by which a mother arrives at her basic caretaking decisions. In the "state" of the infant and in the mutual influence of "state" and "exchange" between infant and caretaker, each acting upon the other, we have a site of adaptive mechanics by which adjustments can be effected between intrinsic subsystems of the infant and between infant as a whole and the extrinsic caretaking environment. Such a site of confluence suggests a kind of analogy to Mason's model (1968) of "overall balance" in which multiple factors, each governed by its temporal structure of phases of maxima and minima, exert influence one on the other, the role of one part at any given time in the interaction between parts influenced by and influencing, in turn, the particular phase of each of the other parts at that moment.

The literature related to investigation of biological rhythms suggests a refinement of such a possibility. It has been reported that over the course of the first 3-6 months of life, circadian rhythmicity is appearing in one physiological function after another, i.e., not across all simultaneously (Hellbrugge et al., 1964). The possibility later on in life of phase dissociation, under particular environmental conditions, between various physiological systems which are ordinarily in phase synchrony, suggests that a primary feature of early postnatal development may be that of establishing and maintaining proper phase synchrony within the infant between his various physiological components. There may be a particularly sensitive period during which a basic regulatory core can jell. There is considerable support for the view that this in turn depends on proper relationship between time structure in infant and time structure in environment.

The significance of temporal organization in physiology is just beginning to dawn upon us, as the literature in the area of biological rhythms continues to mount. Our notions are vague as to the mechanisms by which caretaking interactions relate to the stabilization of intrasystemic coordination and to early temporal organization of infant behavior in its relationship to recurrent environmental regularities.

The literature dealing with biological rhythms indicates a very complex relationship between specific extrinsic signals—*Zeitgeber*—and response curves of a circadian rhythm (Aschoff, 1965). Phase control via inputs from outside would provide an intriguing possibility of a mechanism linking intrinsic infant and extrinsic environmental regularities. It is not possible here to review the adaptive significance of biological rhythms or the kind of models of organization which they suggest. Data from humans in environments free of time cues indicate that the relationship of the parts to each other within the individual may in some way be governed by the time and schedule structure in the relationship of the individual to his environment (Aschoff, 1969). There is some evidence that, for the human, social contingency is a far more powerful synchronizing factor than is a light-dark schedule (Wever, 1970). Aschoff (1969) has summarized these relationships as follows:

> Circadian rhythms are examples of an evolutionary adaptation to time structures in the environment. The process resulted in (a) self-sustained oscillations, the periods of which match approximately that of the environment, (b) species-specific phase relationships between the circadian oscillations and the environment warranted by entrainment, and (c) temporal order between a multiplicity of oscillating systems. Maintenance of the temporal order within the organism seems to depend partly on phase-setting effects of the entraining Zeitgeber. Therefore, lack of proper Zeitgebers may have deleterious effects to the organism [p. 849].

To return to the subject of "primary prevention," one of the problems raised by the recent spate of dramatic new findings in early infancy which are related to single variables or single systems, such as the perceptual, is their impact on the kind of interaction which is focused upon in the infant-caretaker exchange. For those interested in stimulating the generation of early sensorimotor schemata as a means of advancing cognitive development, findings of exquisite sensitivity or responsivity of the infant to visual, auditory, tactile, or kinesthetic inputs can suggest special value in attention to or "training" of the infant in these areas. The general issue of attempting to exploit these capabilities prematurely has been discussed by Wolff (1969), who makes the point that "In all aspects of cognitive and motor acquisition there seems to be a crucial difference between the first qualitative steps—which are relatively independent of controlled environmental input and probably not 'learned' in the usual sense—and the subsequent quantitative refinements" (p. 12). Wolff adds that these first qualitative steps, although relatively independent of "controlled" environmental input, are critically dependent on a certain "background" or "nonspecific" stimulus environment.

Some of the summarizing points which Wolff makes in referring to cognitive development and the issue of what can and cannot be taught infants and young children are the following:

> The over-riding problem in cognitive development is revealed in many facets: from a physically heterogeneous environment, the naïve child is able to extract a set of complex rules for categorizing experiences and for generating new rules of action and thought. The origins and development of this ability are at the core of what we must understand before we can decide what we can and cannot teach young children. . . . Children have at their disposal unlearned, or at least unteachable, acquisition devices for creating order out of random events, and for transforming ordered experiences into generative

principles (Cognitive Structures). The source of such devices does not conform to our current conceptions of how children learn [pp. 11, 18].

The fact is that the "physically heterogeneous environment" is not a random one, a realization which nothing makes more clear than the ubiquitous presence of rhythms and cyclic recurrences in biological systems, orchestrated in symphonic coherence to give unity and continuity to organic existence.

The mechanisms which make a nonspecific stimulus environment essential may be built around the redundancies which are constituted in the recurring encounters attending periodic fluctuations of behavioral states of the infant, during which patterns of exchange are becoming stabilized. This essential redundancy may need to be encountered at the outset of postnatal life, perhaps critically, much earlier than heretofore suspected. Regulation for the infant as a whole may be inseparable from a stable regularity or redundancy in key exchanges between infant and caretaker.

An around-the-clock regulation of infant-caretaker interaction in terms of consideration of "the infant as a whole" has fallen largely to the synthesis provided by a mother's intuition. Much of this synthesis, unconscious or only at the borders of consciousness, is utilizing machinery involved in the temporal organization both of intrinsic infant variables and the extrinsic variables related to events in the dyadic exchange. When infant and caretaking environment can be regarded together as an organic system, research in the area of biological rhythms suggests that the nature of this machinery may include mechanisms of phase control, phase synchrony, entrainment, etc., in the establishing and maintaining of basic regulation.

SUMMARY

We summarize a few of the implications for primary prevention which these data and the experience of collecting them have generated for us. In the first place, we have yet to define precisely what basic mechanisms are involved in the regulation of the cycling infant states, how interaction with the caretaker bears upon these mechanisms, and what relation the particular course of history, through which regulatory processes pass in becoming established, bears to *later* characteristics of regulation, differentiation of function, or organization of behavior. The kind of environment to which the individual may have to adapt later may confer advantage or disadvantage upon the various configurations which are possible.

In the second place, the significance of the first 10 days of life may be much greater than we have realized in the establishing of a basis for temporal organization of infant-caretaker interactions. The nonchalant separation of infant and mother in the first 5 days of life, which we have accepted unquestioningly as part of standard maternity care, needs a thorough reappraisal.

Furthermore, when we consider mechanisms of regulation, day-by-day and around-the-clock data provide a different set of variables by which adaptive processes can be investigated. The information which is available from investigations of biological rhythmicity carried out over the past 40 years cannot be neglected. Characteristics of periodicity, entrainment, phase control, and phase synchrony may play a central role and demand a keener appreciation for the role of time and temporal relationships. Models other than our familiar learning model are becoming available to account, in the immediate postnatal period, for the impact of specific features of extrinsic environment on periodic characteristics of infant states.

In a general way, we have merely been putting our customary language of the infant-mother "relationships" into a new vocabulary. The formulation of more detailed models of "organization" in the infant environment system provides the means of analyzing events at a more detailed level—within a framework that preserves a meaning, a logic connecting them. It is not intended as a substitute for the traditional concept of "relationships" in early development, but as a bridge to underlying processes.

That her infant stops crying when she picks him up is interpreted as "being spoiled" by one mother, and as a sign of her successful mothering by another. The "meaning" this has for us as investigators has customarily been focused upon such alternatives as these maternal interpretations of the events suggest. We pay special attention to any events we can assimilate into our formulations of maternal character or which suggest predictions in respect to qualities of later "object relations." The event itself—the termination of a cry when the baby is picked up—may also be viewed in terms of more complex models, such as the adaptive-regulatory, which envision the event as an interaction of infant, caretaker, and age effects, requiring a consideration of the history of such interactions and its relations to a context of other influences and events.

As we have pursued our research questions, it appears that we have been left with new questions as the best answers we have been able to find to our old ones. Although we may come to "know" the factors, or the mechanisms, which lie behind "simple" notions about relationships and their importance to the human, the existential demand upon the mother in actuality is that of an integration of all such "mechanisms" in her "relationship" with her new baby. The subtle orchestration which optimally can characterize the experience of a mother and infant in their mutual encounter presents us with as great a problem in understanding integration as confronts the biologist in his efforts to understand integration in the single cell. He seems to see this as a problem in understanding the life process itself.

It appears to us that the rather complex perception by the mother of behaviors identifying infant state, ordered in some temporal framework, may be replacing, in the human infant-caretaker situation, the more stereotyped and fixed action patterns that govern maternal and infant behavior at the infrahuman level. The "state" of the baby represents a manifest configuration depending upon a complex synchrony of intrinsic subsystems and may provide an initial site for synthetic function—a sensitive behavioral indicator, by means of which a next level of phase synchrony can be established between infant "as a whole" and recurrent regularities in the extrinsic world. It is conceivable that as we gain a clearer understanding of infant state regulation, a more meaningful comprehension of the postnatal caretaking adaptation will become available, as will a more meaningful comprehension of the nature of what we are trying to accomplish by interventions carried out in the immediate postnatal period in the name of "primary prevention."

PART III

The Developmental Course and Some of Its Variations

15

THE MATURATION OF AROUSAL AND ATTENTION IN THE FIRST MONTHS OF LIFE

A Study of Variations in Ego Development

Barbara Fish, M.D.

The study of individual variations in ego development requires the application of quantitative methods to very complex clinical phenomena. Most quantitative studies of individual differences in infants have been limited to the newborn period. Such studies have demonstrated differences among newborn infants in autonomic response patterns (Bridger and Reiser, 1959; Grossman and Greenberg, 1957; Richmond and Lipton, 1959), activity level (Fries, 1944), and sensory responsiveness (Birns, 1965; Graham, 1956). However, it is more difficult to demonstrate that any of these variations persist into later infancy or childhood. It is still more complicated to show how they affect personality development. Fries (1944) found some longitudinal consistency in individual activity type and described relationships between the extreme variations and certain personality characteristics in later life. Graham (1962) found no clear correlation between increased threshold to pain in the first week of life and neurological damage at 3 years of age. Comparable follow-up data are not yet available for the other variations seen in the newborn period. Their persistence and their significance for later personality must still be demonstrated.

The clinical experience of those who have worked in infant development for the last 15 to 30 years suggests that developmental profiles may be more significant than isolated functions. Single functions such as perceptual sensitivity, motor coordination and drive, and the threshold for irritability may show consistent individual differences (Escalona, 1950; Escalona and Heider, 1959; Gesell, 1945; Shirley, 1933; Wolf,

Reprinted from the *Journal*, 2 : 253–270, 1963.

1953, 1954). However, these workers emphasize that it is essential to study the relationships between several areas of development. Obtaining separate developmental curves for locomotion, visual-motor coordination, language, and social development yields a profile of the child's developing assets and disabilities, which is more meaningful than any average score (Bayley, 1956; Buehler et al., 1935; Gesell, 1947). Escalona looked for particular developmental syndromes involving specific patterns of activity level, perceptual sensitivity, social responsiveness, and the ability to delay impulse expression and need gratification (Escalona et al., 1953; Escalona and Heider, 1959).

These same workers indicated that the amount of spread or scatter between the several developmental functions seen in such a profile is itself a significant individual variable. Gesell recognized as early as 1925 that one must consider not only precocity or retardation but the balance of development, and pointed to the lack of integration and developmental harmony in the idiot savant, certain forms of dementia praecox, as well as in certain types of precocity. It was Escalona's impression (1950) that significant discrepancies among areas (motor vs. language, and so on) may reflect real developmental disturbance, whereas scatter which occurred within any one of these areas was more frequently seen with temporary upsets in the testing situation. She found that excessive scatter on infant tests was frequently associated with manifest clinical disturbances.

In investigations conducted since 1952, I have studied the significance of scatter and variability in infancy as an index of later childhood schizophrenia and personality disorders. The Gesell developmental examination was adapted so as to define differences in the integration of development, as well as individual differences in various capacities. The profile of functioning of each infant was determined by plotting separately the developmental quotients for locomotion, fine coordination and adaptive behavior, language and social development. For this purpose, Gesell's items of fine coordination were considered exclusively "adaptive development," leaving only the locomotor and postural items to be analyzed as "motor development." Poor integration of neurological maturation was said to occur if there was wide scatter between several developmental capacities at any one time, or wide scatter within a single function; if there were marked irregularities in the longitudinal sequence of development over the course of time, or irregularities in the normal cephalocaudal progression. It was predicted that increasing degrees of poor integration in infancy would be correlated with greater vulnerability to stress in later life (Fish, 1957).

This and subsequent studies suggested that there was indeed a variation in the capacity for integration in the early neurophysiological development of infants that could be correlated with the capacity of individuals to maintain psychological integrity in the face of stress. The threshold for later personality disorganization tended to be lower in those cases with greater disorganization of early neurological development (Fish, 1957, 1959, 1960a, 1961, 1964). Studying the integrity of the developing nervous system, as well as the growing organization of motility and perception appeared to yield important information on certain primitive ego functions and the development of ego strength in infancy. The preliminary analysis of the 9-year follow-up data on the children in the first study substantiates the earlier reports.

For the current study, a behavioral continuum of arousal was defined which ranged from deep sleep through alert attentiveness to extreme excitement or crying, with three intermediate steps (restless sleep, open-eyed drowse, and restless wakefulness with slight whimpering). Within this arousal continuum, the infant is most accessible to environmental stimuli when he lies quietly with his eyes open and is alert to visual stimuli. Accessibility is reduced if he is less aroused, being sleepy or drowsy, or if he is more aroused, becoming restless or vigorously crying. This continuum resembles the behavioral continuum of arousal which Lindsley (1960) related to gradations of awareness and to levels of activation on the electroencephalogram in adults.

The ability of the infant to respond at a particular time must be interpreted in the context of his changing sleeping-waking patterns, and the dependence of his state of arousal on hunger, satiety, and perhaps less obvious internal rhythms (chap. 5). I approached this problem by studying the variability itself in the infant's state of arousal, and his growing capacity for maintaining a more stable state of awareness. The study of the organization and pattern of responsiveness was assumed to provide more useful data on the growing integrative capacity of the nervous system than would a study of isolated responses.

Since the earlier studies had shown that it was possible to define developmental deviations in terms of standard developmental norms (Fish, 1959, 1960a, 1961), the study of arousal and alertness was approached in the same manner. An attempt was made, first, to define the usual maturational sequence; the ability of the infant to maintain a stable state of optimal alertness was therefore analyzed as a function of age. The pattern of individual infants was then studied for their deviations from the group trends and for any interrelationships which appeared between deviations in different functions (Fish and Alpert, 1963). Gesell (1945), Kleitman and Engelmann (1953), and Parmelee (1961) have studied the 24-hour pattern of waking and sleep in growing infants, but no comparable standards were available for the shorter periods of time sampled by this examination.

An infant population was examined which was genetically loaded for schizophrenia. This group was expected to show a higher incidence of developmental disorders than would a random sample of newborn infants. Neurological, physical, and psychological development was followed, using the methods of the earliest infant study (Fish, 1957, 1959). Vestibular function was also tested, in addition to the following study of states of awareness and sensory responsiveness (Fish and Alpert, 1963).

METHOD

From March 1959, to September 1960, all infants born to patients in two New York State hospitals were included in the study. All mothers had been diagnosed as schizophrenic by the hospital staffs. They had been ill for 6 months to 20 years. Most mothers had no phenothiazines for 1 to 3 months prior to delivery. Routine obstetrical analgesia was generally given with the onset of severe labor pains. In general, these mothers complained less of labor pains than ordinary mothers, so that less medication was usually given than on a normal obstetrical floor.

All of the infants had normal birth weights, and there were no records of prenatal or perinatal disorders. However, most of the mothers had not been hospitalized during the first 3 months of gestation and adequate antepartum records were not available for that period.

The infants were examined on the first day of life, usually between 12 and 24 hours of age; at about $3^1/_2$ days of age; and again at 4, 8, 16, 28, 40, and 56 weeks, and at 2 years of age. Thereafter, they are seen yearly, as long as follow-up can be continued. Two infants were lost after the initial examination in the nursery. The remaining 13 have been followed for 10 to 24 months; 9 are in foster homes, 3 with their grandmothers, and 1 is in a foundling institution.

Infants were examined between 1 and 2 hours after the last feeding. In addition to the Gesell examination (1947), the responses to a graded series of stimuli were recorded. A continuous time record was kept, on which were recorded stimuli, responses, and the periods of time at each of several levels of arousal from deep sleep through restless sleep, open-eyed drowse, quietly alert, restlessly awake, to maximum arousal, or crying.

Stimuli were usually presented in order of increasing strength from a dangling ring to a voice, light, bell, touch, pain, and finally postural and vestibular tests. The infant was observed following each stimulus for immediate response and spontaneous recovery state. If activity or crying did not spontaneously subside, a pacifier was used in order to achieve a quiescent state prior to the next stimulus. The responses specific for each age were scored according to Gesell's norms, as previously described (Fish, 1959). In addition, the level of arousal produced by each stimulus was noted. The infant's "base-line" state was defined as that level of arousal to which he spontaneously returned after gentle sensory stimulation, sufficient to test visual following. (Except in the sleepy newborns, this required only mild stimulation, or none at all if the infant was already awake.)

The continuous record of the infant's behavioral state made it possible to analyze the fluctuations in arousal which occurred spontaneously and in response to the series of stimuli, as well as the duration of each behavioral state.

The organization of consciousness at each age was analyzed according to (1) the level of consciousness which was spontaneously maintained after initial arousal (i.e., base-line state); (2) the longest period of quiet, open-eyed alertness which the baby could maintain without a pacifier; (3) the relative time spent at the various levels of arousal; (4) the frequency of change in state of consciousness; and (5) the profile of the responses to the spectrum of stimuli presented. These data were analyzed for their characteristic maturational sequence, for differences in this sequence, and for the relationships between any differences which occurred.

RESULTS

From birth to 2 months of age there was a definite progression of the group as a whole toward increased alertness and attention directed toward the environment. The characteristic or base-line state of arousal changed with chronological age (see fig. 1). The majority of infants were sleepy on the first day, but very few remained so after the fourth day, when most had recovered from obstetrical analgesia and the birth process. The number of infants who cried when awake, unless given a pacifier, increased after the first day of life, and then dropped sharply after 4 weeks of age. The number of infants who sustained open-eyed alertness without a pacifier gradually increased to 90 percent by 8 weeks of age. By 8 weeks almost all infants were able to maintain an optimal level of responsiveness to external stimuli, without dropping off to sleep or quickly shifting to sustained crying.

This maturation was also reflected in the maximum time during which the infants could continuously sustain optimal alertness without a pacifier (see fig. 2). The median time for maintaining continuous open-eyed alertness increased from only 2 to 5 minutes between birth and 4 weeks of age to 25 minutes at 8 weeks, and it continued to rise thereafter, to 45 minutes at 16 weeks, and still longer in the older infants. The median trends in this group conform to clinical descriptions of arousal states in the first months of life (Gesell, 1945; Graham, 1956; chap. 5).

By 8 weeks of age, 90 percent of the infants developed the ability to
modulate the extreme excitability or crying which accompanied arousal
in the first month. This meant that they could then maintain optimal
accessibility. This capacity for modulated arousal developed parallel
with the infants' ability to tolerate more strenuous postural manipulation without excess excitation or crying. Figure 3 shows the percentage
of the group which responded with sustained crying to each of three
items on the examination—passive manipulation of the extremities,
jolt, and being placed in a prone position.

There was little crying in response to postural stimuli in the newborn
period, when the infants were sleepy and unresponsive. Crying during
postural tests increased at 4 days and 4 weeks, along with the other
signs of increasing arousal and excitation noted already. After 4 weeks
of age, the infants began to tolerate these strenuous stimuli with less
crying. At 8 weeks, when 90 percent of the infants could sustain open-
eyed alertness without crying, almost all could also tolerate passive manipulation of the extremities. This may be related to their toleration for

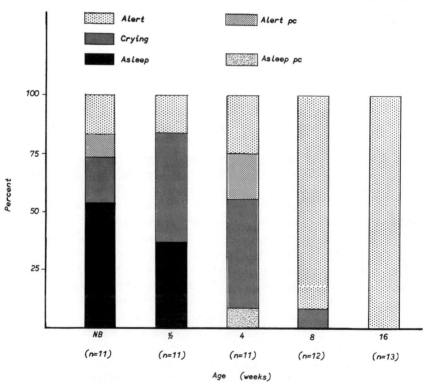

Figure 1

their spontaneous arm and leg movements, with less tendency to shift from activity to an excited, crying state.

The qualitative increase in alertness at 8 weeks reflects the capacity of the central nervous system to organize and maintain stable states of alertness. Another aspect of this increasing integrative capacity is seen in the drop in the median number of fluctuations of the state of arousal during the examination (see fig. 4). Many more fluctuations of state are apparent in the earlier examinations. This gross measure of instability of arousal state gradually declined with age, as the infants developed the capacity for sustaining optimal alertness.

The development of visual following and fixation in general followed the findings of Gesell (1947) and others. Under 24 hours of age, most infants who spontaneously lapsed back into deep sleep did not show any visual following. By 3 days most of the infants could follow a dangling ring, but maintained only fleeting visual attention on a nonmoving object. With the qualitative increase in the organization of alertness and attention at 8 weeks of age and the ability to modulate and inhibit diffuse random activity, there was an increased capacity to sustain visual attention and to respond to details of the external environment. There was longer visual interest in stationary as well as moving objects, and the infants quieted to a bell or voice. Visual or auditory stimuli had

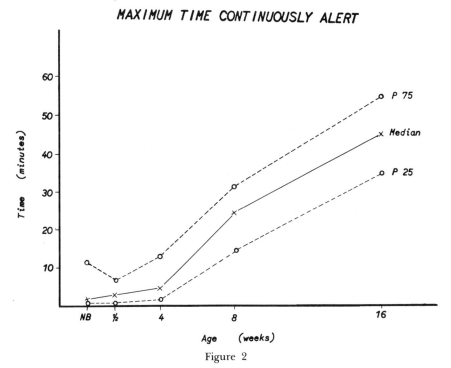

Figure 2

the ability at this age to distract many infants from excitation or crying caused by internal stimuli. Thus, there was a shift from the dominance of internal and proprioceptive stimuli toward increased attention to external distant stimuli of sound and sight. By 4 months, visual fixation had increased up to approximately 1 minute. Random activity could be inhibited briefly from 10 to 20 seconds during visual attention, showing increased control over the overflow of motor impulses and the increased ability to direct attention in an organized manner. By 5 to 6 months of age, organized behavior and goal-directed motility gradually increased and predominated over diffuse motor discharge.

The behavioral expressions of increased organization and differentiation of alertness, crude as they are, made it possible to define those infants who deviated from the group by being excessively irritable or quiet. Three infants showed excessively quiet behavior, with extremes of underactivity, hypotonia, and absence of crying, which are highly unusual for young infants. One infant showed an abnormal degree of irritability. Three infants showed less extreme deviations in the direc-

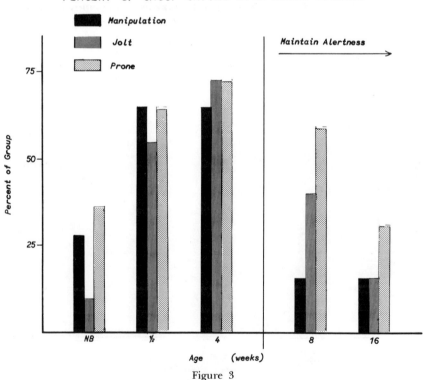

Figure 3

tion of excessive apathy or irritability. These clinical evaluations are based on the examination of large numbers of normal infants, but no exact comparison with an unselected group is possible, since comparable quantitative data are not yet available.

On my advice, the excessively quiet infants were placed with particularly warm and stimulating foster mothers. By 1½ years of age, usually with the onset of independent locomotion, they became more reactive, and to date have shown no serious psychopathology, although the most extremely quiet infant, Charles, is considered to be "rather high-strung." The most irritable infant, Rachel, showed the most severe psychopathology of the group at 2 years of age.

The 3 most extremely quiet infants differed primarily from the rest in their ability to maintain a base-line state of quiet, open-eyed alertness as early as 13 hours of age. One resembled the other infants by 4 weeks, but the other 2 were always quietly alert and never showed the base-line state of crying with arousal. These infants could remain quietly alert for 15 to 80 minutes during stimulation in their first

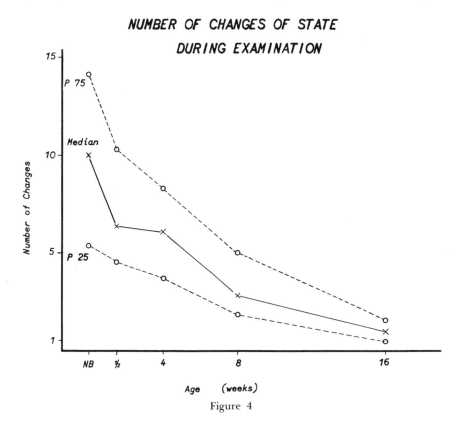

NUMBER OF CHANGES OF STATE
DURING EXAMINATION

Figure 4

month of life, in contrast to the median of 2 to 5 minutes. Unlike the other infants, they also tolerated vigorous manipulation of joints and muscles without crying.

Charles, the most extreme example of this, was excessively quiet for his first 6 months of life. He was markedly underactive, lay still and quietly alert, and tolerated vigorous manipulation of muscles and joints, jolt, and change of position without crying. However, he followed visual stimuli normally as he developed, and was extremely alert to slight sounds and touch. He cried sharply and briefly with a light pinprick. He was therefore selectively unresponsive to proprioceptive stimulation, compared to other modalities. His muscles were extremely doughy to palpation, feeling indistinguishable from soft subcutaneous tissue. Although his head control was normal for his age, his trunk and extremities were so flaccid that he could be folded or twisted like rubber to bizarre, extreme positions without showing any increase in tone or signs of discomfort. The nursing staff spontaneously and affectionately nicknamed him "Floppy," commenting, "He's like a little rubber doll." His poor tone affected his early grasping and reaching, and caused a marked delay in sitting (less than 4-month level at 6 months of age). However, he rolled and pivoted like an 8-month-old when he was only 4 months of age. Unlike hypotonic infants with peripheral neuromuscular disorders (Walton, 1957), his deep tendon reflexes were 3 +, loose and pendular. His hypotonia was apparently of central origin.

Although he was placid and inactive, he became very socially responsive and vocalized after 3 months of age. After 6 months of age, he showed a marked spurt in postural control, and by 7 months he was able to sit and creep like a 10-month-old. Shortly after this, the tone of his legs improved, and locomotor development advanced so rapidly after 10 months that he could walk, run, and climb stairs like a 21-month-old when he was 14 months of age. At 6 months the foster mother felt he "showed no spirit," but his self-assertion increased along with his motility, and she noted at 12 months that she could "hardly keep him down." During this period of his most rapid development around 12 months of age, it was noted that for several weeks he became afraid of all cats, dogs with dark fur, and of people wearing dark clothing. These symptoms, apparently associated with his increased assertiveness, gradually subsided after 13 months of age.

He has been hyperactive and impulsive since 14 months of age. Daytime fears and tantrums and severe night screaming spells, accompanied by head banging, occurred periodically from 12 to 18 months of age, and then gradually subsided. He is still considered "willful" and sensitive, but tantrums are brief and no longer occur daily.

Valerie was the fourth most quiet baby and was considered to show only borderline deviations in this direction. She always tended to be somewhat underactive and rarely cried. However, she tended to be less visually alert and less responsive generally to stimuli, so that her lack of crying in the context of this decreased arousal did not appear as deviate as the unusual quiet state of Charles and the 2 other quiet babies. She was never as hypotonic as Charles and the others; however, her legs did show decreased tone and tended to be maintained in extension, rather than in the normal semiflexion, for the first 2 months of life, with her toes curled under at 2 months.

She tended to be less alert than normal. Visual fixation was delayed and brief through the fourth month. Motor responses and affective responses were delayed, slow, and minimal. Motor landmarks were normal, however, although she continued to be underactive. Her approach to toys was hesitant and slow, although fine coordination performance tests developed at approximately an average rate. She tended to be less attentive to detail and showed little variety and no behavioral evidence of affective pleasure in her exploitation of objects. From 2 to 4 months, she was in a mediocre foster home, with a mother who was not particularly stimulating. She was changed at 4 months to a very warm, stimulating foster home. This family was concerned about her inactivity and underresponsiveness and her tendency to sleep all the time. They gave her all the extra affection, attention, and encouragement that she seemed to need. She became more socially responsive to her foster mother, but her characteristic response to strangers and to new situations was still to become very inhibited and underresponsive.

At 2 years, her development, including language, was approximately normal. However, she was considered to be shy with anyone outside the immediate family and "nervous," i.e., she became very excited over minor frustrations. On examination she continued to show the very slow, tentative approach even to her own toys, as well as when offered toys by others, or given something to copy. She whimpered, looked very anxious, and retreated when approached. She gave up readily if something proved slightly difficult. However, she was able to respond to her mother's encouragement and, with this help, was able to come up to approximately normal performance.

The most irritable of the infants, Rachel, has shown a number of difficulties, despite the ministrations of a very calm and understanding foster mother. At 17 hours of age, she was a small, normally sleepy infant. The only abnormality noted was her slow, stretching motility, resembling a premature infant more than a full-term baby, and her tendency to maintain her legs in extension rather than semiflexion. This posture also appeared at 72 hours. She was unusually responsive to auditory stimuli, showing a precocious quieting and alerting to voice and bell. By 1 month, she had difficulty swallowing, began to vomit, and had to be fed small amounts at frequent intervals. Medical investigation could demonstrate no organic gastrointestinal pathology, and these symptoms subsided after 6 months of age. At 2 months she was hypersensitive to a variety of stimuli; a light touch or a soft sound made her startle, and the smallest change in position made her cry, whereas the other infants had begun to tolerate such events.

Her marked irritability has persisted up to the present time. At 7 months she could sustain attention barely as long as a baby half her age, and her visual-motor performance began to lag. At 14 months when a toy or activity was offered to her, she screamed or ignored it. Sometimes merely looking at her started her screaming. Her anxiety was associated with an erratic and poorly integrated use of her abilities. At 2 years, one could break through this panic reaction if she was approached circuitously and was permitted in a roundabout way to take the initiative herself with the test material. She showed a very low frustration tolerance, but her poorly integrated adaptive performance could not entirely be blamed on anxiety; even when she persisted, for instance, with the form board, she showed severe disturbances in form perception and problem solving. Even at home her manipulation of objects is tentative. Through 2 years of age, she has had excessive fears of strangers, "freezes" in new situations, and is still sensitive to minute and distant sounds.

Conclusions

Alertness and the responsiveness to stimuli in young infants showed changes in organization and differentiation with maturation which can be used as a measure of the growing integrative capacity of the infant. One can conceptualize alertness and attention in neurophysiological or psychological terms. In physiological terms, these functions reflect the integrative capacity of the central nervous system. In the first months of life, at least two skills develop which are necessary for the maintenance of the quiet, open-eyed alert state. There is an increased general level of arousal sufficient to permit responses to minimal visual and auditory stimuli. There is also a gradual modulation of spontaneous excitability and an increase in the toleration of proprioceptive stimuli. This permits a continuing stable state of awareness and prolonged focused attention. These abilities are essential prerequisites for the well-integrated development of specific alerting responses (Lindsley, 1960), which involve differentiated attentiveness, perceptual discrimination, patterns of accommodation, and the more complex functions which modify the accessibility of the central nervous system to different stimuli.

In a psychological frame of reference, the mechanisms underlying alertness and attention subserve important ego functions. These include the perception of stimuli and the protection against excessive stimuli. The increasing "stimulus barrier" may be seen in the infant's developing ability to tolerate fatigue and proprioceptive stimuli without showing overflow excitation, and in his developing ability to focus on and maintain attention to specific aspects of the environment. Ego functions are also involved in the suppression of random motor activity and excitation, and the development of goal-directed voluntary motility.

Deviations in the maturation of alertness and attention can be defined in terms of the normal maturational sequence in the organization of these behaviors. Deviations within a behavioral continuum of arousal may occur in the direction of irritability and exaggerated responses, or apathy and underresponsiveness. Examples of both types of deviation were found in a group of infants born to schizophrenic mothers. These variations in ego development were associated with disturbances in attention, in the preception of external stimuli, and in the organization of adaptive responses to the environment.

Disorders in the development of arousal and attention may have repercussions in many areas of the developing personality. An infant must be able to maintain alertness, to inhibit crying and random movement, and to sustain focused visual and auditory attention before he can develop an organized perceptual experience of the world beyond his body boundaries. Underresponsiveness, or an inability to sustain attention, or an inability to screen out irrelevant internal or external stimuli represent primitive disturbances of arousal and attention. If we can measure such disturbances of these primitive ego functions in infancy, we will be able to study the ontogeny of apathy, irritability, and the complex disorders of awareness, attention, and perception in organic brain disturbances, childhood schizophrenia, and the behavior disorders.[1]

1. Independent psychological evaluations were performed when these children were 10 years old. For analyses of these findings and more recent follow-up data, see Fish (1975, 1976) and Fish and Hagin (1973).

16

ON EARLY INFANTILE PSYCHOSIS

The Symbiotic and Autistic Syndromes

Margaret S. Mahler, M.D.

In private practice here and abroad and as a consultant to the Children's Service of the New York State Psychiatric Institute and Columbia University, I was brought face to face with the problem of children's cases that could not be fitted into the well-established nosological categories of primary behavior disorders, neurotic or conduct disorders, psychopathic character deviations or impulse disturbances; neither would they fit into the "wastebasket" categories of the organic, or brain-damaged group of amentia cases (Mahler, 1947). At that time (in the late 1930s and even in the 1940s) Lauretta Bender's (1942, 1947) pioneering work in childhood schizophrenia was by no means accepted in the child psychiatric field, Bradley's (1945), Potter's (1933), and Despert's (1941) work notwithstanding.

It was in the early '40s that Kanner's concept of "early infantile autism" (1943, 1944) rendered the idea of severe psychotic derangement in young children somewhat more acceptable to workers in the field. This acceptance of the existence of "early infantile autism" had one long-standing consequence, however; any clinical picture of childhood psychosis in which anything resembling autistic mechanisms was detected, and in which the psychotic break with reality occurred in a young child, was henceforth designated as "autism."

Among the 16 child psychosis cases that I had thoroughly studied by 1949, cases where psychosis had begun before the age of 10 years, a closer scrutiny of their histories revealed disturbances that could be traced to two crucial periods of development (Mahler et al., 1949). One was the period which Anna Freud (1952) designated as that of the "need-satisfying object." This is the period which begins when a person in the environment, under the specific condition of the infant's need hunger, is perceived by the infant, transiently and dimly at first, later

Reprinted from the *Journal*, 4 : 554–568, 1965.

more distinctly, as being outside the orbit of his self, and is responded to by the child with the social emotion of "confident expectation," a phenomenon to the importance of which Therese Benedek (1938) has drawn attention. Normal "confident expectation" or "basic trust" (Erikson, 1950a) is derived from the fact that the rhythmically and predictably recurring experience of the accumulation of need tension, of "affect hunger" (Levy, 1937), is just as predictably gratified and relieved by a "good" outside source. In this "need-satisfying" period of object relationship, which coincides with the phase of normal symbiosis, the mother still partakes in the omnipotent orbit of the mother-infant dual unity (Mahler and Gosliner, 1955).

In the past histories of some of the 16 psychotic children whom we studied, we could trace their disorders back to disturbances in the earliest rhythm of alternation between instinctual need tension (expressed in affectomotor discharge phenomena) and the states of saturation expressed in the infant's quiescence and sleep. In the anamneses of those children we often, though not always, found that, during their infancy, they had not passed beyond (or after an imperceptible and short progress, had relapsed into) the earliest infantile mode of perceiving the proprioceptive and enteroceptive increase of physiological tension as diffuse organismic distress.[1] Those children seem to have been unable, as infants, to recognize or to learn from experience that, whereas physiological tension originated within their own bodies, the "confidently expected" relief from instinctual tension, i.e., gratification of needs, came from somewhere outside of the body! They could not develop the ability to wait, one of the first reliable signs of a functioning rudimentary ego. Hence, the response of these infants to instinctual hunger tension remained immediate, violent, and diffuse random activity, reminiscent of affective panic; and if this tension was not immediately responded to (the random activity being the only available undifferentiated cue), then retraction of affective contact, that is, regression, took place, culminating in a few cases in apathetic withdrawal. The tendency to diffuse random activity is reminiscent both of the affectomotor storm-rage reactions of early infancy and the clinical picture of catatonic agitation, whereas the reaction of apathy was in turn reminiscent of the terminal states of psychoses (Mahler et al., 1949).

The second important period of the manifest onset of childhood psychosis seemed to take place later in infancy, at a time when the symbiotic, need-satisfying relationship with the mother should be gradually becoming more mutual and consolidated. This is the time when the mental representation of the mother, the infant's memory traces of

1. For example, very early intractable sleep disturbances were reported in several cases, from as early as 8 months, and earlier.

her, should be in the process of becoming gradually and slowly representations of the whole object and the way be paved to object constancy (Hartmann, 1952), whence the infant's functioning indicates that he is capable of maintaining the mother's mental representation even in her absence for increasingly longer periods of time.

The mental representation of the object is built through identificatory and differentiation processes during the separation-individuation phase. The existence of the established mental representation of the object makes it possible for the toddler to experiment with separation and return (i.e., reunion with the mother) (Mahler and Gosliner, 1955; Mahler and Furer, 1963).

Maturation of the mental apparatuses, of which the maturation of the sensorimotor apparatus may serve as the paradigm, brings with it an increasing awareness of separateness from the mother. *Pari passu* there is an increasing sense of emotional dependence upon the mother arising out of the feeling of helplessness and of the threat of object loss. The predicament of the individuating infant is complicated by the fact that he has to cope with an expanding reality, in the midst of the age-specific psychosexual conflicts. These new requirements seem, in some constitutionally or experientially vulnerable toddlers, to cause undifferentiated, often agitated panic tantrums instead of eliciting signal anxiety. These states of panic seem to be the immediate trigger for psychotic regression or, we might say, for psychotic fragmentation of the rudimentary ego structure. The clinical picture is either dominated by abysmal panic or else it is characterized by the well-known secondary restitutive mechanisms (Mahler et al., 1959).

Let me say at this point that there are two important areas of agreement between the psychoanalytic theory of child psychosis and that of the academic schools. I fully agree, for example, with Lauretta Bender's thesis that the different groups of clinical pictures of childhood schizophrenia depend upon the stage of maturity of the central nervous system at which the psychosis becomes manifest. I believe that psychosis, in adults as well as in children, consists of, or implies, a functional failure of the controlling, steering, integrating part of the central nervous system—in other words, the "ego." In adolescent and adult schizophrenics, the schizophrenic process acts upon a mental apparatus in which the three essential, structurally differentiated components of the personality—the ego, the superego, and the id—have been fully developed. But in child psychoses the organization of each of these structures is still in a state of flux. Thus, the essential differences between the syndrome of the psychotic child and that of the adult schizophrenic would seem to be due to the degree of structural differentiation.

The second area of agreement between analysts and the academic school of childhood schizophrenia is that we too fully believe that child-hood psychosis seems to afflict only constitutionally vulnerable infants, or else very, very young ones, whose rudimentary ego was subjected during the first weeks or months of life to unusually severe, ac-cumulated traumata.

Our differences, I believe, are in the realm of emphasis. We believe that the lack of, or loss of, the ability to utilize the symbiotic (need-satis-fying) object is the core deficiency, which impairs the ego's integrating, synthesizing, and organizing functions. We believe that all other distur-bances are accessory to this absence of the human beacon of orientation in the world of reality and in the inner world. Therefore, we have come to regard the small psychotic child as only half an individual, one whose condition can be studied optimally only through as complete as possible a restoration of the original symbiotic mother-child dual unit. Only in this way can we find out to what extent he can be helped to in-dividuate.

One may protest that this sort of restoration is, in the first place, very seldom possible; and that, even if it were possible, it would not always be, in the practical sense, the best therapeutic method. However, our hypothesis dictates that the natural history, the dynamics, the path-ogenesis be reconstructed, to begin with, by our trying our utmost to reconstitute the mother-child symbiosis of the original dual unit, on the grounds that its alienation or interruption was the primary cause of the psychotic fragmentation of the ego.

In contrast to this kind of reconstructive or regenerative approach, the academic schools, which look upon the child as the carrier of the disease, place their emphasis on dealing with him therapeutically as a separate individual entity, within the limits of what is constitutionally given, and attempting to substitute as far as possible for that which is irreversibly lost.

THEORETICAL CONSIDERATIONS

In the human young, the instinct for self-preservation has atrophied and become unreliable, so that, as Freud (1923) said, the ego has to take over the role of adaptation to reality which the id cannot fulfill. But the neonate appears to be an immature, almost purely biological organism, with instinctual responses to stimuli, not on a cortical but es-sentially on a reflex and thalamic level and with no ego to speak of. He has at his disposal (since cortical inhibition is still undeveloped) only somatic defense mechanisms, which consists of overflow and discharge reactions. The neonate's and the very young baby's mental apparatus is thus not adequate to organize inner and outer stimuli for survival; instead, it is the psychobiological rapport between the nursing mother and the baby that complements the infant's undifferentiated ego (Mahler, 1952; Benedek, 1959).

Empathy on the part of the mother is normally the human substitute for those instincts on which the animal can rely for its survival. In a quasi-closed system or unit, the mother executes vitally important ministrations, without which the human young would in fact be unable to survive. During the postnatal period, the intrauterine, parasite-host relationship has to be replaced by the infant's being enveloped, as it were, in the extrauterine matrix of the mother's nursing care, a kind of social symbiosis. Even this primitive symbiosis must develop as a somewhat more differentiated phase than the neonate's and the infant's postneonatal state.

I think that we may profitably describe the very first weeks of extrauterine life as the stage of "normal autism" of the infant (Mahler, 1958; Mahler et al., 1959). In this "normal autistic" phase, from birth until about the second month of life—a period which Hartmann et al. (1946) speak of as the "undifferentiated" phase—the infant makes no discernible distinction between inner and outer reality, nor does he seem to recognize any distinction between himself and the inanimate surroundings. As he gradually moves into the symbiotic phase, the infant becomes dimly aware that what relieves his instinctual hunger tension comes from the outside world, whereas the painful accumulation of tension stems from within him. However, this recognition requires that there take place, during the symbiotic phase, some rudimentary ego differentiation. In the intrapsychic organization of the infant, the boundaries of his self and of the mother are still more or less confluent and fused; the distinction between them is dependent on the degree of affect hunger, when this distinction fleetingly exists, and its alternation with satisfaction, whence the boundaries are fused again (Lewin, 1950).

We can observe how, from the second half of the first year on, the young infant gradually begins to differentiate from the mother-infant symbiotic dual unit; he separates his own self (and his mental representation) from that of the mother. While the consolidation of the symbiotic phase is by and large achieved within the first year of life, it is from the second half of this first year that it is overlapped by the separation-individuation process, which culminates during the second year of life in gradual disengagement from the symbiosis (Mahler and Furer, 1963).

In the normal autistic phase, as well as in the symbiotic phase, the mother complements the more or less deficient innate stimulus barrier, performing the vitally important ego functions that the infant's primitive ego cannot execute and serving as a buffer against excess stimulation. In the phase of individuation and disengagement, on the other hand, the mother's role should be that of supportive encouragement for the toddler's gradual attainment of ego autonomy. Some mothers function excellently throughout the symbiotic phase; they are able to respond with empathy and skill to the cues that the infant gives. There are mothers who help the toddler gradually to disengage and individuate; but there are also mothers who cannot bear the child's steps toward disengagement, and who thus impede his individuation (Mahler, 1963).

It is undeniable that, in the anamnesis of early child psychosis cases, we often find an accumulation of severe frustrations and traumata within the symbiotic milieu; for example, a debilitating emotional unavailability on the part of the mother because she has a depression. We also find, that the opposite pole, an interference with the infant's gratification-frustration experiences, a stifling of his budding ego, by a smothering disregard of his need to experience gratification and frustration at his own pace. This then results in an interference with individuation which carries over into the second and third years of life and even beyond. But we have found in our study just as many cases of infantile psychosis in which the mother belonged to Winnicott's group (1958) of "ordinary devoted mothers," and we could reconstruct in some cases such extreme, seemingly intrinsic vulnerability on the part of the child which even the most favorable environmental situations could not conceivably have counteracted, thus preventing infantile psychosis.

To repeat my main thesis: I believe that from the genetic, dynamic, and structural points of view, the paramount—namely, that which appears to be the cardinal difficulty—is the inability of the psychotic infant to use the external maternal ego for structuralization of his own, rapidly maturing, and therefore most vulnerable, rudimentary ego. The designation of early psychotic pictures as "symbiotic-psychotic syndrome" rests on this hypothesis. The term "infantile symbiotic-psychotic syndrome" calls attention to the decisive fact that the survival of the human young depends on the sociobiological symbiosis with the mother organism, in the sense previously elaborated.

Disturbances of the symbiotic phase may go unrecognized, so that the psychotic picture emerges at the age when separation-individuation should begin and proceed. In these cases, delusional symbiotic restitutive mechanisms and panic prevail. On the other hand, if defenses are already built up during the symbiotic phase, against apperception or recognition of a living outside object world, then retreat into secondary autism dominates the clinical picture.

In every case of infantile psychosis that has been subjected to prolonged observation and treatment, we have found the basic mechanisms, the psychotic defenses, to be delusional autistic modes of adjustment. The essential aim of the latter is restoration of the omnipotent oneness with the symbiotic mother, although along with this aim goes a panicky fear of fusion and of dissolution of the self. Syndromes may show a prevalence of one or the other, but our research bears out the hypothesis that the autistic picture is a secondary formation.

17

LANGUAGE BEHAVIOR AS A PROGNOSTIC INDICATOR IN SCHIZOPHRENIC CHILDREN UNDER 42 MONTHS

Theodore Shapiro, M.D.

The course of clinical investigation follows a reasonably uniform pattern. Clinical description is followed by attempts to establish natural history; and multiple empirical treatments are tried. Then more molecular features of the disease or disturbance are investigated to establish substructure in the hope that etiology can be determined and rational therapy be instituted. Childhood schizophrenia and early infantile autism have been in the clinical market place since the early 1940s (Bender, 1942; Kanner, 1943). During this interval a progression of clear clinical descriptions (Bender, 1947; Kanner, 1946; Creak, 1961; Rank, 1949; chap. 16) have emerged and attempts been made to differentiate syndromes (Mahler, 1952; Bender, 1956a; Rimland, 1964; Goldfarb, 1964; Fish and Shapiro, 1965). There are also many advocates of empirical therapy ranging from appropriately modified psychoanalytic techniques (Bettelheim, 1967; Mahler, 1952, 1968) to operant conditioning (Hewett, 1965; Lovass et al., 1966), machine teaching (Colby, 1968), and use of pharmacological agents (Fish, 1960b; Fish et al., 1966). These treatments also carry the weight of theory building because they imply concepts of the structure underlying the disturbances treated. Because of the ethical "imperative to treat," there is no account of how such children would develop if merely left to their own devices without therapeutic intervention of any sort. Since concepts of natural history in psychiatry must be practically modified to include the human environment and all its extensions, the current medical environment is as much a feature of the schizophrenic child's world as is his family. Thus, when we say we study natural history, we mean evolution of a syndrome in the existing therapeutic environment. Many therapists sound

Presented at the 1971 symposium in Boston.

enthusiastic about given approaches to childhood schizophrenia. Nonetheless, as I read the literature, it seems to me that no one can be very sanguine about outcome, and no one has reported uniformly better results with one intervention as compared to another. Eisenberg and Kanner's (1956) review of the literature notes that regardless of therapy, 25 percent of these children do reasonably well socially, although they retain rigidities of ego structure which may be remnants of their earlier global disturbance. In discussing prognosis, they and others (Bender, 1956a, 1964) attest to the crucial importance of the child's attaining communicative speech by age 5. It is no wonder, then, that a number of investigators have turned their attention to a closer study of this crucial function (Goldfarb et al., 1956; Cunningham and Dixon, 1961; Weiland and Legg, 1964; Wolff and Chess, 1965; Cunningham, 1966, 1969; Rutter, 1968; Hermelin, 1967; Hermelin and O'Connor, 1967). These studies have contributed to better formulated descriptions of the language defect in childhood schizophrenia. There are, however, only two longitudinal follow-ups of single children (aged 7 and 4½ years [Cunningham, 1966; Ward and Hoddinutt, 1968]) using a consistent method of analysis. Aside from these, there are no longitudinal studies of this condition during the crucial period prior to the age of 5. Gittelman and Birch (1967), Rimland (1964), and Rutter (1965) all attest to the residual disturbances found in the children they followed after 5; in any case, their work did not focus specifically on language.

Our own studies on language development of young schizophrenic children began on a broad base of global clinical evaluation (Fish et al., 1966). Gradually, we focused on language function (Fish et al., 1968). We first presented our work in 1967; we had by then developed a specific method of analysis (Shapiro and Fish, 1969). We contrasted the development of two children with early speech disturbance and withdrawal over a 6-month period. Our method distinguished two aspects of speech, the morphological and the functional. We suggested that by means of the functional scale in particular, the schizophrenic child could be distinguished from the nonschizophrenic child. On this scale the psychotic child's speech showed a high incidence of irrelevant, out-of-context remarks. While both children echoed, the echoing of the nonschizophrenic child was thought to be a feature of a normal developmental burst during the examinations.

Our second investigation (Shapiro et al., 1970) was designed to study the imitative and echoing behavior of 8 schizophrenic children at 4 years, compared to similar behavior in normal controls aged 4, 3, and 2 years. Our results indicated that 4-year-old schizophrenic children produced significantly more rigid imitations than even normally developing 2-year-olds. We related this productive rigidity to the more generalized concept of identification, and suggested that close structural analysis of small speech samples could provide a useful index of ego rigidity and deviance in integrative function. Thus, Freud's (1914) prediction that the study of psychoses would be revealed through closer scrutiny of the ego rather than the drives seemed to be borne out.

In 1971 we presented the case of a childhood schizophrenia whom we had begun to study at age 26 months and then followed for 4 years (Shapiro et al., 1971). Analysis of speech samples during these 4 years of treatment in a nursery school revealed that by age 6 the child had not attained the intelligibility of a 30-month-old. At 6, his peak mean sentence length was 2.6 (30-month level). Our method also provided quantitative measures of his deviance; although he achieved a language DQ of 99 at 4 years (Gesell and Amatruda, 1941), an analysis based on our functional scale showed that less than 50 percent of his speech was communicative (compared to 90 percent in normal 2-year-olds). He continued to "echo" a great deal, and there was much disturbance in the context of his speech. The latter tendency increased as he grew older and acquired a store of phrases and words. In contrast to this, once phonetic storage was established, the echoing decreased as it does in normal development. Moreover, analysis of his communicative speech revealed major rigidities. Simple naming and often heard commands predominated. All his sentences were cast in the present tense and indicative mood; he asked but one question, used the past tense once, and did not employ the future at all.

While he followed the usual sequences of storage and repetition, he failed to develop creative usage. The ego apparatuses necessary for adaptive language to express complex thoughts were either absent or inoperative. The rigidities defined by our quantitative speech analysis are viewed as an index of deviance in cognitive structure, identification, and integration.

Thus our work to date has shifted from longitudinal comparison through cross-sectional study of a specific subfunction to long-term investigation of a single child. Each study in turn revealed a further aspect of the structure of childhood schizophrenia which again raised new questions for study. As clinicians, however, we must not lose sight of essential issues; one such problem is how to make early prognostic distinctions within at-risk groups.

At the present time, we have used our technique of language analysis to study 30 children. Here I present the data accumulated on 11 of those 30 children; these 11 were less than 42 months old at first examination. By investigating the speech behavior of these young children (all of them drawn from an extremely high-risk population), I hope to uncover some of the structural and developmental precursors of poor prognosis. I submit the proposition that intensive study of a single ego function offers the clinician an explicit index of a child's deviance which is only implicit in the more global clinical evaluation.

METHOD

Population

There were 30 children under 7 whose language was studied since 1965. The youngsters were drawn from a treatment and research program at the Bellevue Psychiatric Division Nursery. All the subjects were severely withdrawn and showed gross retardation in speech (most showed less than 70 percent of expected speech for their age). The group includes severely impaired schizophrenic children along with some severe disturbances considered diagnostically borderline.

The children were in the nursery, either as inpatients or as day care patients. During the study, they were treated with a number of modalities including drug therapy, milieu and educational techniques, and, where indicated, psychotherapy. Except for one case with a known history of meningitis, and two cases who later developed transient convulsions, none of the group was considered to have specific central nervous system involvement.

There were 9 males and 2 females with a mean age of 36.7 months (range 27–42).

Of the 11 children, 8 were followed for more than 12 months (average 25.3 months); 2 additional children are known to be in state institutions and have never developed speech; and the 1 child is still in our nursery developing well. Of the original 11, 6 were followed past the age of 5 (mean for group 61.9), which is the index year for past prognostic studies; these plus the 3 children mentioned above bring our group to 9. The 2 additional children not followed past 5 are in schools for retarded children (see tables 1 and 2).

On discharge, there were 7 children with a final diagnosis of childhood schizophrenia, 2 diagnosed as developmental speech lag, 1 child with expressive aphasia, and 1 with an organic mental syndrome secondary to meningitis. The current placement of the group ranges from special schools for psychotic children to normal public schools (see table 1).

Procedure

For our language development studies, each child was seen by the examiner in a playroom at regular intervals. The child played quietly for 10 minutes without interruption and then was stimulated to speech for 10 minutes. The structure of the session was open. The interviewer followed the child's lead and/or introduced material (toys, books) to elicit speech. The child's utterances were taped, and his activities and context were recorded by a second observer (see Shapiro and Fish, 1969 for details).

The tape was transcribed after the session, and each utterance was counted and coded along two dimensions. (1) *Speech morphology* is divided into prespeech and speech as major categories cataloging the clarity of speech from vowel sounds through babbling and jargon and single words through 5-word phrases (see table 3). (2) *Speech function* includes 24 items clustered under major categories which described the difference between *noncommunicative* and *communicative* utterances. The *noncommunicative* section describes *isolated expressive* speech and *echoes* as well as speech which was completely or partially *out of context*. The latter

Table 1

Subject	Sex	Age Exam 1	Age Exam N	Length of Follow-up	Discharge Diagnosis	Current Placement 7/71
6	M	27	74	47	Child schiz.	School for schiz. children
29	M	32	39	7	Withdraw. react. (speech lag)	Bellevue nursery
8	F	34	40	6	Severe retard. child schiz.	State hospital
17	F	35	66	31	Child schiz. with aphasia	School for schiz. child; then spec. school
4	M	36	51	15	(Speech lag) borderline psychosis	School for retarded
15	M	38	55	17	OMS with retard.	Normal child care placement
16	M	38	66	28	Child schiz.	Normal nursery
14	M	39	81	42	Child schiz.	Kindergarten P.S.
3	M	41	101	60	Child schiz.	School for schiz. children
22	M	41	61	20	Child schiz.	Bellevue nursery
9	M	42	47	5	Child schiz.	State school for retarded

Mean   36.7 mos.   61.9 mos.   25.3 mos.
Range   (27 mos. 42) (39–101)   (5–60)

Table 2

First exam ≤ 42 months (range 27–42)   11
Follow-up more than 12 months   8 *
Follow-up past age 5 years   6 †

* 2 additional children in state school and hospital still mute; 1 additional child still on ward doing well,
† 3 as above,* and 2 more in school for retarded.

includes inappropriate rigid remarks for which the examiner could find no referent in the room, or in common experience. The communicative range, on the other hand, consists of *appeals* and *referential speech* of varying quality. The latter includes naming, questioning, or simple sharing of events (see table 4). Thus, each utterance is coded in two dimensions, its morphology and its functional features.

To allow for both short-term and long-term follow-up, each child was tested three times. The first examination established the baseline. The second examination was given within 3 to 4 months; this became the short-term figure. The third examination, ranging from 5 to 60 months later, was utilized for long-term follow-up. Thus, the three examinations provided us with an index of stability and short- and long-term outcome.

Results

The Entire Sample

Of the 30 children in our total sample, 28 were examined 3 to 4 months later, and 26 were given their final evaluation from 5 to 63 months later. These 84 studies over a span of 5 years were used to eval-

Table 3

Morphology

Prespeech

Vowels and Vowel-Consonant Combinations
Babble and Jargon

Speech

Conventional Sequences
Single Words
Two-Five Word Combinations
Disjunctive Syntax

Table 4

Function

Noncommunicative

Isolated Expressive Speech (6 Items)
Context Disturbance (complete) (1 Item)
Imitative Speech (3 Items)
Context Disturbance (partial) (2 Items)

Communicative

Appeal Speech (wish-oriented) (5 Items)
Signal/Symbol Speech (propositional) (7 Items)

uate the general developmental trend of these deviant children during the formative years when they were acquiring language and speech (see fig. 1). As a group, they tended to remain below the norms of intelligibility, compared to their nondeviant age peers; however, the intelligibility of their utterances did increase with increasing chronological age.

There is a similar upward trend in communicativeness with age. However, the mean communicativeness never exceeds 71.6 percent, even in the group over 73 months. Thus, although these children function as retarded and deviant, they are *not static,* and any prognostic statement must be viewed in the light of this potential for progressive development.

Sample Under 42 Months

The two dimensions of intelligibility (morphology) and communicativeness (function) were used to make further differentiations within our target group of 11 children (under 42 months). We first created a category which included those children who had no speech at all and those who were more than 50 percent retarded in intelligibility (Sampson, 1945). We segregated these from those who were not so retarded. We then split the latter group between those who were less and those more than 75 percent communicative. Thus, our first group was grossly retarded (or nonverbal), our second less than 75 percent com-

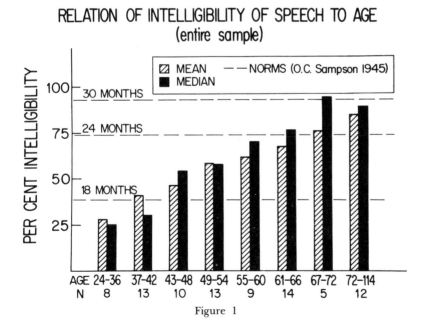

Figure 1

municative, and our third, those whose speech was more than 75 percent communicative.

Our first and second examinations provided subjects in only two of these three categories. Initially, there were 7 (first group) children with grossly retarded functioning and 4 (second group) who were not grossly retarded, but <75 percent communicative. The second examination reversed these figures, with only 4 (first group) who were grossly retarded and 7 (second group) who were no longer so retarded, but <75 percent communicative (see table 5).

Thus, in the 3 months between the first two examinations, 3 children advanced sufficiently in the intelligibility of their productions to leave the most retarded group and enter the speaking but uncommunicative group. In effect their morphology improved, but their functioning (communicativeness) remained poor.

At the final examination, 3 of the 4 children who initially had been grossly retarded continued to function at that level. Only 1 of these children joined the 4 Group 2 noncommunicative children who entered the best category of largely intelligible speech (Group 3, more than 75 percent communicative). Thus, at final examination, the noncommunicative group segregates into a better outcome group and a persistently poor communicative group (see table 5).

Closer analysis of the functioning of the children in each of these groups suggested the prognostic power of the 3-month examination. We divided our population according to school placement (in 1971), which we believe is a rough indicator of social adaptation. By the time each child had been exposed to the ward milieu and offered an opportunity for short-term (3-month) adaptation to the nursery program, we were able to plot his communicative speech score. This provided a perfect sorting on both sides of the median between those who are currently placed in state hospital, hospital school, and school for schizo-

Table 5

Distribution of Types
During Three Exams

Exam	I	II	III
No Speech or >50% Retarded Intelligibility	7	4	3
Less than 50% Retarded but <75% Communicative	4	7	3
>75% Communicative	0	0	5

phrenic children as contrasted to those in regular or special education class in a public school. Interestingly, the one child whose score fell exactly on the median of 52 (median for entire sample of 28 children at second exam was 52.5) was the same child who continued to be retarded at the time of his second examination at age 40 months, but then joined our best group at final exam when he was 66 months old. His development accelerated at 42 months when at a mean sentence length (MSL) of 1.7 he had a burst of echoing and subsequent better communicativeness (see fig. 2).

Thus, as measured by this method, prognosis seems related to communicativeness. Perusal of the third examination, however, offers another fine point of observation to which clinicians should be alerted. All 3 of the children who remained noncommunicative at this point showed more than 20 percent context disturbance on this last examination (which accounted for the rise in the mean score of context problems for the group). Interestingly, the mean percentage of echoing dropped for these children and, indeed, there was a reversal of predominance of echoing and context problems. The latter predominated at the last exam (see table 6).

It would be important to see how early this rise in context disturbances emerges. The data suggest a natural relationship to another index of development, MSL. In none of the 3 children did context-

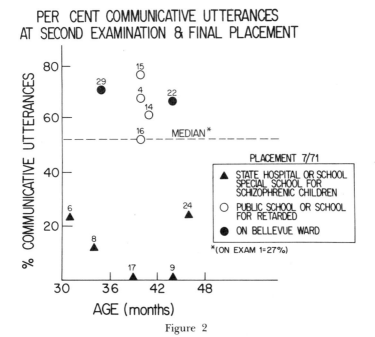

Figure 2

Table 6

Percent Echoed and Context Disturbance in Three Examinations

S	Echoes			Context		
	I	*II*	*III*	*I*	*II*	*III*
4	0	23	12	0	0	1
6	36	16	7	0	0	40
8	0	0	2	0	0	0
17	0	0	2	0	0	0
3	27	24	9	0	2	20
9	0	0	0	0	0	0
14	19	20	4	2	2	23
15	53	21	1	5	0	2
16	14	19	2	5	2	2
22	12	30	14	8	1	6
29	15	24	7	0	1	1
	176	177	68	20	8	95
Mean	16	16	6.1	1.8	.7	8.6
Median	14	20	7	0	0	2

echo reversal occur under a MSL of 1.9, although it may have been rising earlier (to 7–10 percent range). More significantly, by contrast, the 5 children who advanced to the best communicative group showed sharp bursts of echoing at comparable ages and MSL, but then receded. Moreover, they never showed the increase in context disturbance which characterizes the 3 children who remained poorly communicative and had the most deviant school placement.

INTERPRETATION OF RESULTS

Clinicians have been gradually segregating retarded and mute children into varying subgroups with characteristic clinical pictures and specific etiologies, e.g., biochemical defect or genetic chromosomal variation. The psychotic child sometimes shares retardation with these children, *but* he is distinguished from them by his withdrawn and/or bizarre behavior. However, within the psychotic grouping, further differentiation should be possible which might allow clinicians to make a more precise estimate of prognosis and ultimate social adaptation. Our data suggest some clues to this distinction, based on language behavior in its early stages of development.

As has been documented elsewhere (Fish et al., 1966), long-term prognosis seems to be closely related to short-term responsiveness, especially when measured in early childhood. While this is true, developmental measures in these deviant children do not remain static. As we showed in the longitudinal study of a child from 2 to 6 years, there is some increase in function proportional to age. The data in this present study on the children below 42 months suggest a clue to an important prognostic sign. Our method distinguishes gross categories which are easily related to clinical observation and which, when counted and compared, seem to be relevant to prognosis.

In the course of speech development, there is an early phase when verbal forms (morphological structures) are acquired through imitation and stored in memory. A parallel maturation in grammatical form must be postulated which becomes evident only as the child uses early syntactic forms to encode complex ideas. It is at this point that the contextual irrelevance of our children's remarks becomes evident. They seem to use their verbal skills inappropriately, so that the listener is confused unless he is well acquainted with the child's background and life.

For example,[1] each time one of our children entered the hallway, she would shout, "I really mean it!" On the face of it, this verbalization seems bizarre. Given an additional bit of history, however, it becomes relatively understandable. On former occasions she had run down the hall without permission, necessitating frequent reproach from the nursery teacher, who, in desperation would say she "really meant it." This obviously affect-laden remark was then recalled for use each time this child entered the hall. This vignette provides an interesting focus to discuss this child's level of symbol formation in relation to her object representations. She reenacts the affect-laden interaction each time she recognizes the original context of the experience, but she can do it only by simple storage and repetition of the teacher's words. Thus, even in the teacher's absence, the child recathects the object of the experience, but each time as a unique event with uncertain integration to other experiences with that object, and without the predicative language facility which would allow the individual to ascribe to that object any number of attributes.

The rigidities we could measure in the areas of context, irrelevance, and echoing may well be viewed as parallels to the ego rigidity that clinicians describe when they report their impressions of schizophrenic children. They point to the demand for sameness, the panic at separation, the treatment of human beings as objects. Theoreticians such as Bender and Mahler paid close attention to these clinical observations before they discussed the structure of this disorder. Bender utilized a biodevelopmental framework to suggest that one could account for the emerging clinical picture on the basis of maturational lags in central nervous system functions. Mahler (1968) focused on ego failure during

1. I would like to thank our nursery teacher, Mrs. Dale Ehrenberg, for this enlightening anecdote.

the separation-individuation phase and tried to pinpoint the psychic experiences of the child during this process by observations of his subsequent behavior.

Our own work borrows from both traditions. We believe that behavior emerges as a reflection of both psychic structuralization and patterns of interaction. We see development as an ongoing process based on phase-related integrations of maturational biological givens and interactional support and stimulation from the mother and other relevant environment. Thus, at each stage new structures emerge which should be measurable as new techniques become available. Language function offers one behavioral indicator of these structures.

Recent work during the mid-60s in operant conditioning seems to challenge these theoretical models. Psychotic children with limited speech were taught to increase the number and range of their words and phrases through operant and machine training. It is not certain, however, that they increased flexible usage. In fact, our current data suggest that cognitive psychologists and linguists may have a "crucial experiment" in childhood schizophrenia. These are groups of children who appear to defy the premise that reenforcement alone yields "natural speech." It yields rigid echoing and contextural irrelevance along with some natural speech.

Our data suggest that storage over time increases intelligibility, i.e., learning does occur, but structuralization remains remarkably retarded, rigid, and deviant. Moreover, the sequencing of stages is less apparent, and the child continues to show components of the past stage during each new developmental epoch. Thus, these children echo well into later life, they speak out of context, and at the same time they may make *some* good grammatical transformations.

We believe that focusing on language development has provided an early index of prognosis because it is an early indicator of the degree of structural ego deviation.

We wish that we had better understanding of what determinants in biopsychosocial makeup resulted in the better communicative group that we encountered. However, our data are inadequate in this regard. They point toward the ego's structuralizing capacity, but do not preclude the relevance of its support systems, i.e., mothering. However, if this work provides some clues to earlier prognostication, it has been worth the pursuit.

18

HOW CHILDREN COPE IN FAMILIES WITH A PSYCHOTIC PARENT

E. James Anthony, M.D.

The introspections of genius have furnished many psychological investigators, such as Freud, Erikson, Greenacre, and others with hunches that have led to further exploration. It is important to bear in mind that this type of strategy is only prelusive to research and that the ideas generated by a single preeminent mind are as liable to wishful distortion as those formulated at a much lesser level of insight and, therefore, as needful of scientific evidence. Having stipulated this limitation, we can now turn to an autobiographical fragment by Piaget (1952) (which in the service of brevity I have paraphrased) as a preliminary to understanding how children in families cope with a parent suffering from mental disorder.

> One of the direct consequences of my mother's poor mental health [he writes] was that I started to forego playing for serious work very early in childhood; this I did as much to imitate my father (a scholar of painstaking and critical mind who taught me the value of systematic work) as to take refuge in a private and nonfictitious world. I have always detested any departure from reality, an attitude which I relate to this important influential factor of my early life, namely, my mother's poor mental state. It was this disturbing factor which made me intensely interested in psychoanalysis and psychopathology but at the same time blocked any desire I had to involve myself deeper in that particular direction. As a result, I have always preferred the study of normalcy and the working of the intellect to the tricks of the unconscious.

From the age of 7 onward, he became successively preoccupied with mechanics, birds, fossils, and seashells. He invented an "autovap"—an automobile provided with a steam engine, and wrote a compilation on birds. At the age of 10 he decided to become even more serious and became a collector and classifier of mollusks, spending all his free time

---

Presented at the 1971 symposium in Boston.

on this work. By 15 he was already a recognized malacologist, but then the trouble began.

> Between the ages of 15 and 20, I experienced a series of crises due both to family circumstances and to intellectual curiosity. I was able to overcome these crises thanks to the mental habits that I had acquired through my early contact with the zoological science.

Not altogether, however. The emotional pressure continued to build up. When he was 15, his mother, who was a devout Protestant, insisted on his taking religious instruction. His father, on the other hand, did not attend church and, because of his scientific frame of mind, was critical of current beliefs. Piaget tried to solve the incompatibilities between religion and science by reading everything he could lay his hands on, writing down his ideas in numerous notebooks, and attempting in every way to resolve the split in the internalized father-mother image. The inner representations were experienced as parts of the father and parts of the mother in constant and vehement conflict with one another. As a result, his own emotional health broke down and he was forced to spend a year on the mountains completely removed from his frenetic reading and writing. A novel that he wrote at this time delineated this intense inner struggle with its severe identity crisis. At the height of his disturbance, he came upon a solution to this conflict by elaborating a comprehensive system.

> I suddenly understood that at all levels, from the living cell to society, there exists the same problem of the relationship between parts and whole, and I was convinced that I had found the solution to it, which was really very simple. In all fields of life there are totalities qualitatively distinct from their parts but imposing an organization on them. There cannot, therefore, be any isolated parts since parts are necessarily dependent on the whole which pervades them. One can postulate relationships of the whole to itself, each part to itself, of the various parts to one another, and of the parts to the whole. Within the total structure, the parts can predominate over the whole, the whole over the parts, or the two can be related reciprocally. This last form of equilibrium is more stable and desirable than the other two.

This solution emerging almost miraculously out of his disturbance, became the cornerstone of his later psychological system. The fundamental notions regarding part-whole relationships and the equilibria involved in these relationships determined his scientific activities for the next 50 years. The adolescent crisis had served to bring him back to an even keel. He had reorganized the fragments within himself and systematically contrived a representational whole that could incorporate father and mother parts, feeling and cognition, science and mysticism, psychology and biology, in terms of assimilation and accommodation all striving toward equilibrium. The solution was by no means final. Having constructed his system, he could not afford to leave it alone, but was compelled to work on it ceaselessly.

> I have to go faster for fear I might not finish in time before the world situation becomes troubled . . . I am fundamentally a worrier whom only work can relieve. I have a perpetual reservoir of anxiety that I have to transform into a need for work. This takes the form of a dionysiac excitement that ends in intellectual activity.
>
> [Moreover, he also saw himself as split in two: one side socially responsive and forthcoming and the other retiring into himself.] It is this *dissociation*, this double aspect of myself which has enabled me to surmount this permanent fund of anxiety and turn it into a need for working.

The creative synthesis of adolescence was therefore not once and for all. He continued to work at it all his life in a way suggestive of what Erikson has described as "self-chosen therapy."

What then did his mother's mental disorder do to his internal representational world? First of all, it split it down the middle so that the father-generated parts of the totality were at variance with the mother-generated parts. During early childhood, by turning his back on the split and preoccupying himself constantly with new intellectual pursuits, he managed to achieve a lopsided, rather precocious development that served as an escape from reality, from feeling, and from any pressure of psychological insight. Predictably, the situation flared up at adolescence when the internal maternal demands were overtly manifested in the "religious problem." It seemed as if he had to choose between father and mother, between reality and unreality, between affect and intellect, and between rationality and irrationality. The need to bridge the gulf, to integrate the incompatible parts, and to bring them into a meaningful relationship to the whole and to a state of equilibrium led not only to a resolution of his inner dissociation of which he speaks with such understanding, but also to the erection of a magnificent theoretical edifice—one completely comprehensive, self-contained, internally consistent, without loose ends or unfilled spaces, and rigorously freed from affect: no place at all for anxiety to permeate. The gradual building of this affectless monolith helped to mitigate the constant rub of anxiety that persisted in haunting him. His work habits were also directed toward closure. Every moment required to be filled with thought; each space of paper completely covered with writing; everything had to be included and nothing left out. Once again, there was no place for anxiety infiltrations.

This was one man's method for coping with mental illness in a parent, and since he also happened to be a genius his coping became creatively transformed, the vast system in 25 volumes was a monument to the child that died early in childhood and was replaced by an intellectual paragon. The defense mechanisms—intellectualization, splitting, isolation, asceticism, manic activity, withdrawal—are all familiar maneuvers by which adolescents respond to a variety of stresses. It is the coping mechanisms that are novel and innovative and idiomatic in relation to the individual and his circumstance. Piaget was not better defended against the overwhelming anxieties induced by parental mental illness than any of the 200 subjects in our research, but his techniques for coping were infinitely greater. We have had some examples of creative coping, but not of this order.

The Coping Situation of Psychotic Stress

In this research, so far, we have seen 200 children, one of whose parents has needed to undergo hospitalization for psychosis (Anthony, 1968). The classical diagnosis of the parent threw little light on the stresses to which the children in the family were exposed; a rating on a process-reactive scale and an assessment of the mental health of the nonpsychotic spouse proved better indications of the family's predicament; however, in the final appraisal, it was the child's-eye-view, of being involved or not involved, supported by a rating of the helpfulness or harmfulness of the so-called well spouse that gave the best impression of the coping situation. An involving psychosis, therefore, came to mean one that incorporated the child into the psychotic system of the parent, making him an integral part of the disorganized thinking and feeling of the parent as expressed in delusions, hallucinations, and bizarre moods and behavior. The child becomes at one and the same time the love-hate object of the parent, transformed by psychotic transference, manipulated by wayward psychotic impulses, and subjected to chaotic sexual and aggressive transactions. In the noninvolving psychosis the parent undergoes a kind of psychic death and is largely unavailable to meet any of the child's needs. As far as emotional interchange is concerned, he is a nonperson for the child, although a premorbid internal image that may reveal in day and night dreams, suggesting that the child is keeping alive his otherwise lost parent within himself.

The disturbances in the children are heterogeneous and range from apparent normality to gross disorder. Almost every diagnosis in the standard nomenclature has been seen in the 200 subjects in our sample, with a few unusual ones in addition. In the latter category, there has occurred extreme primitivization following massive developmental regression; in some children transient episodes of psychosis that increase in frequency with age; various degrees of *folie à deux* with the strength of conviction depending on concomitant reality factors; and an unusual variety of Ganser syndrome in which the children play at lunacy (Anthony, 1969a).

With these wide variations of normality and abnormality in the parents and the children of the same family, the basic question immediately arises as to what factors determine the vulnerability of the child. The invulnerability of a large number of children immersed in the same pathogenic environment has gradually become the most intriguing research question of all.

Genetic factors undoubtedly play a part and we have tried to disentangle this in other papers (Anthony, 1972a). Here, the emphasis will be on the defense and coping mechanisms used by the children in response to psychotic stress. Our data have been derived from psychotherapy, projective tests, and living-in experiences with the family. It was this latter encounter that led us to appreciate the variety of coping techniques used to counteract external objective anxiety.

DEFENSE AND COPING MECHANISMS IN RESPONSE TO PSYCHOTIC STRESS

Murphy (1970) has discussed the difficulty of separating defense and coping mechanisms. She concluded that coping was a broader concept than defense in its classical connotation. In this context, the ego takes defensive measures with regard to intrapsychic operations relating to affect and instinct and although not necessarily pathological in character, they are generally assumed to be so. Coping has had its meaning amplified within the last two decades to imply something over and beyond intrapsychic defensive maneuvering. It has come to include the overcoming of objective anxiety, the mastering of subjective anxiety, and the tolerating of increasing doses of frustration and suffering. There was an implicit suggestion that whereas defenses must be analyzed, coping had to be taught and learned. The former tended toward stereotypy, whereas the latter could be creative and innovative. The main difference lay between habitual and spontaneous behavior, between the fixed and the flexible, the internally determined and the externally responsive.

We were chiefly interested in three aspects of this problem. (1) Were the children that we reckoned to be at greater risk and the more vulnerable more inclined to the use of rigidly applied defenses than a wide-ranging deployment of coping mechanisms? (2) Did the intrapsychic defense pattern bear a relationship to the overt coping behavior elicited by objective disturbing experiences? (3) Did habituation begin in time to block out catastrophic events within immediate sight and hearing? We have talked to children who have been in a room where violent psychotic interactions, both verbal and physical, have been rampant, and who will still deny, in the manner of the three proverbial monkeys, that anything untoward has occurred. I feel convinced that such survival techniques are internal, automatic, and no longer conscious. Some of our "invulnerables" seem expert at "turning off" at the first hint of disturbance. Here is a summary statement from an 8-year-old boy: "I thought first she was going to kill me—then I thought she'd hit me, just hurt me, and that scared me—then I thought she'd sort of holler at me and nothing else—and then I didn't really mind anymore. I just don't think about it." In one house, there was a group of children watching TV with apparently intense concentration while behind their backs their mother was undergoing a severe psychotic decompensation. We were constantly surprised by the way in which these children continued to function, both at school and at home within the normal range, while they were undergoing experiences that would seem devastating and disintegrating to adults (Anthony, 1969b).

There were a number of related questions: did these horrendous experiences actually register in the psychological life of the child? Did he understand them in the way that the adult observer understood them? If there was anxiety, what disguises did it assume, and if the child was coping, what normal or abnormal outlets did he use (Anthony, 1972b)?

Our investigations in fact disclosed that the apparent imperceptiveness of the children by no means precluded a complete registration of disturbing events that could be brought to light by therapeutic and projective methods, and that the children not only understood what was happening but could differentiate and categorize the events, and were able to distinguish between mental and physical illness, although often fobbed off with inadequate or erroneous explanations. They also were able to recognize the premonitory signs of psychosis and, after several parental relapses and remissions, developed an uncanny expertise with respect to diagnosis, prognosis, and treatment.

The relationship between defense and coping mechanisms often underwent changes over a period of time. Initially, the defensive system as portrayed in therapy and projective tests and the coping as observed in living-in observations on the family bore a striking resemblance to each other; external avoidance was reflected in internal denial, external intellectual preoccupations in internal isolation, external canceling behavior in internal undoing, and so on. As time went on, coping mechanisms tended to become repetitive and stereotyped and were gradually incorporated into the character defense structure.

I have already indicated that it is more difficult for the child than the adult to isolate and insulate an involving psychosis that disorganizes his life and backs him into chaotic transactions. The sex of the parent is also important. It is especially hard for younger children to cope with a psychotic mother since their daily rituals and hence their comfort are so tied up with her. Where mothering fails, these small ones fall back on one another or learn to mother themselves so that they become solicitous and protective of themselves and their siblings. When the father becomes psychotic, the children may also learn to father themselves and the sons especially may assume protective and supportive roles.

The age of the child at the time of exposure is also crucial. In the case of the younger ones in whom the internal inhibitions against aggression, for example, have not been fully established, there may be a greater acceptance of psychotic violence. The early latency child who is still struggling with defenses against destructiveness may have these reactivated by the external aggressions. On the other hand, the preschool child's animistic fears may be intensified by the objective anxieties to which he is exposed. We have observed an outpouring of objective anxiety resulting from murderous psychotic behavior lead to subjective anxiety and nightmares linked to ghosts and monsters (Anthony, 1971).

From our data, it would seem that a high degree of involvement with the psychotic parent and a strong identification with him, combined with personality traits tending toward suggestibility, submissiveness, and a generally nonrealistic orientation, make for increased risk during childhood. The child becomes submerged in the parental psychosis and develops some variety of *folie à deux*. Genetic and constitutional factors become more significant with regard to the risk of development of adult psychosis.

The struggle against involvement is waged along many different fronts. For example, there is the child constantly practicing counter-suggestibility ("My mother is still ill. She says it might affect me—that she was like me at my age. She says, 'Look what happened to me.' But I won't let it happen to me. I'll never get sick like her"). There is the child showing increasing tolerance ("I've had all I can take of this madhouse. I can't stand it anymore." Leaves room but returns later. "Perhaps I can stand it. I didn't think I could"). Then there is the wide variety of avoidance reactions ("When my mother starts, we kids all get together in a room by ourselves and shut the door—we shut her out. If she wants to be crazy, she can, but that way we can't see her and hear her, and so we're not upset"), distancing mechanisms ("I always find something to do. When he gets that way I read and play music and make my models and write essays. The teacher says that I am the busiest child she has ever met"). The alertness of the children to the earliest manifestations of psychosis has, at times, almost a clinical quality about it. ("I know when my mom is going crazy, because her B.M.s smell different. We all go and smell it, and we know it's different, and we know she is going to be different." Or. "My mother becomes so dirty so that she leaves everything about the place. That always happens before she goes to the hospital." Or. "My mom starts shaking her leg, that's the start of it always.")

The children in this milieu are obsessed with fears of becoming ill, of going crazy, of developing brain tumors, of becoming suddenly stupid, of losing their memories, and of dying (Anthony, 1969b). Like Piaget, they may resort to a flight from affect or a flight from insight; become preoccupied with hobbies, inventions, model making, writing, and reading; spend a lot of time learning about their parents' illness and talk of majoring in psychology or becoming therapists; or live their lives within a huge margin of safety, seldom taking risks, always making sure, constantly checking for danger, and hoarding all their possessions just in case they might ever come in handy. (This was also typical of Piaget.)

A few of these children are stimulated to creativity under the pressure of anxiety and may even produce naïve systematic expositions to explain their world. Like the child Piaget, they can fill their lives with ruminations and preoccupations which do not entirely offset the cycles of anxiety provoked by interchanges with the disturbed parent. A number, like Piaget, have bypassed the better part of their childhood by becoming premature and overserious adults with little inclination or ability for play. Again, like him, they may become internally dissociated as a result of profound discrepancies between the paternal and maternal elements of the personality, leading the child to a total rejection of the emotional world and to the construction of a world of his own. The "family romance" is magnified into a "world romance" that may not altogether tally with reality but is the most realistic under the circumstance.

CONCLUSION

Every child seen in the research is rated along two scales: his likelihood of developing an emotional disorder during childhood and his likelihood of developing a mental disorder in adult life. The two are not necessarily correlated and we are still in doubt about the relationship. For example, we have rated many children high on the one and low on the other. It has been found retrospectively by several researchers that 30 percent or even more schizophrenics have undergone a childhood that is indistinguishable from the ordinary, and we ourselves are becoming aware that many of the children we see reacting pathologically to the psychosis of their parents may ultimately become functioning adults, although not too stable and far from certain of themselves, but not necessarily psychotic. We have been studying the childhood risks at close quarters and with a high degree of intensity; the grown-up children of psychotics need a similar study to be carried out on them. It is only then that we will know something about the whole spectrum of risk, the different degrees of vulnerability involved, and the range of devices manufactured by the children to cope with the disastrous misfortune of a psychotic parent.

PART IV

Clinical Considerations and the Challenge of Intervention

19

PARANATAL STRESS, COGNITIVE ORGANIZATION AND EGO FUNCTION

A Controlled Follow-up Study of Children Born Prematurely

*H. Caplan, M.D., R. Bibace, Ph.D., and
M.S. Rabinovitch, Ph.D.*

Human behavior must be seen as reflecting a constant interaction and reciprocal interplay between several groups of variables. These can be classified as constitutional forces, inherent maturational or developmental factors, and the impact of object relationships. Another grouping would be biological, social, and psychological forces. Although the literature has contributed to a study of these variables, insufficient attention has been paid to the interaction between variables, particularly within a controlled research setting.

In the case of children, the biological aspect has prime importance and biosocial forces are frequently in rapid transformation. Many workers have focused attention on the role of parents, mostly the mother, as the main determinants of the child's psychological development.

Working in a psychiatric clinic at The Montreal Children's Hospital, we have been impressed by the frequency with which problem children had a history of paranatal complications and developmental instability. This was reflected in disorganized motor integration, language and learning disorders, and problems of organization of space and time (Caplan, 1952, 1956).

The relationship of these findings to the pattern of intrafamily dynamics proved interesting. The stresses on family life occasioned by the child's deviant development often seemed reflected in severe parent-child conflicts which had feedback characteristics.

In keeping with our own findings, clinical and epidemiological stud-

Reprinted from the *Journal*, 2 : 434–450, 1963.

ies have been reported which demonstrate that a comprehensive understanding of psychopathology necessitates a consideration of constitutional and maturational as well as psychodynamic factors (Bender, 1956b; Fries and Woolf, 1953; Pasamanick et al., 1956a, 1956b).

While we are ultimately concerned with a wide variety of paranatal and neonatal factors, we limited ourselves in this phase of study to a relatively easily definable subgroup, namely, to children born prematurely. This research may therefore be designated as an investigation of the interplay of parturitional prematurity, intrafamily dynamics, and the "idiogenetic," [1] cognitive organization of the child.

Since our own clinical concepts had emerged from studying a psychiatric population, we felt it was essential to control this factor and select children who, as far as we knew, had no problems and were not attending psychiatric clinics. We wished to collect a group of children who would most likely have been exposed to "minimal brain damage" fitting into the lowest end of Pasamanick's "continuum of reproductive causality" (Rogers et al., 1955). A search of hospital birth records indicated great difficulties in trying to select retrospectively prenatal and paranatal stresses, such as toxemias and birth anoxias. We expected that every baby would be weighed at birth. From these birth records we could then go on to select a population that could be studied methodically.

In addition to our clinical findings, our research was stimulated by the following questions:

1. What is the relationship between birth experience and subsequent cognitive organization? How are cognitive deficits related to behavioral and learning difficulties? (By cognitive deficits we mean deficits in sensorimotor behavior, in perception, and in formal thought processes.)

2. What is the relationship of these cognitive deficits to the patterns of intrafamily psychodynamics? How do parents and siblings deal with or accommodate to a family member who is developing in a deviant manner? Does such a family member tend to bring out latent anxieties in other family members? Do certain types of families tend to aggravate, while others tend to ameliorate, the consequences of cognitive deficits?

3. In what way do disorders of cognitive organization influence the personality structure of the child?

4. What is the natural history of a disorder of cognitive organization? What happens to the pattern of maturation over a span of years? Do cognitive deficits observed in childhood remain fairly static or do they change? Do children really "grow out" of these so-called developmental disorders of cognition?

1. With regard to this term, we are not using the ordinary dictionary definition but rather are defining "idiogenetic" very specifically to mean those consistent variations that characterize the individual's patterns of cognition within the overall ontogenetic sequence.

Our general plan was to study cognitive organization and family interaction in a group of 50 "normal" prematures and a control group of 50 "full-term" children. These were selected from previously existing birth records of English-speaking hospitals in the City of Montreal. All subjects were male and drawn from a population whose basic language was English. Subjects were limited to children whose mothers had received semiprivate or private hospital accommodations for their delivery. This was an attempt to control for socioeconomic status (Pasamanick et al., 1956a).

Prematurity was defined as a gestation period of at least one lunar month short of full term and a birth weight between 1,500 and 2,250 grams. Multiple births were excluded. All children were normal on pediatric medical examination and had IQs ranging from 90 to 140 on a weighted score on the Wechsler Intelligence Scale for Children Vocabulary Subtest.

Controls were matched as closely as possible from identical sources with birthdays on the same day or within a few days of the test subject. They differed only in that their birth weights were above 2,600 grams. The subjects chosen were then located via telephone and city directories and approached with the help of the attending obstetrician and the family physician. In the premature group 23 percent of the parents refused to cooperate, while among the controls we had a refusal rate of 37 percent. Of the 40 cases of refusal, about half gave reasons relating to time and transportation difficulties. In 6 instances, the father refused to become involved with the psychiatrist; and in 12 instances the parents were unwilling to subject the child to the various tests. It may be of note that over 20,000 records had to be searched in order to find the 50 experimental cases meeting the above criteria.

This was a rather surprising finding and is largely explained by the following considerations. Hoping to find birth weights, we began with the obstetrical register. Unfortunately, many infants were merely labeled "premature" and the records had to be rejected because the birth weight was outside the 1,500- to 2,250-gram range. A large number of cases had to be rejected because the actual hospital file did not in fact have a written record of the birth weight at all. In a number of cases the information available in the hospital file did not facilitate contact with the family. In general, hospital records left much to be desired for research experimental purposes. Further, many cases were excluded because the families were French-speaking. The other main causes for exclusion were positive pediatric and neurological findings on physical examination, and low testing on the IQ scale. Not the least of our problems was the arduous task of tracing the names via annual telephone and city directories, and motivating the parents to participate in a study which meant about ten visits to the hospital and absence from school on these occasions.

The experimental and control groups consisted of two age ranges, 7–8 and 11–12 years. We wished to know whether any of the effects of prematurity apparent at an early age were still present at a later age. The specific age groups (7–8 and 11–12) were selected because there is evidence from the work of Werner, Piaget, and the University of Montreal Scale of Mental Development that these age ranges are often periods of transition from earlier to later stages of cognitive development (Pinard and Laurendeau, 1955).

Each child was given a thorough medical examination which included a careful pediatric and neurological examination, skull X ray, electroencephalogram, blood and urine analyses, tests of vision, and audiometric tests. An exhaustive developmental history was obtained. To study cognitive organization, we selected three modes of functioning—motor behavior, perception, and thought. With regard to thought, we chose three categories—time, space, and number. The battery of psychological tests included the following:

Wechsler Intelligence Scale for Children (Wechsler, 1949)
Lincoln-Oseretsky Test of Motor Development (Sloan, 1955)
Bender Visual Motor Gestalt Test (Bender, 1938)
Durrell Analysis of Reading Difficulty (Durrell, 1955)
Marble Board Test (Werner and Crain, 1950)
Werner's Test of the Perception of Verticality (Werner and Wapner, 1955)
A Test of Size Constancy (Beyrl, 1926)
Three Groups of Items from the University of Montreal Test of Mental Development [2] (Laurendeau and Pinard, 1962)

In assessing intrafamily dynamics we attempted to cope with the problems of methodology by using the Parent Behavior Rating Scale (Baldwin et al., 1949) developed by the Fels Institute, and psychoanalytically oriented psychiatric interviews. The psychiatrist carried out individual interviews with mother, father, and child; part of these were joint interviews with mother and child, husband and wife. The Fels Rating Scale was done by a social worker in a series of home visits. All the members of the research team worked independently until all the data were assembled. None of the research workers except the coordinating secretary knew which case was a premature and which was not. However, it did happen, despite advice to the contrary, that occasionally the parent in talking to the psychologist, psychiatrist, or social worker did reveal that they believed their child was born prematurely, or had had difficulties at birth. The latter was also found to be true of children who in this report fall into the "control group." There-

2. This scale is "process" oriented within the context of a standardized test. Twelve items were used relating specifically to notions of space, time, and number.

after, the data became available to all team members for purposes of evaluation and statistical processing. All the psychological and laboratory tests were done within 1 year; the psychiatric interviews over a 2-year period. A very competent and prudent secretary served as coordinator of the project, compiling files, etc.

The Parent Behavior Rating Scale was thus used as an index for evaluating the home influence or, more specifically, the mother-child relationship. This technique for collecting information is expressed in a standardized vocabulary and includes a prescribed list of variables. Of the 30 variables described, only 18 were selected as most appropriate to our study. Every subject was rated numerically on each of the 18 variables.

In addition, "cluster analysis" was used. A cluster is a group of variables which are closely related and which define and measure some common aspect of parent behavior. The clusters which it was possible to utilize within the limits of our 18 variables were:

1. Warmth (including the variables child-centeredness, acceptance, affectionateness, and rapport)
2. Indulgence (including the variables babying, protectiveness, and solicitousness)
3. Intellectuality (including the variables accelerational attempt, readiness of explanation, and understanding)

A profile was developed for each mother on which each rating was charted; by this means a composite picture of the relationship and a comparison between subjects were made possible.

After considerable discussion the psychiatrist and social worker pooled their findings and agreed on 4 groupings: (1) well-adjusted children; (2) problem children; (3) growth-stimulating families; and (4) growth-inhibiting families.

It is of note that the enthusiasm of the research group changed significantly when the phase of collecting data moved into the phase of compiling and integrating the findings. The problem of eliciting trends from the multiple variables studied proved to be a research project in itself.

Only some of the data are reported here.

RESULTS

General Findings

We were impressed with the cooperation and interest we received from the obstetricians, pediatricians, and family doctors who facilitated our case finding. We found that there were shortcomings in hospital records regarding the descriptions of the birth processes and observations of infants neonatally.

From the psychiatric point of view, it became apparent that psychoanalytically oriented interviews offered a dynamic understanding of forces within a family, yet it was most difficult to attempt a comparison of families. It was only after a scale was evolved to rate such variables as overall functioning, school behavior, interpersonal relationships, anxiety, passive aggressiveness, and others, that comparisons could be made from the interview data. In many ways the Parent Behavior Rating Scale data on the mother-child relationship proved more useful in delineating mothers as growth-inhibiting, growth-tolerating, or growth-stimulating. The problem of assessing the impact of two parents on a child proved most difficult, especially when we had to weigh, for example, the effect of a growth-stimulating mother and a growth-inhibiting father. In the end, this remained a clinically subjective value judgment, shared by the social worker and psychiatrist.

It is noteworthy that the psychiatrist had more difficulty assessing the younger children than the older ones. Apparently, as more factors in the personality undergo differentiation, the easier it becomes to make comparisons between children. It may also be of interest that the assessment had a therapeutic impact on a number of families, although efforts were made to avoid therapeutic entanglement.

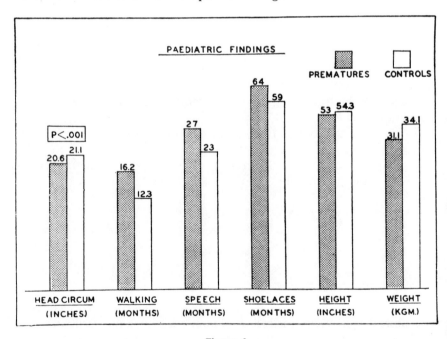

Figure 1

Specific Findings

There is evidence that a lag in cognitive development is related to parturitional prematurity as one birth variable. Further, it seems that such lags in development may affect personality development and, particularly, school achievement. Moreover, such lags extend far beyond the commonly accepted concept that the prematures catch up within the first 2 or 3 years of life. In fact, one of the more unexpected findings was that, in a number of tests reflecting cognitive ego functions, the older 11–12-year-old group showed greater significant differences than the younger age range of 7–8 years.

Pediatric Findings. No special differences were found in the skull X rays, blood and urine examinations, and visual and audiometric tests. A routine analysis of electroencephalograms did not reveal significant differences either. However, the EEGs require more careful study with statistical methods. Thus, when we compare the 12 dullest normals with the 12 dullest prematures, we find that the latter group has a significantly higher proportion of abnormal EEGs. The prematures were an average of $1^{1}/_{2}''$ shorter and $2^{1}/_{2}$ kg. lighter than their matched controls. It was, however, of interest that the mothers of prematures were $1''$ shorter and 1 kg. lighter on the average than the mothers of the controls. The head circumference was an average of $20.58''$ as opposed to $21.1''$ for the controls. The differences have a significance at the .001 level of probability. Older prematures were $1''$ shorter and $3^{1}/_{2}$ kg. lighter than the controls. Their head circumference was $20.9''$ as opposed to $21.4''$ for the controls, again significant at the .001 level (see fig. 1).

Psychiatric Findings. The developmental milestones indicated a constant trend in favor of earlier mastery of day-to-day tasks by the control

Table 1

Personality Findings

Age	Number	Prematures	Controls
		Well-adjusted Children	
7–8	8	4	4
11–12	8	2	6
Total	(16)	(6)	(10)
		Problem Children	
7–8	21	12	9
11–12	13	9	4
Total	(34)	(21)	(13)
		Growth-stimulating Families	
	7	1	6
		Growth-inhibiting Families	
	33	20	13

group in both ages. The mean age of walking was 16.2 months for the prematures and 12.3 months for the controls. Use of sentences was mastered at 27 months for prematures and at 23 months for the controls. Ability to tie shoelaces was accomplished at 5 years, 4 months for prematures and at 4 years, 11 months for the controls. Ball catching, bicycle riding, and swimming have all revealed differences, always in favor of the controls. Admittedly, this type of datum is retrospective and subject to many sources of error, but the consistency is very striking.

We found a clear preponderance of well-adjusted children and growth-stimulating families in the control group and a preponderance of problem children and growth-inhibiting families in the premature group. The differences for well-adjusted and problem children are clearer in the older than younger subjects. In general, problem children (34) outnumbered well-adjusted children (16). This statistic is clearly related to the criteria used. It is easier to tag problems than to define mental health. The same applies to growth-stimulating families (7) and growth-inhibiting families (33) (see table 1).

The ratings seemed to reveal a larger number of abnormal ratings for children and families than is expected. As already indicated, the judgments were made by the psychiatrist and social worker from the raw data available. Essentially, these are very subjective, but the clinical

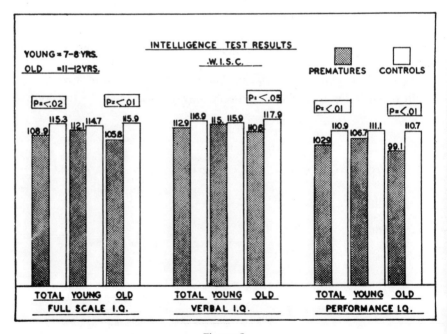

Figure 2

observers were constant throughout the study. Possibly we were geared too much to look for pathology and perhaps we saw more than was really there. Also, it has been pointed out how difficult the task was to take a recorded interview of either parents or child and attempt to make a comparison between subjects. Further, although, for example, there were 8 well-adjusted children and 21 problem children in the young 7–8-year-old group, there were 21 children who would be considered "average." If we add the "average" populations to the "well-adjusted" and "growth-stimulating" groups, we reach figures closer to what is more usually expected, i.e., 66 children out of 100 would be considered "average" youngsters (16 well-adjusted children plus 50 average children) and 67 families out of the 100 would be considered "average" families. In any case, this whole issue begs the question of what is a "case," what is normal and abnormal.

A comparison of means and medians on the Parent Behavior Rating Scale revealed no striking differences. However, there were definite findings on the "Intensity of Contact" and "Coerciveness of Suggestion" variables, i.e., mothers of the premature showed more intense contact and less coerciveness in their suggestions than the mothers of normal children. When we studied the distribution of the subjects on each scale, there was a decided tendency, on many variables, for the mothers of the prematures to get more extreme ratings than the mothers of full-term children. Thus, considering the variable of "Child-centeredness," of the 10 highest ratings on this variable, 8 are in the premature group, only 2 in the control group. On the variable of "Intensity of Contact," 17 of the 20 highest scores were in the premature group. On the variable "Clarity of Policy, of Regulations, and of Reinforcement," 9 of the 10 poorest ratings were prematures. On the

Table 2

WISC Results

	Prematures	Controls	
	Total—100 Subjects		
Full scale	108.94	115.28	P = <.02 *
Perform.	102.90	110.92	P = <.01 *
Verbal	112.84	116.84	P = <.10
	Young 7–8 50 Subjects		
Full scale	112.12	114.68	P = >.10
Perform.	106.68	111.12	P = >.10
Verbal	115.04	115.84	P = >.10
	Old 11–12 50 Subjects		
Full scale	105.76	115.88	P = <.01 *
Perform.	99.10	110.72	P = <.01 *
Verbal	110.60	117.90	P = <.05 *

* Statistically significant.

"Friction" variable, 8 of the 10 high ratings were prematures, similarly for variables like "Babying, Solicitousness, Protectiveness, and Acceleration Attempts."

Analyzing the data in terms of the clusters of scales, we found that the homes of the prematures were characteristically more saturated with worries and anxieties about their children. There was more indulgence, less decisiveness, and a general lack of confidence, as well as doubt on the part of the parents in their own ability to manage their children.

Psychological Findings. (a) In the total sample of prematures and controls, the prematures are less intelligent than the controls on the whole full-scale Wechsler Intelligence Scale for Children. This difference is mainly accounted for by the performance IQ (see fig. 2).

(b) In the 7–8-year-old group (50 subjects) the controls are consistently but only slightly superior to the prematures. None of these differences is statistically significant (see table 2).

(c) In the 11–12-year-old group (50 subjects), the controls are significantly superior to the prematures. This difference is again more marked on the performance IQ than on the verbal IQ (see table 2).

Other Psychological Test Findings. In test situations which required physical coordination and the integration of perceptual and motor skills, it was found again that the controls were superior to the prema-

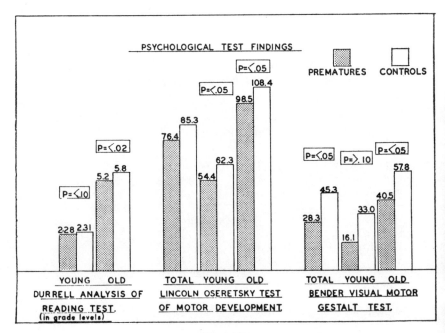

Figure 3

tures. On the Bender Visual Motor Gestalt Test the performance of the control group is significantly better than that of the prematures. The older subjects showed the more significant differences. Similar findings are seen on the Lincoln-Oseretsky Scale of Motor Development and the Durrell Analysis of Reading Test (see fig. 3).

Perception of Verticality. For this test the child, who is in a dark room, is asked to say when he sees a rotating, luminescent rod as vertical. The rod is started from four positions, 30° and 10° to the left and 30° and 10° to the right of true verticality. The subject makes his judgments from three sitting positions, upright and tilted 30° left and 30° right. The results are evaluated according to two possible effects: (a) rod-starting position, and (b) body tilt.

With regard to the perception of verticality, our results show that the premature group as compared to the control group was more strongly influenced by the rod-starting position in their reports of when they saw the rod as vertical. This finding is interesting in view of Werner and Wapner's (1955) studies which have shown that this effect is characteristic of early developmental levels. They report that the starting-position effect is greater on younger than on older children, and with psychopathological as compared to normal groups, and with primitivizing agents such as lysergic acid. These authors explain the starting-position effect by what they call "stimulus boundedness." This is a form of lack of differentiation between self and outside object typical of less mature stages of development, and this is what the data on perception of verticality suggest about the premature group.

Discussion

Our findings indicate that the follow-up study of children suffering paranatal stress (prematurity) showed a greater incidence of cognitive disorders. These deficits in children seemed to occur more frequently in homes that were growth-inhibiting. Our results indicated that cognitive difficulties became worse with time and our older subjects showed greater differences than our younger ones. This of course may also reflect that the various measuring instruments are more effective and accurate in the older age range.

This study throws some light on current concepts of ego psychology. Freud (1926, 1937) in his later years, Rapaport (1951), Hartmann (1939, 1950a, 1950b; et al., 1946), and Kris (1951) have evolved the concept that the ego itself has an innate biological tendency toward organization, regulation, and adaptation to the environment. In 1937 Freud stated: "We have no reason to dispute the existence of primary congenital variations in the ego." Hartmann (1950b) speaks of the ego as "a substructure of personality defined by its functions," which include the organization and control of motility, perception, and thought. There has been considerable discussion in the literature whether innate neurophysiological patterns are exempt from the influence of the environment.

We have found in a controlled study that there are wide variations in the maturation of apparatuses which may be considered, in Hartmann's terminology, the neurophysiological bases for certain autonomous ego functions. These differences were found in children who were judged to be normal, healthy subjects. The children who were born prematurely had significant deficits in cognitive organization and were found more likely to show personality disturbances than the controls. It was also found that the prematures came from growth-inhibiting homes more frequently than did the controls. It seems to us that the older subjects showed greater differences in cognitive development because of the impact of psychological stress factors which resulted in inhibition of development. It would appear that inhibition exerts its influence in the direction of the inherent defect of the ego. It is not yet fully clear what the nature of the relationship is between the deviantly developing ego and the growth-inhibiting home environment. Nevertheless, the evidence is in favor of a reciprocal interaction. In some cases studied, one felt that the deviant child affected the home in upsetting a delicately balanced dynamic system which then exerted feedback influences. In other cases, pathological forces in the home could be seen as aggravating and reinforcing deviant cognitive development. Thus the reciprocal interaction between organism and object is seen.

Our findings are perhaps of interest not only to the psychiatrist but also to the obstetrician and pediatrician. In the presence of paranatal stress, attention must be given to the detailed observation of the developmental process and the dynamic structure of the family unit. Strengthening personality forces within the family and guidance in specific training procedures of the young child can facilitate the progression of one state of development to another. For many years experts in education have been interested in the development of techniques of training and rehabilitation, especially with the blind, deaf, spastic, and subnormal child. Many of these skills can be adapted to strengthen ego structure in the areas of sensorimotor organization, language, motility, and integration in time and space.

By way of summary, we have described a research project which throws some light on current problems of ego psychology and personality development. We have shown in studying a premature and control group that there are definite differences in regard to certain ego functions, notably the so-called "autonomous conflict-free spheres of the ego." Some of these differences are clearly related to central nervous system variables, which in turn seem to relate to differences in birth patterns. These ego variations reflect overall ego functioning which can be seen in the growing child to be very closely linked in a reciprocal manner with the personality structure of the family unit.

20

INTERVENTION IN INFANCY

A Program for Blind Infants

Selma Fraiberg

The program that I describe is concerned with a special group of at-risk infants, the infant blind from birth. But I believe that some of the methods we have developed in work with this group have general applicability to other groups of disadvantaged infants.

Our work in infant intervention is the outgrowth of a series of longitudinal studies of infants blind from birth. The research began out of our deep concern for the very large number of blind children who show gross abnormalities in ego development which are closely related to autism. If we separate from this group the children with known brain damage or multiple handicaps, there remains a very large group of blind children who are condemned to something like a sensory void for the rest of their lives.

Typically, these children appear to have no significant human ties. Language, if present at all, is echolalic. There is no definition of body boundaries, of self and other. There are motor stereotypes of the trunk and the hands—such as rocking, lateral rotation of the head and trunk, empty fingering. Many of these children have not achieved mobility. These children constitute approximately one quarter of the population that is defined by "total blindness from birth," excluding children with known brain damage.

Within the same population, blind from birth, a very small percentage of children achieve adequacy in ego development with stability in human object relations, demonstrably good speech, good adaptive hand behavior, free mobility, and a stable concept of self and of "I." This means, of course, that under the most favorable circumstances, blindness need not obstruct vital currents in ego development.

Between the two extreme groups is the very large group of congenitally blind children who demonstrate great unevenness in their devel-

Reprinted from the *Journal*, 10 : 381–405, 1971.

opmental achievements and in general functioning and who will have limited educational possibilities.

In all three groups, the developmental histories show certain similarities. Apart from the wide range of economic and educational backgrounds, apart from the qualities of mothering which were available to all of these children, there were certain areas of adaptive functioning that were impeded to a greater or lesser extent in all three groups. Adaptive hand behavior, gross motor achievements, and the constitution of a body and self image were delayed by sighted child standards for a perilously long time.

We considered that the characteristic delays for all blind babies in these sectors of development in the sensorimotor period might tell us that these areas were largely organized under vision. If this were so, then the blind baby must find an adaptive substitution for vision in order to get back onto the developmental path. How does he find it? How does his mother assist in finding the adaptive solutions? And if he comes to a developmental impasse and cannot find the solution, would he then remain there, frozen in the postures of the early sensorimotor stages with inutile hands and a motility that is fixed in empty rocking? And if the bridge to an outer world cannot be found in blindness, would we see a child who remained on the level of body-centeredness, without connections to an outer world and with echolalic speech that testified to the last failure in human connections?

To find the answers to these questions we have conducted a series of longitudinal studies of infants blind from birth. Babies who qualified for the research were totally blind or had light perception only, were neurologically intact, and had no other handicaps. To date, 9 of our 10 babies have passed their second birthdays, with the oldest child aged 7, and these children constitute the sample on which I am reporting. We have also seen a total of 43 infants and preschool children in our consultation and education program which have given us a range of developmental problems in the larger blind child population against which we can assess our findings. Our methodology and some of our findings have been reported elsewhere (Fraiberg, 1968; Fraiberg et al., 1966). A detailed report of our education program and technique appears in Fraiberg et al. (1969).

As our research expanded, we began to see the unique developmental patterns of a blind baby. There were typical developmental roadblocks, which could not be clearly seen as impediments due to blindness itself. Two exceptional mothers and their babies found the adaptive routes; most could not without help. And as we began to understand the developmental problems, we were able to find ways of translating this new information into a home guidance program for these babies and, eventually, for a larger group of babies and young children in our educational program. This program represents both research and applied research in our work with blind babies and their families.

HUMAN OBJECT RELATIONS

The absence or failure of human connections was the most morbid sign among the children in the deviant blind population. Even among the blind children who have achieved some degree of coherence in ego organization, there are many who show grave instability in their human object relations or give the appearance of "lost children" in moments in which they are not in direct contact with adults or other children.

Psychoanalytic studies of the development of human object relations provide us with compelling evidence that the love bonds between child and parents are established during the first 18 months of life. Was it possible, then, that congenital blindness was an impediment to the establishment of human ties? Yet, there was evidence from the study of some exceptional children blind from birth that the capacity for love and attachment need not be impeded by blindness. What was it, then, that transpired between a mother and her blind baby that led to a failure in human connections in a considerable group of blind children and demonstrably good human ties in another, small sector of that population?

In our twice-monthly observations of the baby in his home we recorded detailed notes on all aspects of mother-child interaction and examined these data in relation to criteria for human object relations available in the psychoanalytic literature. Décarie's Objectal Scale (1963), which employs psychoanalytic criteria in a sequence with age norms, was available to us for comparison of our blind babies with a sighted population. When we excluded visual responses, we still had a range of differential responses to the mother; smiling, vocalization, tactile discrimination which afforded comparisons between our blind babies and sighted babies.

As the data emerged, we began to see that under the most favorable circumstances, when a mother and her blind baby found a tactile and vocal dialogue, all the milestones for human object relations were met without significant differences between that blind baby and a normal sighted baby. The response smile to the sound of mother's or father's voice was elicited in the first quarter; differential vocalizations and differential responses to holding in relation to mother and strangers appeared in the second quarter; stranger reactions to voice or touch appeared in the third quarter along with demonstrations of affection to the words, "Give Mommy a kiss," or "Give Mommy a hug." Separation anxiety, testifying further to valuation of the mother, appeared at the end of the first year, with one major difference in comparison with the sighted child: separation anxiety in certain cases was sustained for a good part of the second and third year.

How can we explain, then, that certain mothers were able to establish a tactile and vocal dialogue with their babies and others were not? Were there extraordinary qualities of motherliness in the successful mothers? Yes, and no. We learned that even a mother who had demonstrated adequacy in mothering her older sighted children might not be able to find her way into a blind baby's experience without help.

The rearing of a blind infant is not a fair test of motherliness in a woman or fatherliness in a man. The birth of the blind baby was a disaster for each of the families we have known. The defective baby opened up old wounds in the femininity and masculinity of the young mother and father. Three of our fathers developed potency problems soon after the birth of the baby. There may have been others too shy to tell us. Unconscious revulsion in mother or father took the form of avoidance, of not touching the baby except when it was necessary. In several cases, babies were brought to us for consultation at 6 months, or 10 months, or 12 months, with bald spots on the back of the head, which gave mute testimony to long hours spent supine in a crib. They were described as quiet babies who never complained. For most of their 24-hour day these babies lived in a sensory desert. The unspeakable thought, "He would be better off dead," was translated, "as if he were dead."

At the time we met them, nearly all of our young parents were depleted of their own emotional resources, without hope, without expectations, and often without comfort or support. Visitors to the house, even grandparents and relatives, were caught up in a conspiracy of silence. No one said the baby was adorable, or cute, or any of the other things that are uttered upon seeing a new baby. Apart from anything else we did in our work with the families, we were often the first people who entered these mourning households who could say such things as "He's a fine baby," "He's a beautiful baby," or "Look how strong he is! He's all boy!" We do not underestimate the role we played as the baby's advocate; we were reclaiming his human rights for his family.

We spoke of ourselves as the baby's advocate. Our most important task after this was to become the baby's interpreter. The blind baby spoke a foreign language. We might add that sometimes sighted and intact babies speak a foreign language with parents, too. We mean, of course, that many inexperienced parents do not understand the language of babies, the signs and the signals of the first year of life. But, since intact babies employ a universal language, most parents can pick up some of the major signs and, if they miss a few things, there is always an alert grandmother or a neighbor who knows the language and can act as interpreter. But if you are a blind baby, it is just possible that not only your mother, but your grandmother, and all the neighbor ladies, too, never had a chance to study your language.

Let's consider one component of the basic vocabulary of an 8-week-old sighted baby, the love language. If mother or father or grandmother or the lady next door leans over the crib and smiles, the 3-month-old baby will immediately respond with a smile. This smile is the universal greeting sign of our species and everybody knows what that means or thinks he knows what that means. Once the baby produces his smile in response to the configuration of the human face, we begin to carry on a complex and highly differentiated sign language with the baby. We interpret the exchange of smiles as "I love you." "I love you, too." "You're marvelous." "I think you're great, too." Around 7 to 8 months the smile acquires a differentiated vocabulary. It becomes an exclusive smile, for mother, for father, for the select few. "I love you and only you. Never mind the lady with the red hat and the guy with the mustache who wiggles his ears. *You* are the one. Only you." When this happens to a baby's smile, we are hooked. Let's admit it. Even a misanthrope would melt.

If we take only the smile, then, we can see how much the sign vocabulary of infancy is a *visual* vocabulary. But, when the parents of a blind baby lean over his crib and smile (without speaking), the blind baby does not respond with out tribal greeting sign. It feels curiously like a snub.

"How will he know me?" is one of the first questions parents may ask us. We could tell the parents because we know the blind baby's language. Some parents were amazed to learn that the blind baby would smile in response to mother's or father's *voice* at around the same time that sighted babies smile at the *sight* of the human face. And, when the smile emerged, as predicted, the baby's parents were slightly more delirious than the parents of sighted babies at the same stage. Then, because we had information from our research on differential smiling in the first quarter, we could initiate a small experiment which was very impressive to parents. We would ask mother and father to speak to the baby and the smile would appear. Then one of the investigators would speak to the baby. No smile. We could repeat the sequence. The baby responded selectively to the sound of mother's or father's voice. It was an eloquent demonstration. The baby "knew" his parents.

As we should expect, the baby's response to his parents became the first rewards of love between baby and parents, and once we achieved even this much reciprocity we could begin to count on something else happening. The baby would woo his parents! No matter that unconscious revulsion, guilt, or impotent rage at fate were present in the parent. Once the vocabulary of need and love brought rewards for parents and baby, the baby knew his job and became our collaborator in the educational program for his parent.

At around 5 months of age, we offered another demonstration to the parents. One of the observers would pick up the blind baby and hold him for a few moments. He would begin to squirm, strain, and complain. Here we were testing differential responses to holding, of course, but it became a useful demonstration for the parents. "*You* want your mother!" we would say. And, when we returned the squirming baby to his mother, he snuggled down, comforted.

At 8 to 12 months of age, if all went well, the blind baby began to take a dim view of the University of Michigan research team. He might sober or cry when we entered the room and he heard our voices. "He doesn't take to strangers like he used to," his mother might say apologetically. Sometimes a mother was surprised to learn that this was an important sign of his attachment to mother.

At around the same age, if all went well, the blind baby could match the sighted baby in language development. He was imitating sounds, had a few "words," and spoke a gibberish that sounded like English. We had told the parents long ago that this would happen, that the baby would indeed learn to speak at about the same time as sighted babies. But when it happened, because this was a blind baby, it appeared like a miracle to his parents.

It was not only the language of love that required us to be interpreters for the blind baby. The very large vocabulary of facial expression in a baby was restricted in the case of the blind baby. Apart from the universal expressions of emotion, "joy," "rage," the range of pleasure-unpleasure, there is a large group of expressive facial signs which are differentiated through vision and even the musculature of the eyes, and are reinforced through visual experience, literally seeing another face. The expressive look of longing, or the expression that we call "quizzical," or the expression that we call "coy," and many, many expressions that have sign value to us are absent in the totally blind child. When we see a sighted baby of 4 months stare unwaveringly at a bright object, thrust his head forward and drool, we need no interpreter to tell us what he wants. In the absence of such a sign language the blind baby appears to have no modulated vocabulary for expressing need or wish before speech appears.

We became "hand watchers" in our research program because we were studying prehension among many other aspects of development; and as we developed expertness in hand watching, we became sensitive to another vocabulary of emotion, the expressive motor signs in the hands themselves. If a toy was dropped or removed from the hand, there might be a fleeting pursuit movement or a grasping-ungrasping motion which could be interpreted as "I want." Not that the baby could conceptualize it in these terms. But if the gesture connoted "I want," we could give it meaning through our response, which, after all, is the way in which all language is built. Sometimes a game between observer and baby ended and a moment later the observer felt the touch of the baby's hand, so lightly and fleetingly that if we were not "hand watchers," we would not have been aware of it. The gesture could be interpreted as "More," "Again," and if we responded to the gesture, you can see that the gesture would acquire sign value.

From all this you can see that the most important part of our work centered in promoting the love ties between the blind baby and his parents, and in helping the parents find a dialogue with their baby who communicated in another language or, better perhaps, another dialect, which is not easily accessible to those who live in the world of sight. And in the 9 cases in our research sample each baby demonstrated at the end of the first 18 months that stage-by-stage he had fulfilled all the criteria for human object relations that we expect of a sighted child.

Now, of course, when we promote the human object ties of a baby, we are also promoting adaptive capacity and cognitive development. But in the case of the blind baby we must take into consideration another very important fact: one of the central organs of adaptation, vision, is not present. This means that the blind baby must find adaptive substitutions for vision in order to achieve a coherent sensorimotor organization. With all the love in the world the blind baby may not find the adaptive routes by himself.

THE HANDS

We are all familiar with the cliché, "The hands are the eyes of the blind." If we examine a large population of school-age blind children, we will encounter a terrible irony. Among those children who are totally blind from birth, a very high percentage of children will have blind hands, too. These are the blind children who have never achieved coordinate use of the hands, whose hands bring them little or no information, who may, in fact, retain the hands at shoulder height in the neonatal posture, the fingers fixed in inutile postures or empty grasping. If we exclude all the children in this population with known brain damage, we still have a very large group of blind children with "blind hands." What we see in these children is an adaptive failure in the sensorimotor period. We now know through our research the complex and hazardous route of adaptive hand behavior in the absence of vision. We also know that if we can reach such a child even as late as the second year of life, we can bring those hands into a coherent sensorimotor organization.

A moment's reflection will tell us that everything that we know as adaptive hand behavior in the sighted child is predicated upon the coordination of eye and hand schemas. Vision mediates. In the absence of vision the sequence that leads to coordinate use of the hands may not evolve. Sustained mutual fingering at 16 weeks normally brings the hands into the field of vision. In the absence of vision there may be chance engagement of the fingers but no sustained fingering. And if the hands do not engage at midline, a complex sequence leading to hand reciprocity and coordinate use of the hands may not evolve.

When we understood this, we began to experiment. The experiment was actually an educational intervention; the intervention was in itself the testing of a hypothesis. We encouraged our mothers and fathers to play games and to employ strategies that would bring the hands together at midline. And since vision would normally provide the pleasure bonus for mutual fingering, we substituted other rewards. We encouraged the mothers to place both hands upon the bottle during feeding. We suggested patty-cake games, hand-clapping games with songs. In supine, we employed cradle gyms and dangling toys. In supported sitting, we encouraged the presentation of objects at midline. The result, in every case in which we intervened, was motor equivalence in coordinate use of the hands to that of the sighted child.

If we were successful in bringing the hands together at midline, we helped the baby along one part of the route in adaptive hand behavior, but there was still a hazardous stretch beyond. Between 5 and 6 months the sighted baby can attain an object "on sight." He has been practicing this feat for many weeks, and we consider it unremarkable when he achieves it. In our early innocence, we had assumed that in the blind baby an adaptive substitution of sound for vision would take place at the same point. But no baby in our series, not even the most precocious blind baby, was able to demonstrate reach on sound cue with equivalence to the sighted child's performance. Through twice-monthly testing of each baby during the first year of life we established that *the modal age for reach on sound cue alone was 10 months!* We must remember that we are speaking of a highly selected sample of blind babies and a group which had had educational assistance from us. Again, after we made this discovery, it became evident to us. Localizing an object on sound is normally mediated by vision. Reaching for an object on sound cue alone requires a level of conceptual development other than reach on sight. Vision insures that the thing seen is a thing "to be grasped." But sound alone does not confer substantiality or "graspability" on an object; the blind baby must actually acquire a concept of an object in which the sound connotes "the thing." For a perilously long time in the first year of life the blind baby behaves as if the musical toy in his hand is one object and the sound of the musical toy "out there" is another object. These findings have been summarized and explicated in other papers (Fraiberg, 1968; Fraiberg et al., 1966).

We can well understand, then, that many parents of blind babies are confronted with another set of worries in the second half of the first year. Is the baby mentally defective? Is he also deaf? He doesn't reach for objects. Naturally, it was of considerable help to parents that we were able to explain the long and difficult problem for a blind child to reach for an object on sound and to give the necessary reassurances. But there was also no guarantee that the baby would find the adaptive solution if we did not build in the necessary hand and ear experiences for him in the first year of life.

We had to educate the baby's hands. We had to build in rich tactile experience and tactile differentiation through toys and other interesting objects. If we could feed tactile information into the fingers, create interest in things, the first notions of substantiality would appear and a kind of pursuit of and search for tactile objects would follow. Toys that united tactile and sound qualities were sought out by us and the parents to encourage a sound-touch identity for objects. We created the conditions under which a blind baby could reach at midline and regularly encounter interesting objects. Through the devices of a special play table and a playpen we created "an interesting space" in which a search or a sweep of the hand would guarantee an encounter and an interesting discovery. You see, even the motor patterns for reaching may not appear in a blind baby who has no incentive to reach. Many blind babies live in something like a sensory void in which the hands grasp at air and a flung-out arm touches nothing more than the crib bars or a blanket. Our parents themselves became marvelously inventive in providing toys and games which would invite search and grasping and which would assist in the coordination of tactile and sound experience.

Then, one day, we, the hand watchers, would see an idea emerging. The sound of the bell would activate the hands. A grasping-ungrasping motion would appear, or, even more marvelous, a hand gesture that looked like the motor pattern for bell-ringing. There was not yet reach, but we knew the idea was emerging. A few days later, a few weeks later, the baby would make a discovery which ought to win him a scientific award. Without vision, he discovered that the sound that we call "bell sound" was an attribute of an object that we call "a bell," and the bell which he could not experience in his hand was "out there" in space. Since it took us several years to figure out how the blind baby worked out this difficult problem, we hope that the world at large will not casually employ the term "retarded" for the blind baby whose science is not equal to the task at 10 months of age.

As the coordination of sound and grasping emerges, the blind baby is on his way. Within a few months he will become very good at tracking objects on sound. Most important of all, of course, is that he now has the rudimentary conceptual equipment to begin the construction of an object world. The blind hands of the deviant blind child tell a tragic story. When the hand must substitute for vision, it becomes the bridge between the body ego and the objective world. Without this bridge the personality may remain frozen on the level of body-centeredness and nondifferentiation of self-not self.

LOCOMOTOR FUNCTIONING

If we are able to provide minimum guarantees for ego development in the spheres of human object relations and adaptive hand behavior, there will remain only one other major hazard in development during the sensorimotor period. Typically, in the large population of blind infants and young children we will find that mobility through creeping and walking will be delayed by several months, or even several years. In what ways, then, can blindness be an impediment to locomotion? Our longitudinal studies told us a story. In normal development when control of the trunk is achieved in a stable sitting posture, there is a smooth transition to bridging and creeping. In our sample, most of our babies achieved stability in sitting well within the range for sighted babies. Most of our babies demonstrated the ability to support themselves on hands and knees within the range for sighted babies. Then, something that should appear on the developmental timetable did not appear. The baby did not creep!

Do we have the picture? In each case, there was postural readiness for creeping, judged by all the signs. In one eloquent film sample, we see Robbie at 9 months rocking back and forth on hands and knees. At one point we see him balancing himself acrobatically on his hands and one leg. But he cannot propel himself forward. We offer him enticing sound toys and soundless toys a few inches from his hands to lure him forward. He continues his futile rocking on hands and knees. You must already have guessed why Robbie could not creep. He had not yet learned to reach on sound cue alone. Since locating and reaching a toy on sound cue is the only way in which the blind child can find equivalence for reaching and attaining an object on sight, there was no motive for reaching. The sighted child, in the same posture, will reach for the out-of-reach toy which propels him forward. It is the visual incentive that initiates the creeping pattern. At 11 months and 1 day, Robbie demonstrated his first reach on sound cue. At 11 months and 3 days, Robbie's parents called to announce that Robbie had begun to creep.

As the data came in from all the babies in our series, the links between creeping and reach on sound were firmly established. *No baby learned to creep until he first gave evidence that he could reach on sound cue alone.* If a baby had maturational readiness for creeping and demonstrated reach on sound cue, he would either find the creeping pattern soon afterward or we could "teach" him through offering lures. Once the baby had mobility on hands and knees his world began to open up to him in a new way. There would be still another delay between the first steps and walking freely, which we can easily understand. For the blind child, walking freely may represent stepping out into the void. There are also no models, normally provided by vision, for independent walking. Yet each of our babies attained walking freely, a little late by sighted child standards but far in advance of most babies in the blind population. The modal age for free walking in our group was 17 months.

"Will he walk?" was one of the most urgent questions that came to us from our parents throughout the first 18 months. Since we knew through our research where the impediments to locomotion would appear, we were able to help our parents step-by-step before parental anxieties led to pushing tactics. (In spite of everything, this did happen in one case.) We also helped our parents to understand and to build in all the steps in motor development that would lead to good control of the trunk and experimentation in prone posture. Most parents of sighted babies do not have to know how a baby achieves control of his trunk and moves toward the upright posture. "It just happens." Given minimum adequacy in the environment, the sighted baby will practice endlessly without any encouragement. But the parents of a blind baby need special education in the area of locomotor development. At every point where vision would normally intervene to promote a new phase in locomotor development we had to help the baby find an adaptive solution. The prone position, for example, is not an "interesting" position for the blind baby. The sighted baby spends long periods in prone, with head elevated, "just looking around." The blind baby, without such incentives, may resist the prone position. We build in "interest" in prone through speaking to the baby, through dangle toys or other devices. Sitting with support is "more interesting" for a blind baby if he is seated at his little three-sided play table with toys within reach. Practicing pulling to stand and cruising will be "more interesting" in the familiar space of a playpen with favorite toys offering sound-touch incentives. And one day, sometime between 13 and 19 months, the blind baby steps out into the vast black space to his mother's voice across the room and the news is telegraphed to us that he is walking! A year later, he can outrun his mother. One of our most cherished memories is that of a small boy of 2 with the devil's own light in his blind eyes, racing down the slope behind his house, while his fat mama panted 50 feet behind him and screamed his name hoarsely.

From this sketch you can see something of the design of the educational work. From the clinical evidence we deduced that blindness was an impediment to development in three central areas of development:

human object relations, adaptive hand behavior, and gross motor development. We can add, "body and self image." In the 9 cases that constitute our original research sample we have seen that if we can provide minimum guarantees for development in these three areas, a stable body and self image will emerge, adaptive solutions will be found in cognition, and a coherent ego organization will result. The performance of these 9 children places them in the upper half of a blind child population as measured on the Norris Scale; all of these children are educable.

Some Case Illustrations

Since this presentation is also concerned with some of the larger and more general problems of intervention in infancy, it might be interesting to examine our educational work with the parents and baby in still another light.

Five of our 9 babies would have qualified as high-risk babies if they had been sighted. In these families, poverty or near poverty, unemployment or irregular employment constituted the economic risks. The educational level of the parents did not exceed grade 10 and, in two cases, the parents were barely literate. Two of the blind babies were born to unwed mothers. Three of the mothers were clinically depressed. Here I am not speaking of reactive depressions to the birth of a defective baby. I am using strict clinical criteria in defining depression. These were also cases where depressive symptoms had been present prior to the birth of the blind baby. We can see, then, that our sample was heavily weighted on the side of human ills. There is no reason to believe that our selection played any part in obtaining this distribution. As we know, blindness and other birth defects fall unevenly upon the poor, the uneducated, and the families that cannot obtain good medical care.

Yet none of these factors in family background or family illness proved to be an impediment to our work on behalf of the blind baby. The one family that proved least accessible to our education was actually one of the three families at the top of our group in economic and educational status. While this proves nothing in itself, it does tell us that the capacity of a family to mobilize itself on behalf of a child should not be measured by standards of economic or social stability or education alone.

Becky

There was Becky, for example, the illegitimate child of a 17-year-old girl. Becky lived with her child mother in a household that was so chaotic we spent weeks trying to get straight the family composition.

There was a grandmother and a grandfather, migrants from Appalachia, and their 8 children, without exception school failures and school dropouts. Those older children who had jobs never seemed to get to them or keep them, and when Morton Chethik of our staff visited the home at 11 o'clock in the morning, the working as well as the nonworking members staggered out of bed. There were miscellaneous male boarders and visitors in the household, some of whom slept in the same bed with Becky and her mother. It took some insight to see that within this chaos there were family bonds, and that the illiteracy of this family would not prevent them from learning from us about the needs of a blind baby.

This was a family in which babies were not specially cherished, in which no child grew up feeling valued as a person. The cement that held this family together was never apparent to us except in moments of crisis at which time everyone rallied round and closed a circle around the afflicted member. (Oscar Lewis [1961] seems to make the same point about a number of families studied by him in his work on "the culture of poverty.") We recognized this as a genuine strength in an otherwise disorganized family. We could use this strength in mobilizing the family around the needs of the baby.

The blind baby whom we valued became a special person in her own family. Something of our staff's affection and caring, and concern, and interest in every detail in the baby's day-to-day progress carried over to grandmother and mother and to all the other members of the family, too. There was an investment in Becky's growth and development as a baby, as a person, which was, we suspect, very different from that which was given all the older children in this family. Through Morton Chethik and, later, Winnifred Connelly of our staff, the family acquired some understanding of developmental expectations for a healthy blind child and a feeling of their own importance in nurturing and providing experience for the blind child. Yet, some of our good plans were never carried out by the family. And many of the toys that we brought to Becky fell into the hands of the older aunts and uncles or disappeared into the general family debris. This was not important, in the end. What mattered is that we were able through our work and counseling to insure at least adequacy in the family nutriments for a baby's development.

Even in matters of health care and visits to our hospital for pediatric and ophthalmological examination our staff had to take central responsibility. In a family where no one saw a doctor except in an emergency ward, neither preventive health care nor following a medical regime made any sense. To drive Becky and her mother to the hospital for examination, to help the family carry through on medical plans became simply part of the overall service of our program to the family.

In the end, Becky thrived. Family pride in her achievements was shared with us, and our own pleasure in Becky's progress enlarged this pride. At the age of 3, Becky's developmental achievements place her well in the upper half of a blind child population. She is a lively, winning, imaginative, talkative little girl. She is unquestionably the smartest child in her family. She is, we reflect, the first baby born to this family who has benefited from the psychological and medical advances of the twentieth century.

Robbie

Robbie's mother was a young woman who lived perilously close to a severe depression during the entire 3 years we knew her. At the age of 19 she was grossly obese (she had gained 40 pounds during her pregnancy and 40 or more pounds since the birth of her blind baby). When we first met her we were privately alarmed at the signs of imminent illness. She was eating compulsively, she was garrulous and overexuberant with immoderate bursts of hilarity. She was a compulsive housekeeper. She did not acknowledge to us or to herself how much pain and disappointment there was in the discovery that her baby was blind.

And what of the baby? He was one of the most adequate blind babies we had ever seen at 4 months, sitting attentively in the midst of household commotion, smiling a gorgeous smile, and cooing when we leaned over to talk to him. His mother was constantly in touch with him, bouncing him, roughhousing with him, and filling the room with her nonstop talk. We reflected, to ourselves, that this poor mother would have worn out a sighted baby of the same age. But for the blind baby the amount of physical contact with his mother and contact with her voice afforded vital nutriments in sense experience. He was flourishing. No doubt about it. This meant to us that as long as Mrs. Perrin could ward off depression through eating, and through denial of pain, she might continue to function as a mother. We took great care not to disturb this equilibrium in our work.

But at one point when Robbie was 10 months old, a well-intentioned resident in internal medicine placed Mrs. Perrin on a strict diet. As Mrs. Perrin tried to comply with the diet, her depression broke through. She lost contact with her baby and for the first time we saw listlessness in Robbie and a developmental impasse in both language and prehension. We understood what was happening. We urged Mrs. Perrin to give up her attempts at dieting and gave her all the support she needed in reestablishing her relationship with Robbie. Mrs. Perrin's old defenses were restored; she moved back into contact with her baby and Robbie began to flourish again.

We followed Robbie regularly until the age of 3 and, after the family moved to another community, we saw him twice in school at the age of 6. There was never a sign of an ego disturbance in Robbie and no depressive features in his personality! Were there *no* effects of his mother's disturbance upon this child's personality? Yes, at least one that we know of. He had an eating problem. For although Robbie had always eaten a full range of foods, and never had trouble masticating, his mother had always complained that he did not eat enough, and battles over eating continued for years. We were never able to bring about any changes in this area, the center of the mother's own conflicts. But an eating problem is something we can all live with; an ego disturbance, which is the fate of many blind children, can lead to an irreversible freezing of personality. So, we think Robbie has come off well even though the child of a disturbed mother.

Jackie

Jackie's mother was almost as severely depressed as Mrs. Perrin, but by the time we first met Mrs. Tenney her own defenses were no longer available to her. Jackie was 7 months old when we first saw him and his state was alarming to us. He smiled rarely, seemed unresponsive to voices or touch, did not seek contact with his mother, and lay stiffly in her arms. He could not control his trunk even in supported sitting and collapsed in the testing chair. We could elicit grasping with great difficulty and we saw that the thumb was folded into the palm and the fingers were rigidly extended. There were almost no vocalizations. The question of brain damage remained with us during the early weeks of our work. Yet, our observations of baby and mother showed that for the greatest part of the day Jackie lay supine, in his crib, asleep or awake, without human contact or toys. Unlike Mrs. Perrin, Mrs. Tenney's depression had led her to withdrawal from her baby. Later, as we saw improvement in Mrs. Tenney, we understood that even under the most favorable conditions she did not spontaneously enjoy or seek tactile experience with her children and "talking to babies" was not her mode. For a blind baby this meant that there was no way of experiencing his mother or her presence.

Marguerite Smith and Ralph Gibson of our staff worked together as a team for the family, putting everything we had into the education of the mother and the baby. Dr. Smith worked with the mother supportively and educationally, using her clinical training to sustain the depressed mother and help her toward adequacy, using her knowledge of the development of blind infants to interpret Jackie's needs to his mother. Dr. Gibson used part of every observation session with Jackie in what might fairly be called "an education of the hands." The whole family, including Jackie's older brother of 4, became engaged in the work of helping Jackie.

Within the first 3 months of work, Jackie began to climb toward adequacy in every sector of development. The family began to feel reward beyond all expectations. At the end of a 6-month period Jackie was functioning well within the norms for blind children and his adaptive hand behavior was, if anything, more precocious.

Both Mrs. Perrin and Mrs. Tenney taught us something we had never fully realized. With help, even parents with severe pathology can be enlisted in the work of saving their babies, and it is possible to contain the parental neurosis so that the baby's development is not caught up in the parent's illness.

Karen

A few months ago, we were watching Karen. She was 3 years old, absolutely alive and intoxicated by some new and interesting toys she had found, walking when she couldn't run, but running mostly. Her little sister was present, and I nearly said Karen was keeping a sharp *eye* open for any invasion of her territorial rights, but of course she was keeping a sharp *ear* open. That little sister didn't stand a chance. Any time she swiped a toy from Karen, there was a swift and noisy rebuttal in plain and good English and a well-aimed paw snatched the toy back to its rightful owner.

When Edna Adelson first saw Karen at 10 months of age, she sat slumped in a little jump seat, face impassive and dull, hands tightly fisted, uttering no sounds. Karen slept 22 hours out of the 24. Her mother said she was a very good baby. It was impossible to test fairly the capacities of this baby who seemed not to respond to any stimuli. But, twice during the observation period, when Mrs. Adelson played games with the mute and unresponsive baby, she saw a fleeting gesture. When the game ended or was interrupted, there was a ghost of a gesture, the baby's hands returning ever so lightly to the examiner's hands, a sign that we interpret with blind babies as meaning "More," "Again."

Karen's parents were without hope for their baby. We could not even guess the mother's capacity to work with us on behalf of her baby. She was, herself, phlegmatic, inarticulate, and not welcoming of the help offered her. If we did not know that this baby was in deadly peril, we would have taken the mother's clear sign, "You are not welcome," and withdrawn.

The work with Karen and her mother was very slow at the beginning. There are some mothers who do not enjoy cuddling babies and who literally do not know what to do with a baby after he is fed and diapered. During the early sessions in the home, the mother watched without obvious interest as the psychologist played with the baby or talked with her. When Mrs. Adelson saw interesting signs in the baby's behavior, she interpreted these signs to the mother. But how to get this baby into her mother's arms, how to get these two to know each other? It did not happen at once, but it happened. As interpreter of Karen's foreign language to the mother, Mrs. Adelson began to translate the signs "I want my mother" from a piece of squirming and straining and one day bodily delivered Karen and a basket of toys to her mother's lap. The mother was surprised and the baby was perhaps surprised. Then, shyly, very self-consciously, the mother began to do what Mrs. Adelson did—she played with her baby.

This was the beginning. Now, ever so slowly, the two strangers became acquainted. And very slowly, too, signs emerged in Karen that mother was important to her, that she preferred her mother. Her mother did not, at first, recognize these signs. Mrs. Adelson, as interpreter, translated them. Again, we saw the shy, almost unbelieving look on the mother's face. We found this deeply touching. We were beginning to understand Karen's mother. She was a woman who owned so little self-valuation, so little sense of her own worth or lovability, that she could not recognize the signs of love and valuation in her baby. But when they appeared and when she came to believe in them, her own motherliness was stirred, too. Karen's mother never became a warm and ebullient woman; she will never be a woman who is exalted by the feel of a baby in her arms, but she learned to find pleasure in her blind baby and in her sighted baby, too, and babies are wonderfully adaptable to the styles of love that are offered to them.

During all these months while Mrs. Adelson was introducing Karen's mother to Karen, a very large and important aspect of the educational work was proceeding apace. Those tightly clenched hands would need to unfold or Karen might become one of the children with "blind hands." Toys, games, educational strategies were introduced at each session. And when, at 13 months, the hands began to open up and the fingers began to explore, we all sat back after a film review and sagged with relief.

In the end, as you can guess, Karen has become a most gratifying child to her parents and to us, one of the superior children in our group, according to our recent developmental assessment.

RELEVANCE TO OTHER TYPES OF INFANT PROGRAMS

From these sketches we can see the degree to which such variables as parental style and parental neurosis can be accommodated in a program of early intervention. In this work we have not dealt directly with the parental neurosis, but have focused on the baby and the interaction between baby and parents. We chose this approach on clinical grounds.

We are all trained clinicians. If it had been appropriate for us to do psychotherapy with these mothers, we would have had among us very experienced and expert psychotherapists. But these were our considerations: first, these parents did not come to us for psychotherapy but for educational guidance on behalf of their babies; second, even if the conditions had altered and one of our parents had requested psychotherapy, we would prefer that this work be done with someone outside of our unit. These are the clinical grounds upon which we based our position:

A baby in hazard during the first 18 months of life is a baby in crisis. No baby can wait for the outcome of his mother's psychotherapy which may not be beneficial until he is 3 years old. A baby who is moving toward autism will have arrived there at the age of 3. As crisis intervention, then, we choose to work supportively with the mother, finding the intact areas of her personality, eliciting the best in her mothering capacities, reducing, where possible, the impingement of her neurosis on her baby. In so doing, we obtain a different kind of transference from that of the psychotherapeutic transference. So far as possible, we maintain the transference on a positive level and deal with resistances on an educational level. This is not to say that we evade negative transference manifestations; it is only obvious that the most productive educational work will be obtained within the positive transference. We also believe that such a transference will elicit a positive identification with the counselor—the new, uncritical, patient, teaching mother or father figure—who can serve as another model for parenthood where the original objects have created conflict in parenthood. We have good evidence that in several cases this is exactly what took place.

From this sketch of our work we can see that while some of our problems were unique for blind infants and their families, there are many areas in which our experience has direct relevance to work with any infant population in which normal development is in danger.

The educational approach to parents with a wide diversity of personal and social problems can, we believe, have broader applicability. The visits to babies and their families *in their homes* are essential for the conduct of such a program and make it possible for the trained observer to make a continuous diagnostic assessment on the basis of direct observation in a setting which is conducive to informality and an easy exchange between mother and the guidance worker. A noncritical, nonjudgmental approach on the part of the guidance worker is also essential in any such program of intervention. And, while the problem of making a tactful entry into the home for educational purposes is one that must be worked out for each case, we should remind ourselves that there is nothing like a baby to provide common ground.

Among all the things we thought we brought to our parents, we feel that our caring about the baby, our pleasure in him, our sharing his progress and his problems, created the necessary bond between ourselves and the parents of our babies. This is so banal as to be unworthy of mention, except that it had tremendous implications for our parents, and particularly for those parents who were already overwhelmed by poverty, failure, depression, and hopelessness. Many parents who fail as parents were once themselves children who were not valued, children who received at best obligatory parental care. Throughout their lives in school, later at work, there must have been rare occasions, if any, in which someone valued them or anything they produced. For such parents, our affection for the baby and for them, our praise when merited, our sympathy and support through troubles were a form of nurture which they had rarely known. Even this small amount of nourishment from someone outside made it possible for some parents to invest themselves in their babies, to value themselves and the baby we valued; and, when the investment took place, they experienced rewards they had not known were there for them.

Earlier, I spoke of ourselves as "interpreters" of the blind baby's language. There are analogies in work with other groups of disadvantaged babies. There are parents who have no stable traditions in infant rearing, or parents whose model of infant rearing in their own families was one of perfunctory care, in which a bottle is put into the baby's mouth by anyone handy or a diaper is changed when someone thinks about it. Out of such traditions a young mother or father cannot learn the language of babies either; and the subtle expressions of need, the social signs of greeting and response, the differentiated utterances of the baby will all be lost on parents who do not "speak the language." And since all of this is the substructure for symbolic thought and speech, this baby, whose parents cannot "speak the language," may suffer a permanent deficiency in cognition.

We gave no lessons in baby language, no course of instruction, but in the course of our work, in observing the baby, playing with him, talking to him, we interpreted the signs and the signals and the vocalizations and our parents began to learn the language and to bring observations to *us*. We gave no course in child development, but as we observed the baby, we shared our observations with our parents and explained what we were looking for, what meaning a piece of behavior might have, how a certain behavior observed now would be linked to another behavior which would appear in 2 or 3 months. For example, "Just look at those hands, Mrs. Dexter! He wants his squeaky fish back, but he doesn't know where to find it yet. In a few months he'll connect the sound with the toy and we won't be able to hide it from him. He'll outsmart us every time!" Or, "Did you see how he clammed up and reached for mommy when we came in? He knows who is really important in his life, don't you, Billy?" And we sketch a story of development for the parents as we play with the baby or test him. One mother with two older children said to us, "I never watched my other babies this way. I never knew there was so much going on with a baby." Periodically, too, we load a projector, a screen, and some cans of film into our car and give a special show for mother and father in which they can see the progress of their baby on movie film.

The monthly progress of the baby is followed by us in staff conferences using notes and film analysis. As we watch we are sketching for ourselves a developmental profile. Robbie is way ahead of the game in prehension and gross motor development, but his language development is 2 or 3 months retarded. What's happening at home? What suggestions can we give his parents for promoting language?

A last point and a most important one. What constitutes the training and qualifications of the guidance workers who have been involved in our program? We came originally from many fields, from psychoanalysis, psychology, social work, education, and pediatric nursing. Only two of our staff members had had extensive work or training in infant work. Baby workers are so rare that we could never have found personnel to staff our project. But each was chosen for expertness and extraordinary qualifications in his own discipline. To educate ourselves for specialized work with the blind infant, we employed the most rigorous training in infant development, which included the study of normal and intact infants. Supervision, apprenticeship, weekly seminars, and many hours a week of film study went into the first year training period and the period beyond. Only senior staff members, our most experienced people, have had the responsibility for educational work with the infants.

If we are to extend the work of intervention to many groups of disadvantaged babies, one of our most pressing needs will be the training of professional workers on a scale that we cannot yet imagine. At the present time, the professional equipment of psychiatrists, psychologists, social workers, and educators does not usually include enough intensive training in infancy and early childhood to assess development and developmental lags, to identify the early signs of emotional and cognitive disorders in the early months and years. As for the work of educational intervention, none of these professions has yet a corps of experts in infancy and early childhood which can be dedicated to this work. The specialists, I would hope, would come from all of these disciplines, bringing expertness and specialized knowledge from the discipline itself, but with intensive postdegree training in the field of infancy.

All of us who are engaged in infant intervention are caught up with the excitement and joy of this work, which is rewarding beyond description. There is only one danger. The need is so great, the number of qualified specialists so few, that we may not move swiftly enough to set standards, to set up qualifying postgraduate programs. This work is arduous and demanding of the highest professional skills. For the baby it is in a sense "lifesaving" and unless we agree that a "lifesaving" profession deserves nothing less than the best, this work may fail.

21

A MULTIHANDICAPPED RUBELLA BABY

The First 18 Months

David A. Freedman, M.D., Betty J. Fox-
Kolenda, B.A., and Stuart L. Brown, M.D.

In the years since Engel and Reichsman (1956) first described Monica, a number of infants with significant somatic handicaps have served as subjects for developmental studies. In general these have proved of relevance to the student of development because the limited adaptive capacities of such infants tend to throw into relief aspects of the developmental process which are obscured by the greater flexibility of the normally endowed. This report deals with the first 18 months of a multiply handicapped rubella baby. We first saw C. when he was 3 weeks old. Since then he was observed by one or more of our team on some 31 occasions. We have visited him at home 23 times and one of us (B.J.F.-K.) kept him in her home for 48 hours. With rare exceptions at least two of us have participated in each visit. Each recorded his observations independently. Motion pictures detailing aspects of his behavior were made on 20 occasions.

The complexities of the problem presented by the infant with congenital rubella have been reviewed by Desmond et al. (1969). The severity and persistence of the prenatal infection, as well as its effect on particular organs, vary from patient to patient. In addition, it is difficult to predict from the infant's behavior how his capacity to adapt and mature psychologically will ultimately be affected. A recent 25-year follow-up study, for example, reports that most "rubella" babies adjust well to young adult life. Originally the parents of many of these children had been given extremely pessimistic prognoses (Menser et al., 1967). Despite these uncertainties, some of the observations made by Desmond and her associates appear to be of more than passing significance for the student of psychological development. They found that 40-week-old infants with multiple handicaps and those with bilateral

Reprinted from the *Journal*, 9 : 298–317, 1970.

cataracts scored lowest on the Gesell scale and on other tests of neuromuscular development, whereas those with only auditory defects scored highest. The authors characterize 8 of their multiply handicapped subjects as autistic, isolated, and out of communication. In considering the relation of these infants to their environment, they note that in some instances—indeed almost unavoidably in cases of multiple system disease—sensory deprivation is associated with a decrease in environmental stimulation. In addition to the absolute reduction and qualitative alteration of sensory input consequent upon the presence of defective end organs, the children are physically ill and difficult to handle and feed. Often, because the baby is considered contagious, responsibility for his care falls exclusively on the mother. Inevitably, her protracted social isolation, as well as fatigue, affects the manner in which she handles the child. Other aspects of the infant's behavior may further complicate the problem. Many of these babies, for example, have predilections for particular postures. It is difficult, as Desmond et al. observe, to carry, let alone cuddle, a baby who persists in keeping his head retracted and his back arched.

MEDICAL HISTORY OF C. K.

C. K. is the youngest of four boys born to a lower-middle-class working family. The older siblings (ages 9–5) show no evidence of deviant development. During the first trimester of an otherwise uneventful pregnancy, the mother had a mild skin rash which was considered to be allergic in origin. Up to the time of delivery, she had no reason to suspect she had had rubella. C. was born at full term without complications. He weighed 5 pounds, 4 ounces. Bilateral cataracts, a cardiac murmur compatible with patent ductus arteriosis, hepatosplenomegaly, and a hemorrhagic eruption were noted at this time. His platelet count was 6,000/mm^3. The diagnosis of congenital rubella was confirmed by virus culture. During a 3-week period of hospitalization, he was digitalized. The parents were informed that his chances for survival were very limited.

Between 4 to 8 months, C. underwent cardiac catheterization, repair of the patent ductus, and, in successive operations, extraction of the two cataracts. During this time he was given Diazepam (Valium, Roche) for a period of 7, and later a period of 18 days. It was discontinued at 8 months "because he slept too much." Virus cultures were negative at 4 and 9 months. Both his liver and spleen gradually decreased in size, and the thrombocytopenia improved. When he was 11 weeks old, his platelet count was 224,000/mm^3. At 6 months, gammaglobulin levels and antibody titers were considered adequate. Electroencephalographic studies at 1, 4, and 16 months showed normal overall patterns. In the last tracing, however, a parieto-occipital spike focus was noted.

By the time he was 8 months old, according to those indices we had available, the ongoing infectious process appeared to be over and its obvious effects on the involved organ systems had been contained or corrected. In addition, when he was 8 months old, it was determined by the criterion of "evoked cortical potentials" that he had "adequate hearing." Nonetheless, the development of this youngster has continued to be both retarded in pace and atypical in pattern.

In view of her earlier successful experience in the rearing of children, it can be said with assurance that Mrs. K. is able to operate effectively in the "average expectable mother-child relationship." The task of mothering a rubella baby, however, added complications for which she was not prepared. We have already alluded to some of the frustrating characteristics of the early neonatal period of such infants. In addition, as he grew older, C.'s somatic problems made it necessary for Mrs. K. to devote a considerably greater proportion of her time to him than would have been the case were he a normal infant. Because he ate poorly, he had to be fed every 3 hours during the first 3 months of his life. Although the interval between feedings increased, and she propped his bottle with increasing frequency, he continued to be nursed in his mother's arms until he was 14 months old. At 18 months he still has to be held in his mother's lap when he is fed solid foods. In addition, approximately twice a week Mrs. K. brings him to one or another of the clinics which participate in the rubella program at the Texas Medical Center. By them she is instructed in a variety of regimens addressed to aspects of his problem. In terms of what Spitz (1945a) has characterized as the coenesthetic mode,[1] all of these activities have insured that C. received a relatively greater than usual amount of stimulation.

From very early in our observations, however, it was clear that the care of C. was carried out in a perfunctory manner. We did not see evidence of an active affectional involvement with the baby such as one might expect in a more typical mother-child relationship. Mrs. K. always attempted to do what was asked of her. However, when C. failed to respond to her ministrations or opposed them with irritation, she was quickly discouraged. It seemed to us that much was done *for* him, but little was done *with* him.

C.'s response to his mother's attentions, of course, provided her with no incentive to act otherwise. Early in his life she described some efforts at play with him and some evidence of response on his part. Very

1. According to Spitz, during the first 6 months of life and to some extent beyond this period, sensory experience is in the coenesthetic mode. Unlike diacritic sensation, which predominates later, this is poorly localized and diffuse rather than discrete. The signs and signals to which the infant responds belong to the following categories: equilibrium, tension (muscular or otherwise), posture, temperature, vibration, skin and body contact, rhythm, tempo, duration, pitch, tone, resonance, clang, and probably a number of others of which the adult is hardly aware.

quickly, however, these dropped out. Well before he was a year old, she characterized him as "one of those children who don't like to be bothered." We have no reason from our own observations to doubt the validity of this description.

DEVELOPMENTAL OBSERVATIONS

During his first 9 months C.'s developmental progress was both slow in pace and meager in results. We were able to note so little difference in his behavior from visit to visit that we were inclined to be very skeptical of the reports of even minimal maturational change we received from his mother.

When he was 6 months old, he drank 4 ounces of milk every 4 hours but refused solids. (Six weeks later, however, at 7 months, 17 days, he accepted strained baby foods without difficulty.) It continued to be necessary to hold him for all feedings. At 9 months, 3 days, 6 weeks after the last surgical procedure, he weighed 10 pounds, 12 ounces, i.e., approximately twice his birth weight, and well below the third percentile for his age. He slept most of the day but was awake a considerable portion of the night.

He was able to roll in either direction from his back to his stomach at 8 months, 8 days, but was not able to turn from stomach to back. At this time he could neither raise his head from the prone position nor support it horizontally when he was held prone on the examiner's palm. He could not sit unsupported. Random movements of the extremities, which were infrequent during the earlier months, gradually increased in amount. At 8 months, 8 days, there was still no evidence of purposeful locomotion. Predilection for particular positions was noted at 4 months, 3 days, when he refused to sleep on his left side.

Evidence of a response to other than oral stimulation was first noted at 1 month, when he startled to a light stroking of the skin. At this time he also startled in response to loud noises. At 7 months, 10 days the mother reported that he followed her voice as she moved about. Repeated attempts by us to elicit a response to a sound stimulus were, however, unsuccessful. We have used, in addition to our voices and bells and rattles, a Ling Stimulator (Ling and Ling, 1967), which delivers a 100 decibel mixed tone at the external meatus. At 8 months, 8 days he would not hold onto objects such as a rattle, a pacifier, or his bottle, but 1 month later, at 9 months, 3 days, he grasped and held a favorite pacifier and rattle while rejecting all other objects.

Facial expressions which could be interpreted as smiles were noted as early as 1 month, and at 2 months Mrs. K. reported smiles in response to attention from members of the family. However, evidence of a pleasurable affective response to an identifiable environmental stimulus was not seen by us until 4 months, 3 days, and was not clear-cut until 5 months, 2 days, when he smiled in response to persistent tickling. At this time he also laughed aloud when he was bounced up and down on his mother's knee. At 9 months Mrs. K. reported that when the family returned from a 4-day trip and C. was put to bed, he began to laugh, kick, and coo. She said, "He really was glad to be in his own crib again." On the other hand, at this time she was much less certain of his ability to discriminate among or react to members of the family. Our own observations failed to elicit evidence of any interest in his human environment.

He spent increasing amounts of time engaged in "blindisms." These were first noted at approximately 5 months, 14 days, when they consisted of occasional manual exploration of his orbits and mouth. In very short order, however, this evolved into a repetitive, rhythmical form of self-stimulation. He used either hand for this purpose. By 7 months, 10 days, he appeared to be less concerned with the somesthetic stimulation of his orbits; he would simply wave his hand in front of his eyes whenever he faced a light source. At times he would evert his lips and protrude his tongue so that as his fingers passed before his eyes, the heel of his hand and his flexed thumb brushed both lips and tongue (fig. 1).

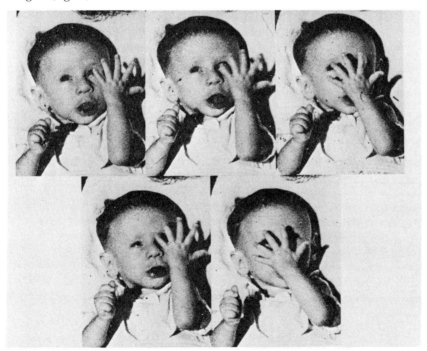

Figure 1

Vocalization in the form of crying was first noted when C. was 2 months old. Two months later, at 4 months, 3 days, he was reported to coo and babble. While the crying appeared to be in response to discomfort and would stop when a noxious stimulus could be identified and removed, we have no data to indicate that the cooing and babbling were influenced one way or the other by the environment. We have never heard this infant vocalize in this fashion. For the most part, his mother described him as very quiet. More recently, at 1 year, 4 months, 14 days, he has engaged in the making of noises by forced expiration through his pursed lips.

At 9 months, 7 days, psychological testing placed C. at the 14-week level. A program of active physical stimulation was initiated.

Three weeks later, at 9 months, 27 days, 2 months after the cataracts were removed, the blindisms continued unchanged. He was unable to sit even with support to his back and had made no effort at horizontal locomotion. Rocking movements emerged whenever he was held either seated or supine. At this time, however, when one of the examiners allowed C. to grasp his finger and then removed it from his grip, he made some searching movements with his hand. His mother reported he appeared to be fascinated by the Christmas tree lights.

At 1 year, 1 month, 4 days, Mrs. K. reported that he would stare at

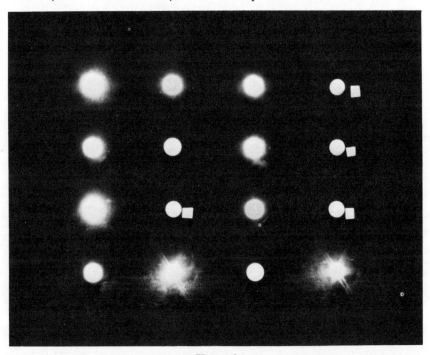

Figure 2

lights for long periods of time. As he did so, he would engage in the blindisms. He now reached for and manipulated a variety of objects. Some of these he mouthed or incorporated into the blindisms with which he occupied most of his time. He showed no evidence of a response to auditory stimuli. At no time he did he evince any desire to be held or cuddled. Although it was noted at this time that he molded to one of us when he was held, the mother repeated that he did not enjoy either being held or played with.

Two modifications of the environment were introduced at 1 year, 1 month, 4 days. Mrs. K. obtained a baby walker in which C. could sit, and the authors provided a new source of visual stimulation. In the hope that it would facilitate a transition from the self-stimulation of the blindisms to concern with stimuli from without, a device was constructed which consisted of 16 varicolored bulbs set into a rectangular panel approximately 18 by 24 inches (fig. 2). It was so wired that the bulbs flashed on and off in a random sequence. C.'s interest in this "visual stimulator" [2] was prompt. About this time the mother had also begun to place C. in front of the television set.

Following the introduction of the stimulator, the amount of time C. spent in self-stimulation appeared to decrease. He continued, however, to wave his hands in front of his eyes and mouth. Not infrequently he would combine this activity with looking at the stimulator.

At 1 year, 1 month, 21 days, while sitting on the floor in front of the stimulator, he was able to support himself for brief periods by placing his palms on the floor. In playing with a teething ring, he now used both hands. When he dropped it out of sight, he groped about with his hands until he could locate it. He had begun to move himself about when he was placed in the walker.

Three weeks later, after he fell down, he seemed to respond to efforts to comfort him. This observation, molding at 1 year, 1 month, 4 days, and his response to vigorous stimulation aside, there was no evidence of interest in or involvement with his human environment. Whereas during his early months his mother had occasionally reported that the older siblings played with him, at this time she indicated their interest had waned. She observed that he was "one of those children who don't seem to want other people." When he was frustrated in an objective, he did cry and whine, but his response was without relation to the individual who would ultimately be the agent of his satisfaction. Mrs. K. reported that it was impossible for the family to watch television when he was awake. Because she was concerned about radiation, she tried to keep C. away from the TV set. His response was to cry so bitterly that no one could watch.

2. This device will be referred to as the "stimulator" for the remainder of this report.

Five weeks later, at 1 year, 2 months, 14 days, he was able to move about in his walker with considerable ease. Interspersed in his wanderings from room to room were frequent visits to the stimulator. His mother reported that he would spend as much as an hour at a time watching it. He continued to show no interest in either his mother or the other members of the family. Except as they might interfere with his movements, their presence or absence seemed irrelevant. At this time he was observed to explore the contours of a chair with his hands. More typically, however, he would go up to a new object and both lick it and explore it with his tongue. Although he would reach for and retrieve objects, when his propped bottle slipped from his mouth, he simply cried until it was reinserted.

At 1 year, 3 months, 17 days, when he was placed prone on the floor and an attractive object was placed out of his reach, he squirmed toward it. His movements were consistent with those described by McGraw (1943) as typical for a 6-month-old infant. Manual prehension was often accompanied by an oral gesture which consisted of puckering the lips and protruding the tongue. The mother reported that he would grasp small pieces of her skin between his fingernails and pinch hard.

Despite the increasing number of objects and other inanimate stimuli to which he responded, he continued either to ignore or to reject actively the efforts of his family to engage him. Evidence of anything resembling reciprocal human relations remained limited to laughing and chortling in response to vigorous stimulation.

He continued to sit in front of the stimulator for extended periods of time and to follow the random pattern of blinking lights with his eyes. Not infrequently as he watched them he would engage in blindisms. At times he seemed to be experimenting with the lights; he would bend his head so as to change the angle from which he viewed them.

One month later, at 1 year, 4 months, 7 days, when he spent a 48-hour period in the home of one of us (B.J.F.-K.), it was not possible to infer that the new people and surroundings had in any way affected him. His mood and manner were not different from those which characterized him in his own home. He was not content to sit, lie, or be held in one's arms unless there was some form of continuing movement. At no time during his stay did he either show concern or make an affectionate gesture. He would, however, lean forward and scan very closely the face of anyone who attempted to engage his interest.

One week later, at 1 year, 4 months, 14 days, his mother reported that as he watched the stimulator, he occasionally took hold of a bulb so that his hand was transilluminated. He seemed, she said, fascinated by this. He continued to show no concern for his mother, his siblings, or ourselves. The only vocalization which could be regarded as a communication occurred when some person or object obstructed his path. He then whined until he was freed. With the aid of his walker he moved about with considerable agility. He also walked well when his hands were held. The only evidence of participation in play occurred when one of us placed him on her lap and pulled him from the supine to the erect position. He then both tightened his muscles in anticipation of being pulled up and, when in the erect position, leaned back as though to invite a repetition of the procedure.

At 1 year, 5 months, 9 days, we removed the stimulator from C.'s home. We were led to do so because we felt his fascination with it was at the expense of concern with other stimulus modalities. We did not, however, anticipate the events we shall now report.

Five days after the stimulator was removed from the home, Mrs. K. called to report the following: C. cried practically all the time. He followed her around the house crying and pulling at her to be picked up. Periodically he would go back to the place where the lights had been kept, stare at the wall, and cry. He slept poorly and woke crying several times during the night. He had, she said, been a different baby since the stimulator had left. She went on to report that he seemed very anxious to go out of doors. On the previous day he had for the first time been interested in watching his brothers and some pet dogs at play.

Two days later, at 1 year, 5 months, 14 days, we returned to C.'s home with the stimulator. Although we had concluded that it would not be in his interest to leave the device with him, we were interested to observe and record his response to it. Mrs. K. reaffirmed the details of her telephone report. C. continued to follow her about the house crying and whimpering until she picked him up. At such times she said he had even used the syllable, "Ma." He continued to be very anxious to go out of doors. She reported he now (i.e., since the stimulator was removed) had begun to play some games with his siblings. Much in the manner of a 10- to 12-month-old, he would throw a ball or other object and wait for it to be returned to him only to throw it down again.

For the first time since we had been following this baby we were able to record on film evidence of an interest in his mother. When she picked him up, he snuggled to her, smiled at her, and at times reached out to touch her face. When either of us took him from her, he squirmed, cried, and reached for her.

When C. saw the stimulator, he went directly to it. He leaned over it, bent his head forward, and watched the blinking lights. After a few minutes he wheeled away in his walker, turned around, and again returned to the lights. He repeated this on several occasions. When we disconnected the system, he first simply sat in front of the box. Then he moved away briefly and returned as though waiting for the lights to come on again.

When finally we picked it up to take it away, he followed it for some 15 to 20 feet. He moved in front of the observer as though to block her path. He then seemed to lose interest and began to wander about. Occasionally he would look up at the sun. For the first time during this visit, he passed his hand in front of his face. He then returned to the spot where the stimulator had been standing and stared at the wall for several seconds. Finally he moved to his mother, raised his hands, and put his head against her skirt. At once, when she picked him up, he cuddled against her shoulder. After a few moments, as she talked to him, he looked up at her face and smiled.

Three weeks later, at 1 year, 6 months, 7 days, he weighed 16 pounds and measured 30½ inches. His attachment to his mother was more marked. He snuggled against her shoulder and smiled when she held him. She reported that he would turn to his siblings for help, e.g., to be taken out of his walker, but would then turn to her to be held. He became upset when either of us took him from her. For the first time during our observations he quieted to the sound of his mother's voice. He could now walk, albeit with difficulty, when he was supported by one hand. Repetitive self-stimulation of his mouth and orbits was, however, much more frequent than on our previous visit. It occurred whenever he was not being held by his mother or otherwise actively stimulated.

DISCUSSION

Escalona (1965) has pointed out that most research problems of behavioral development has implied use of the conceptual model shown in figure 3. The uniqueness of behavior and personality is seen as derived

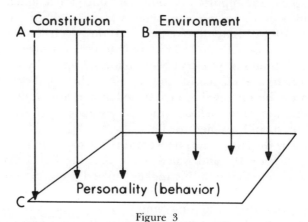

Figure 3
Model 1. Personality (behavior) as resultant of all relevant environmental and intrinsic variables.

from a combination of constitutional (A in the figure) and environmental (B) factors. While they are conceived of as varying in their relative significance from person to person, a direct relation is assumed to exist between the resultant personality and the operation of these factors. She suggests that a more accurate representation of the relevant relations is provided by figure 4. According to this scheme, neither "organismic," i.e., intrinsic in the sense of inherited or already acquired, nor environmental factors directly affect either the developmental process or the ongoing personality organization. The resultant of their interaction, however, constitutes an intervening variable which she designates "patterns of concrete experience"; personality and behavior in turn are determined by the interaction of new patterns of concrete experience with the preexisting psychic state. This concept has the obvious advantage that it introduces considerable flexibility. Within very wide limits the pattern of concrete experience and its effect on personality development may remain constant if variations in A factors are complemented by appropriate changes in B factors.

To illustrate the heuristic value of her model, Escalona considers the problem of the autistic child. Kanner's (1943) original description of the parents of such children and the assumptions made by him and others (Eveloff, 1960; O'Gorman, 1967; Rimland, 1964) concerning the role they play in the development of the syndrome will not account for the fact that autistic behavior also occurs in youngsters from radically

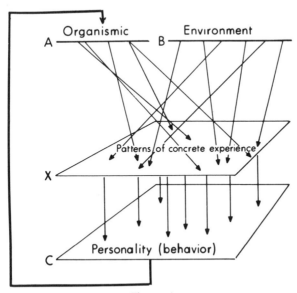

Figure 4

Model 2. Personality (behavior) as the function of concrete experience, which, in turn, is the resultant of all relevant environmental and intrinsic variables.

different backgrounds. If, however, one postulates the operation of "organismic" factors which alter responsivity in an appropriate direction, it could follow that the pattern of concrete experience would correspond to that of Kanner's patients, even if the characteristics of the parents were quite different from those he describes.

Observations made in the congenitally blind lend direct support to this proposition. In at least two communications (Fraiberg and Freedman, 1964; Norris et al., 1957), autisticlike patterns have been noted in 25 percent of congenitally blind youngsters. The authors of both reports have found that the etiology of the blindness was irrelevant. Not only were various etiological agents present in the afflicted group, but also not all children blinded by a given etiological agent became deviant. The assumption seems to be appropriate that the organismic factor "congenital blindness" serves to create a strong tendency toward patterns of concrete experience which result in autistic behavior. The statistical evidence (75 percent nonautistic), coupled with the case material included in one of the reports (Fraiberg and Freedman, 1964), however, indicates that appropriate environmental factors can counteract this tendency.

We agree with Escalona that use of a conceptual model which includes patterns of concrete experience as an intervening variable should prove most fruitful in longitudinal studies. Indeed, a similar concept has been implicit in all the major developmental theories derived from psychoanalysis as well as in Piaget's work. Inherent in the zonal libidinal theory, for example, are assumptions concerning cognition, i.e., an organismic factor which affects perception and therefore ultimate adaptation. From this standpoint the toddler can be characterized as perceiving the world through the filter of his "anal" preoccupations. Otherwise stated, no one would anticipate that a 2-year-old will perceive a given stimulus in the same way as either a neonate or a 10-year-old. In general, it can be said that at any given point in a child's development, the possibility exists of a wide variety of combinations of organismic states and environmental vicissitudes which will yield equivalent patterns of concrete experience and, therefore, have equivalent effects on subsequent personality development.

We feel our observations are best understood in the context of Escalona's intervening variable. C. fulfills most of the behavioral criteria Rimland (1964) lists as "necessary but not sufficient" for the diagnosis of infantile autism. Simply to label him as "autistic," however, is to beg the question of the determinants of that syndrome both as we observed its emergence in C. and as it is described elsewhere. At least one major etiological possibility proposed by Rimland, i.e., hyperoxia, is specifically excluded by C.'s history. This child was hyperoxic during the first 6 months of his life, i.e., until the patent ductus arteriosis was corrected. We cannot, of course, dismiss the possibility that C.'s cerebral vasculature was affected by the rubella virus in a manner analogous to that which Rimland feels may ordinarily follow excess oxygen. Rorke and Spiro (1967) as well as Singer et al. (1967) report extensive degenerative disease of the cerebral blood vessels in infants with congenital rubella who died at under 1 year. The defective blood supply hypothesis, however, does not account for the ultimately successful adaptation of many severely afflicted rubella babies, nor, for that matter, does it explain the 75 percent of youngsters blinded by retrolental fibrous dysplasia who do not become "autistic." At most, it seems to us, Rimland's hypothesis may have relevance to one of the "organismic" factors which contribute to the nature of the child's patterns of concrete experience.

For C. specifically, organismic and environmental factors operated in concert to produce atypical and maladaptive patterns of concrete experience. That in the circumstances he should have developed markedly deviant behavioral characteristics is not surprising. Freud (1914) has described the reversion to narcissistic preoccupation with the body which characterizes the physically ill. Despite C.'s having received considerably more stimulation in the coenesthetic mode than would be made available to a normal baby, the patterns of concrete experience which he developed did not include differentiation of the "mothering one." As an agent for the relief of discomfort, she provided a necessary but not sufficient experience for the development of affective attachment. He failed to differentiate her as a special object.

At least two "organismic" factors, in addition to his precarious cardiac state, militated against the development of a more typical interchange between C. and his environment.[3] Like so many "rubella" babies, he responded to being held and cuddled with irritation and evidence of discomfort. His mother was therefore thwarted in her efforts to engage him in the mutually gratifying kind of interchange which usually accompanies coenesthetic stimulation and, we assume, ultimately lends specificity to the individual who provides it. The resentment Mrs. K. felt and expressed at being tied down during this infectious period was compounded by his failure to make a gratifying response to her subsequent "maternal" overtures. Although she continued to take appropriate care of his bodily needs and to carry out the various prescribed regimens, she did this in a perfunctory and "expeditious" manner which further reduced the possibility of the development of appropriate cathectic ties. Coenesthetic stimulation was not supplemented by age-appropriate diacritic experience.

C.'s blindness further limited his ability to receive stimuli from the

---

3. We have noted, but hesitate to evaluate, the significance of his having received a depressant for two relatively long periods between 4 to 8 months.

environment. The appearance of the blindisms at 5 months, 14 days is of particular significance. According to Gesell and Amatruda (1941) and Griffiths (1954), reaching for an object appears in the sighted child at 5 months. Because of this coincidence in time we suggest that the onset of blindisms is evidence of maturational readiness for hand-eye coordination. At least in this respect we feel justified in assuming that the development of C.'s nervous system was proceeding "on schedule." The blindisms, on this basis, can be regarded as the expression of an innate pattern in the absence of an appropriate external stimulus, i.e., as equivalent to what ethologists call vacuum activities. In more traditional psychoanalytic terminology we suggest they represent the expression of instinctual energy in the absence of an external object appropriate to the satisfaction of the instinctual aim. From their monotonous persistence we infer that they were accompanied on the one hand by not unpleasurable sensations and on the other hand by a failure to achieve the experience of resolution of tension, i.e., of mastery.

Glover (1932) has observed that, "An instinct excitation that can be gratified on the individual's own body is *a priori* to some extent manageable. An instinct that requires a true external object . . . is unmasterable unless with the collusion of the real object." We regard the blindisms as representing a persisting instinctual excitement which C. attempted unsuccessfully to master in Glover's sense. However inappropriate in terms of larger problems of human adaptation, the stimulator was an external object with which C. could "collude."

The introduction of it and the walker were accompanied by evidence of increasing awareness of the world of objects. Yet he continued to show no evidence of interest in or even awareness of human objects as such. He would cry if he was thwarted or uncomfortable. But once he was satisfied, he showed no interest in the individual who had helped him. It was, therefore, most impressive to us, as well as quite unexpected, that he should have responded as he did to the removal of the stimulator. We propose that both his response to this device while it was in his home and his behavior upon its removal suggest that he developed an affective attachment to it. Certainly, his behavior following its removal had the quality of a period of mourning. It was in the context of his distress over its loss that he turned to his mother and expressed interest in her.

Schechter et al. (1969) have proposed that the autistic defense may originate in a withdrawal from overwhelming inner or outer stimuli. In these cases they feel that the defense, which may have had its origins in particular susceptibilities of the infant, has come to be used in response to any and all types of stimuli. From this hypothesis they postulated that placing autistic children in a situation of prolonged perceptual isolation might serve to reduce their need to maintain withdrawal. They report good results in the treatment of 3 autistic children by prolonged periods (up to 73 days) of sensory isolation. Although our observations do not support these workers' theoretical point of view, C.'s response to withdrawal of the stimulator certainly seems to have qualitative characteristics analogous to the results they report. We suggest that the use of Escalona's model may serve to resolve the theoretical differences. Just as we must assume the existence of a primordial physiological stimulus barrier, i.e., one which cannot be considered defensive in a psychological sense, so must we postulate infantile patterns of concrete experience which both precede and, from their nature, determine the character of later psychic defenses. It would not be possible to say, for example, that C. failed to cathect his mother on defensive grounds. At the age when such a cathexis is ordinarily made, he was still "preoccupied" with the problem of remaining alive. By the time his cardiac disturbance was corrected, he had long passed the critical period for the smiling response and was well into the age period at which, a mothering person having been differentiated, stranger and separation anxieties ordinarily appear. Discriminating vision was made available to him only at that time in life when these indicators of differentiation among human objects are normally at their height (Spitz, 1959). Having passed these critical periods without age-appropriate environmental input, he continued to experience the constant objects in his world according to the coenesthetic mode. In Glover's sense, the stimulator made available a greater degree of gratification of C.'s need for visual and visuomotor experience. Here was an external object which "colluded" with him in providing gratification. The pleasure he derived from its contemplation led him to seek it out repeatedly. Much as a normally developing child will interrupt his play periodically to return to his mother, he would from time to time return to the stimulator. The evidence, we propose, indicates that his cathexis of this object was analogous to a more typical child's cathexis of the "mothering one." It was only after the attachment was disrupted by our removal of the stimulator that he sought out new objects.

This proposition requires, however, that we account for his selection of Mrs. K. and his ability to respond to her as he did. Two factors seem to us to be relevant. In the first place, Mrs. K.'s constant presence made her the agent for the gratification of his needs who was most likely to be available. We suggest he turned to her in this sense, i.e., as an object to be used to attain a specific gratification. Her response to him, while it did not satisfy his aim, was in itself pleasurable. Secondly, since the stimulator did not reappear, the cathexes which had bound him to it were now available to be turned to her. We have already described the scene when, having brought the stimulator back very briefly, we again made it disappear. He stared briefly at the place where it had been standing and then moved over to his mother, raised his hands, and buried his head in her skirt.

22

INCEPTION AND RESOLUTION OF EARLY DEVELOPMENTAL PATHOLOGY

A Case History

T. Berry Brazelton, M.D., Grace C. Young, M.A., and Margaret Bullowa, M.D.

Developmental pathology is not unusual, but the opportunity to observe it closely from birth is rare. This child came to the attention of these observers, members of three different disciplines, in the course of a longitudinal developmental study of language acquisition (Bullowa et al., 1964). Our intent was to observe and document "normal" language development beginning at birth. For this reason, prospective parents were recruited for the study several weeks before their babies were due, using criteria designed to minimize the probability of abnormal development. Since this baby came under observation under such constraints, the developmental pathology which occurred was unexpected. Because of our having entered the situation as observers, we were not in a position to provide "therapeutic" intervention. But just because of our "observer" status, we were able to maintain continued surveillance at times when the family was angry with the medical attendants and unwilling to utilize available services. During the phase of the child's most severe difficulties the suggestions we did offer were disregarded. Later, when the child had already shown spontaneous improvement, our advice was sought.

PROCEDURE

The case material cited comes from four sources:

1. The child, or rather the mother's pregnancy, was, even before we became interested, under observation by the staff of the Boston Lying-In Hospital augmented by special staff in connection with the Collabo-

Reprinted from the *Journal*, 10 : 124–135, 1971.

rative Perinatal Research project on cerebral palsy, a study of the Perinatal Research Branch of the National Institute for Neurological Diseases and Stroke.[1] We have had access to all of the pre-, peri- and postnatal records of this group, including an EEG taken during the neonatal period.

2. Our own child development team consisting of pediatrician and developmental psychologist, assisted by an audiovisual technician,[2] observed the child. Following 4 observations during the neonatal period, this team visited the child at home monthly for 30 months and has made occasional observations since. The latest observation was made shortly before the child's seventh birthday. At each visit the child was observed in spontaneous activity and in test situations using the Gesell Developmental Scales. The mother was interviewed. One hundred feet (about 4 minutes) of 16 mm. black and white cinema film was taken under room lighting at each visit, and the sessions were taped. The material was worked up as a summary using a standard format. This material, especially that from the first 2 years, is the major source of the ensuing case history.

3. A "vocal" observation team, consisting of observer-psychiatrist and audiovisual technician, visited the home once a week during the first 30 months and every second or fourth week for another $3^1/2$ years. Each $^1/2$-hour session was recorded on tape, including an ongoing description of the child's behavior and interaction with others dictated into a shielded microphone, and on film by a robot camera at 2 frames per second. The tape and film can be synchronized during playback in the laboratory. The observer-psychiatrist also conducted interviews with the parents from time to time. Eventually, when school adjustment became an issue, the parents appealed for advice and were able to make use of appropriate professional investigation of their daughter's problem.

4. Dr. M. L. Scholl, a pediatric neurologist at the Massachusetts General Hospital, saw the child in neurological consultation at 4 to 7 years of age.

Case Report

Mary was born at term after 10 hours of mild labor to a primiparous mother. Marginal bleeding of the placenta and prolapse of the cord

1. NIH Grant No. BP 2372-C4: Collaborative Perinatal Research project on cerebral palsy, mental retardation, and other neurological and sensory disorders of infancy and childhood. Formerly entitled Collaborative Project on Cerebral Palsy: A Study of the National Institute for Nervous Diseases and Blindness; locally referred to as Maternal-Infant Health Study (MIH).

2. We here acknowledge the intelligent assistance of Mr. Edward Basinski and Mr. William Weiner, at the time undergraduate students at Northeastern University, who served in this capacity during the period under discussion.

were indications for emergency caesarian section. There was no evidence of fetal distress before or during delivery (e.g., changes in fetal heart rate or fetal movement and meconium staining after delivery). Premedication was routine (200 mgm. pentobarbitol p.o. 9 hours prior to delivery). Intravenous sodium pentathol and gas (ether and oxygen) were administered for the section. The infant was alert, responsive, and seemed entirely normal on delivery. Apgar scores [3] were 9-9-9 at 30 seconds, 1 minute, and 5 minutes—optimal scores except for acrocyanosis.

The baby was an alert, wide-eyed newborn who looked vigorous and mature. She was entirely normal in all neurological and behavioral responses on the delivery floor and on frequent observation in the ensuing week (Brazelton and Young, 1964). Her movements were free-flowing and seemed quite mature. She sucked her right fist in the delivery room and during repeated observations during the week. At birth she seemed more alert and responsive than babies born by elective caesarian section. She maintained a constantly alert state for 30 minutes during our observation soon after delivery. In this period she showed good muscle tone of her extremities with wide, free, smooth cycling of her arms and legs. When she was pulled to sit, she responded by maintaining her head in midposition with excellent neck-muscle control. She mouthed her hands repeatedly and managed to suck down mucus by sucking on them on two occasions. Her eyes were wide and alert, and she fixed on a red ball and followed it back and forth in lateral excursions. She responded to the noise of the camera with cessation of movement and turning toward the camera. We felt that the preceding labor had alerted her.

For the next 36 hours following delivery she seemed quieter and less responsive. By 48 hours she responded to auditory and visual stimuli with head turning and alerting accompanied by suppression of random activity. She showed a wide range of states, varying from deep sleep when she was first approached to alert responsive states when she was handled. She moved smoothly through the range of states, and her alert states could be maintained by handling and visual and auditory stimulation. When she was allowed to, she quieted down by putting her hand to her mouth and curling up in fetal position. Neurological examinations performed by members of the BLI study group (pediatricians and a neurologist) in this first week supported our impression that this was a normal baby. An EEG taken at this time gave additional evidence of normal function.

Mary was seen at home when she was 10 days of age. Her mother seemed quiet and unresponsive to us, but said that Mary was a "good"

3. Apgar scores, when entirely satisfactory, give two points each for color, cardiac rate, respiratory rate, muscular effort, and reflex activity, and are a measure of the infant's response to delivery.

baby who cried only for feedings. She was wrapped in several layers of thick blankets in spite of hot summer weather. She was curled in fetal position in the blankets and moved very little as we handled her. After stimulation she responded with startles, but quickly resumed the flexed fetal position of arms and legs. Her responses to auditory stimulation were facial grimaces and slight startles. She quickly damped responses to auditory and visual stimuli and maintained a semisleeping state throughout most of our visit. She was visually alert to a red ball and followed it with head turning and a slight smile. She sucked her right fist which was free.

At 3 and 10 weeks she was still a heavily swaddled, subdued infant whose response was limited to brief startles followed by sucking on her fist. Stimulation did not markedly change the semialert state of consciousness in which we found her. Her mother said that her intense gaze "scared you." The mother seemed very inept in handling her, and not attuned to her needs. She held Mary away from her body at all times, and handled her as if she were a stiff, lifeless object. When Mary became upset with this insensitive handling and turned for comfort to sucking on her fist, her mother pulled the fist out of her mouth roughly. As she fed the baby she held her stiffly at arm's length, and Mary turned away from her mother's face to gulp down food from the bottle. Feeding was perfunctory and businesslike with no evidence of pleasurable communication between mother and baby.

By 3 months of age Mary's head was flattening on the left occiput. It was our impression that she lay most of her day swaddled and face turned to the wall to her left as she lay in her crib. She lay on her back in layers of pink clothes dressed like a doll, with only her arms free. Even when she was fretful, her fretfulness had an even tenor and she never seemed to become very upset. When she built up tension from any cause, she turned her head to the left and watched her hands. She seemed to prefer watching her own hands to any of the stimuli we offered, such as a large red ring, our faces or her mother's, a rattle or a bell. Her face brightened briefly to mother as she talked and made faces to her. Even then Mary put up her own hand between her eyes and her mother's face. She watched the butterflies of a mobile over her crib for long periods and, as she watched them, she moved her mouth and tongue intensely. When we uncovered her, she became more animated and began to kick with tense vigorous thrusts of both legs together, but with no sign of pleasure. Her hands remained tightly closed and her face tense and frowning as she kicked. All other responses lacked vigor, were immature, and showed poor adaptation to change in position, as on being pulled to sit or stand, and being placed in prone. Her response to sensory stimulation was brief alerting, quickly damped. There was no apparent pleasure in any of this activity.

She had a dull, unresponsive quality when supine. As she was handled she responded briefly with increased tone, but her body movements were rigid and she seemed to lose interest in any stimulation. She invariably returned to watching her hands as if this were her most important source of gratification.

By 4 months the occipital flatness of her skull was more accentuated, and it seemed obvious that she still was immobile on her back most of the day at home. She was still heavily swaddled in clothing so that arms and head were the only free parts of her body. Her face showed little animation throughout the entire observation. She smiled briefly to her mother as mother talked to her and attempted to elicit response at our request. Once she smiled with more animation to us, but briefly. This led her mother to say, "She always prefers strangers to anybody."

When we visited at 5 months, Mary was sitting in her infant chair with her hands restrained under her diaper and her bottle propped. As she sucked glassy-eyed, she kicked mildly. None of our stimuli interested her. She showed no discrimination between test objects. Her gaze wandered from one observer to another without show of interest and, as her mother approached her, there was no affective response, unusual at her age. Her mother again commented that she preferred strangers. We were impressed with the lack of differentiated response to her mother and to the observers which would be expected from most babies at 5 months.

At 7 months Mary's grim mouth and unresponsive face impressed us. She showed little interest in toys or test objects, putting her hand over her face or mouthing her fingers as objects were presented. She did not attempt to reach out for them. She looked serious and grunted or yawned when we or her mother presented our faces. There seemed to be no differences among her responses to any of us. Her mother handled her at our request. She pulled her into a sitting position in a very clumsy way. The baby looked sober, yawned, eyes became glassy, and she slumped into a ragdoll flop as mother handled her. As she became floppy, her mother became more inept. She quickly relinquished her to us and we felt the tension that had mounted between them. As we handled her, Mary subsided, put one widespread hand over her face and the other thumb in her mouth to suck on. Her mother called her "fresh" for sucking her thumb and tried to remove it. Warding off people with her hands had been present throughout our observations. She usually lay watching her hand for long periods when we were present. She maintained isolation in preference to test objects, to people, and to any kind of motor activity.

After this observation Mary was seen for neurological evaluation at Boston Children's Medical Center as part of the Maternal Infant Health (MIH) study. The neurologist considered her "neurologically suspect" and listed the following abnormalities: (1) head 4th percentile in circumference with flattening on the left occiput; (2) hypotonia of all extremities, especially her legs; (3) some asymmetry of muscle tone with left side of her body greater tone than the right. She seemed immature for 8 months in both motor and social development. Her mother was told by the neurologist that her brain was not normal and that her prognosis for ultimate development was probably poor.

At our next visit at 8½ months the mother was quite upset and told us that she had been told that the baby was retarded and would never change. This seemed to mobilize her efforts to bring out the best in her child. Whereas previously she had to be called in to participate in our observations of her child, now she remained in the room with us and often spontaneously interjected her ideas, and handled Mary to show what she could do. Her handling of the baby was no longer tenuous, and she had definite ideas about how to produce response. This was in marked contrast to her behavior even the previous month. Mary seemed, only 2 weeks after the confrontation at the hospital, to be more active, was rolling around in a playpen, attempted to creep a bit, and sat unsupported with rounded back. She played actively with our test objects, rang the bell, and pulled the string with her left hand to get the ring. She successfully picked up a 1-inch cube with wide open hand. She held the cup briefly and mouthed it. We were struck by the increased vigor of her motor responses and by her new interest in test objects.

By 10 months there was a marked change in social behavior. She was gay and playful with the observers, and with her mother she was playful but actively resisted doing what was expected of her. For example, she put out her hands to be pulled to stand, but when her mother pulled her up, she folded in the middle. She stood up more readily when no one seemed to care. She was now able to creep, roll over, get up on hands and knees, and to respond to voice by vocalizing something like "meh meh." However, she gave up quickly at tasks she could not accomplish easily and put her hands over her ears or face whenever she was frustrated. We felt that she had made considerable progress in the weeks since our last visit, particularly in the social area.

At 12 months fine motor coordination seemed to have advanced almost to the norm for her age. She picked up the pellet with thumb and finger, dropped a cube into the cup, and drew a linear mark. Her leg activity was stiff and awkward, but she was able to pull herself to stand when offered a cookie. She attempted to use a spoon, pat-a-caked, vocalized "da da" and "ba ba," and tried to put on her sock.

She was seen again for the MIH study around this time and was still considered mildly retarded despite normal neurological findings. This judgment was based on lack of affective response, a social score of under 8 months, and a low rating in motor development (8 to 9 months). Our interpretation was that the findings at the hospital represented her response to the pressure of the test situation, whereas by now we were seeing quite a different child at home.

By 14 months she was able to step out awkwardly when supported by her arms, and she lurched along on her own as she crawled. The range of play with objects was still limited to the level of rattling the spoon in the cup, but otherwise her social behavior approximated that expected at her age. She made her wants known by pointing, tried to carry food to her mouth on the spoon, and positioned her arms and legs when being dressed. She now expressed her feeling of pressure during the examination by vocalizing jargon to her mother in a scolding tone which seemd to imitate her mother. In the test situation she was unpredictable and her performance still varied.

At 18 months she walked alone with stiff-legged halting gait, her arms extended. She seemed unsteady and balanced precariously. She achieved a tower of 3 blocks and was able to hold 4 cubes in her hand. She followed directions attentively. For example, she dropped the cube into the cup and onto the plate on request. She grasped the cubes with poor adaptation of her hand and was awkward in large motor activity, yet it seemed that she had concepts about play with objects which she could not yet achieve with these awkward movements. She gave a creditable performance for a child of 1½ years.

By 20 months Mary handled her cup and eating utensils adequately and managed her own feeding. Her fine motor control had improved markedly and gross motor control seemed to be better coordinated. Her mother reported that toilet training was complete and that she seemed much less negative and destructive since beginning to walk. She also said that Mary never allowed herself to fall even though she walked awkwardly.

At 21 months she played with dolls during our observation and several things about her emotional development became clear. The doll was used as an object which she alternately kissed and hit, calling it "bad." She had a wry comical quality which seemed like a deliberate caricature of herself. We felt she saw herself as devalued. There was a hollow quality to relationships as demonstrated in doll play. However, we saw this as moving in the direction of positive interest, a step toward wider interest in her surroundings and in people in particular.

By 2 years there was more open warmth between Mary and her mother. Mary reflected this in the way in which she greeted us by meeting us with more openness and discrimination. She was receptive to complicated demands. Her play with dolls showed concern and interest. For example, when we asked, "Is the dolly asleep?" she said, "Sh" with appropriate gestures. Alternating with such tenderness was heavy-

handed aggressive behavior which was expressed in banging the up-
turned doll on its head when we showed interest in her tender play.

DISCUSSION

We have described the course of development of a child who, as a
neonate, had appeared adequate but who rapidly slumped until she
presented an alarming clinical picture by 8 months of age, a trend
which was reversed, apparently by a dramatic change of emotional
climate.

From the very beginning this young mother was unusually awkward
in handling her baby and in learning the usual techniques of caretaking
such as giving the bottle and burping, and in sensing the baby's needs
as distinct from her own. In the bleakness of this impoverished emotional environment, Mary developed isolated signs suggestive of the autistic children described by Kanner (1935): detachment from her surroundings, stereotyped body movements, and preoccupation with her
own body. She was not, however, wholly detached from human contact
as are the children who are considered autistic. Rather it was the tenuous quality of the relationship which impoverished Mary's affective and
cognitive growth.

Putnam (1955), commenting on the agreement among clinicians on
the diagnosis of child psychosis, stated, "There is a core problem which
manifests itself in lack of clarity in the child's perception of himself as a
person separate from his environment" (p. 521). As clinicians, none of
us would have classified Mary as psychotic. Her responses to people
and to toys were always appropriate though tenuous. As verbal communication developed, she showed no evidence of mental confusion.
We noticed that she was socially responsive with the members of her
extended family, including grandparents and aunt, who played with
her and "made over" her, offsetting the maternal deprivation. With her
grandfather, who lived in the same building, she developed imitative
games. Even the observer who visited weekly could always, albeit with
difficulty, coax a smile from her.

Escalona and Heider (1959) discuss the effects of maternal behavior:
"Those infants whose mothers tended to maintain a good deal of distance from their children, both physically and emotionally, furnished
the most extreme examples of infants who rely on motor habits and,
more narrowly, autoerotic behavior for reestablishment of equilibrium"
(p. 77). The children referred to are not considered psychotic by these
authors, but do resemble psychotic children in some respects, as does
Mary.

Mary, like Daphne described by Kaplan (1964), found satisfaction in
autoerotic activity, seeming thus to make up for the lack of closeness

with her mother. Both of these children showed milder pathology than seriously disturbed autistic children. Both children resumed progress when their mothers turned toward them when given support by professional people. In neither case was extensive therapy instituted.

This baby, who as a neonate appeared well integrated and satisfyingly responsive in the hospital, rapidly became minimally responsive, constricted, and even defensive at home. A situation was set up between mother and baby which kept each from responding satisfactorily to the other. Although this seemed to develop from the mother's anxious, inept inability to stimulate her baby appropriately, the baby's rapid subsidence into inactivity and apathy led to poor circular feedback between mother and baby. The baby's unresponsiveness played into the mother's distance from her child, and resulted in the perpetuation of mutual maladaptation. It seemed to be a sparseness of mutual gratification, rather than distortion of it, which led to the baby's delayed development.

Mary's restitution at 8 months began after the mother had been confronted with the neurologist's dire prognosis. This shook the mother out of her apathy. Her reaction was to focus attention on her child and to set to work suddenly and anxiously eliciting responses from her baby whom she had previously seemed to disregard. The result was rapid mobilization of the child's energy speeding up the developmental tasks which had been arrested. This was accomplished in the context of very negativistic behavior toward her mother. The mother, who had previously seemed indifferent, suddenly became aware of Mary as a person from whom she wanted something. The more mother demanded of Mary, the more Mary resisted, but, at the same time, the more she accomplished. No longer did the mother leave the observers alone with Mary when they came for weekly vocalization records, but instead she remained and was an active participant. The mother had our full support in her all-out effort to rescue her child and disprove the neurologist's prognosis. Undoubtedly our support was a source of strength for her in maintaining a positive approach to reaching the child.

As we watched Mary's development over the critical early months and on through the period of recovery, we were impressed by the poorly modulated staccato quality of her movements, the raucousness of her voice, and a sharpness in the way she would suddenly shift between affective states. These same qualities were reasserted in the awkward manner in which she related when she began to reach out to people.

We have wondered all along whether or not this irregular quality reflected poor integration at the level of the central nervous system. Whether this lack of smooth integration is based on a subtle organic neurological defect, or was the result of early pathology in environmental stimulation, remains the important unanswered question. Our experience with her in the neonatal period suggests the latter, as does the report of the consultant neurologist, Dr. M. L. Scholl. As she grew, her impulsiveness and distractability interfered with the use of cognitive ability which she demonstrated during psychological examinations from time to time. With the acquisition of language she seemed to use speech to express her feelings, and this offered her a method of impulse control which she sorely needed. Along with this control, she became more receptive to learning and demonstrated some pleasure in mastery.[4]

This report of the inception and resolution of developmental pathology in a child continuously observed by an interdisciplinary team has become possible as the study of "normal" child development turns to intensive longitudinal studies. As in the case reported by Kris (1962), an unforeseen turn of events occurred. The child reported here, like the one described by Kris, came from an intact middle-class family. These children were born into situations which, viewed superficially, would not have called for apprehension. Such cases are particularly instructive, even when they raise more questions than they solve, since they alert us to possibilities we might not otherwise consider.

4. We are indebted to Selma H. Fraiberg for her discussion of the use of language in a child's achieving control of his impulses and freeing him for intellectual development (1959, p. 157).

EPILOGUE

Louis W. Sander, M.D.

In this volume we have suggested that the time is right for the child psychiatrist to develop a special interest in the problems of early infancy. We have tried to cover by illustration and example some of the major areas of new information, clinical experience, and additional skills which are relevant to such an interest. At the same time, we hope that some of the unknowns have also been made clear: the gaps in understanding and information which characterize a new frontier. We want to underline again the contributions which the child psychiatrist can offer to reduce these gaps; such contributions should accompany the mastering of the clinical and conceptual challenges which will emerge from more active involvement of the clinician in the problems of earliest infancy. We hope that the reading of this volume will have helped some become aware of areas to which they can or wish to contribute.

The proposal of an Infant Psychiatry requires something of an about-face from the traditional reductionist viewpoint of the research investigator or the search for the cause which the psychopathological syndrome can provoke. The focus is, and increasingly will be, on determinants of ego strengths, on the facilitation of mechanisms of synthesis and integration in the face of recognized handicap and deficit. In general, it is easier to spot deviance than to be sure of normality. We have tended to approach developmental events in terms of seeing in them the genesis of conflict rather than the developing of potentialities or the shaping of adaptive strategies and alternative routes. In contemplating early intervention, we have in mind a discipline which must capitalize on potentialities and the plasticity of the infant organism. Although the enterprise of *primary prevention* has scarcely been launched, intervention into the earliest stages of the child's development already has raised many questions and fundamental concerns. Just where the opportunities lie in early intervention, or what the hazards, the complications, and the special consequences for later life, remain largely unknown at the present. The reader has been left with many of the current issues and urgent questions undiscussed. More could be said of a great many topics: for example, the contribution of the infant to the interactive process—the infant's role as a determinant of maternal behavior—is only beginning to be appreciated. The subtlety of the interactive process itself can be better defined, as well as its sensitivity to contextual influences. The place of biorhythmicity in infant physiology and in the determination of infant state is just coming into view, as is the appreciation that such phenomena as entrainment and phase synchrony between mother and infant contribute basic regulatory mechanisms in bringing about early interactional coordination. Only now is attention being directed to empirical investigations of the role of the father; perhaps systematic attention some day can be given to the role of countertransference in the "helping" professional, the place of the goals, biases, and expectations of the intervener.

For the psychiatrist who has been trained in the tradition which gives a central role to "object relations," both in development and in later dynamics, new awareness is needed of the *multiplicity* of variables determining organization of behavior and of early personality. Much effort is being devoted to sorting out from among these variables those which represent the more stable infant characteristics and those which tend to become modified and thus reflect mutual adaptive processes. In the face of this multiplicity of determinants and their changing features with increasing age of the infant, new ways of thinking about "organization" in early infancy are in order, perhaps shifting from the traditional view of organization as the property of the individual to a conceptualization of organization as the property of the infant-environment system. In development, organization is viewed in longitudinal perspective. From the systems point of view, requirements for regulation of functions at each chronological level determine the necessary interactions between infant and caretaking environment. Coordinations acquired via the adaptive process in the infant-caretaking system at each level involve mutual modification in new variables as interactive regulations of relative stability are reached. Relationships between the multiplicity of variables can then be traced longitudinally through levels of regulation and adaptation to characteristics in the organization of exchanges within the system. Finally, in becoming internalized, adapted strategies which first characterized regulatory relationships with the interpersonal surround will now function as features of self-regulation and eventually characterize personality idiosyncracy.

There is an interaction between the kind of environment that the individual must cope with as an adult and the kind of rearing environment he first must learn to cope with. We know we are in a process of rapid change in our social environments, but we are unable to say what this implies for the kind of experience our infants should encounter in their first years of life. What kind of world must they be ready for 20 years hence? What kinds of experiences should they encounter in rearing to prepare them best?

The adaptive viewpoint supports the conviction that there are many different pathways in child rearing that can lead to the same ends. The diversity of culturally determined rearing practices is defended as a necessity in the preservation of social and cultural idiosyncracy. It is unworkable to think of intervention in the parenting situation as being guided by generalizations and simplistic conceptualizations, which do violence to natural variation and to individual uniqueness. Merely introducing the necessity to think in terms of temporal organization in the infant-caretaking system tends to insure an individual specificity in attaining and maintaining the coordinated interactions necessary for regulation. Differences in characteristics of rearing practices along the most obvious lines, e.g., black vs. white, represent only the grossest delineation of major categories of cultural variation, each major category being comprised of numerous subvariations. How can we distinguish experiences for the infant which will contribute to individual idiosyncracy, to cultural idiosyncracy, or to that with which evolving society will require the infant be provided to meet the demands of the future? As these variations become specified in greater detail and are taken more and more into account, what will happen to the boundaries between the continuum of normal and pathological?

The remarkable number of at-risk infants now being saved, who formerly would have perished, require a correspondingly remarkable "good enough" mothering through which the deviant functions and impaired regulatory capabilities of the infant can be adequately facilitated. If additional caretaking requirements exist for these infants at the outset of postnatal life, will there also be additional requirements at later stages of development—when will the "special" in their caretaking no longer apply? On the other hand, for infant and caretaker who fall into the normal range, what are the risks and complications for the uniqueness of individual development which will attend what appears to be an oncoming mass enthusiasm for early intervention, "expert" help, parenting classes, or child-rearing groups?

If we revise our emphasis in comprehending the dynamic process of personality organization from one which has been involved with a meticulous analysis of the effects of component influences and their interactions, to one oriented about mechanisms and processes of synthesis, synchronization, and integration, the order of importance in our perception of behaviors of both infant and caretaker may shift—along with a shift in our hierarchy of interpersonal values. It is interesting to anticipate the view of human nature and personality development which will predominate in the year 2000—only 25 years from now. There is no reason to believe that our perspective will change any less than it has in the past 25 years since 1950. The door is now open, and we are stepping over the threshold to enter that short corridor of time.

BIBLIOGRAPHY

ABRAHAM, K. (1924), The influence of oral erotism on character formation. *Int. J. Psycho-Anal.*, 6 : 247–258.

ADER, R. (1969), Early experiences accelerate maturation of the 24-hour adrenocortical rhythm. *Science*, 163 : 1225–1226.

———— & DEITCHMAN, R. (1970), Effects of prenatal maternal handling on the maturation of rhythmic processes. *J. Comp. Phys. Psychol.*, 71 : 492–496.

AHRENS, R. (1954), Beitrag zur Entwicklung des Physiognomie- und Mimikerkennens. *Z. exper. angew. Psychol.*, 2 : 412–454.

AINSWORTH, M. D. S. (1959), The development of security and attachment in East African infants. Read at Amer. Psychol. Assn., Cincinnati, Ohio.

———— (1963), The development of infant-mother interaction among the Ganda. In: *Determinants of Infant Behaviour*, ed. B. M. Foss. New York: Wiley, 2 : 67–104.

———— & BOWLBY, J. (1954), Research strategy in the study of mother-child separation. *Courrier*, 4 : 1–47.

ALDRICH, C. A., NORVAL, M. A., KNOP, C., & VENEGAS, R. (1946), The crying of newly born babies. *J. Pediat.*, 28 : 665–670.

———— SUNG, C., KNOP, C., STEVENS, G., & BURCHELL, M. (1945), The crying of newly born babies. *J. Pediat.*, 26 : 313–326, 27 : 89–96, 27 : 428–435.

ALPERT, A., NEUBAUER, P. B., & WEIL, A. P. (1956), Unusual Variations in Drive Endowment. *P.S.C.*, 11 : 125–63.

ANDERS, T., EMDE, R., & PARMELEE, A. H. (1971), *A Manual of Standardized Terminology, Techniques and Criteria for Scoring of States of Sleep and Wakefulness in Newborn Infants.* Los Angeles: Brain Information Service, UCLA School of Health Sciences.

———— & HOFFMAN, E. (1973), The sleep polygram: A potentially useful tool for clinical assessment in human infants. *Amer. J. Ment. Defic.*, 77 : 506–514.

ANTHONY, E. J. (1964), Communicating therapeutically with the child. *J. Amer. Acad. Child Psychiat.*, 3 : 106–125.

———— (1968), The developmental precursors of adult schizophrenia. In: *Transmission of Schizophrenia*, ed. S. Kety & D. Rosenthal. New York: Pergamon Press, pp. 293–316.

———— (1969a), A clinical evaluation of children with psychotic parents. *Amer. J. Psychiat.*, 126 : 177–184.

———— (1969b), The mutative impact on family life of serious mental and physical illness in a parent. *Canad. Psychiat. Assn. J.*, 14 : 433–453.

———— (1971), *Folie à deux.* In: *Separation-Individuation*, ed. J. B. McDevitt & C. F. Settlage. New York: Int. Univ. Press, pp. 253–273.

———— (1972a), A clinical and experimental study of high risk children and their schizophrenic parents. In: *Genetic Factors in Schizophrenia*, ed. A. R. Kaplan. Springfield, Ill.: Thomas, pp. 380–406.

———— (1972b), The contagious subculture of psychosis. In: *Progress in Group and Family Therapy*, ed. C. J. Sager & H. S. Kaplan. New York: Brunner/Mazel, pp. 636–658.

———— (1972b), The contagious subculture of psychosis. In: *Progress in Group and Family Therapy*, ed. C. J. Sager & H. S. Kaplan. New York: Brunner/Mazel, pp. 636–658.

APGAR, V. (1953), A proposal for a new method of evaluation of the newborn infant. *Curr. Res. Anesth. Analges.*, 32 : 260–267.

ARAI, S., ISHIKAWA, J., & TOSHIMA, K. (1958), Psychomotor development in Japanese children. *Rev. Neuropsychiat. Infant*, 6 : 1–7.

ASCHOFF, J. (1965), Response curves in circadian periodicity. In: *Circadian Clocks*, ed. J. Aschoff. Amsterdam: North Holland, pp. 95–112.

———— (1967), Desynchronization of human circadian rhythms. *Jap. J. Physiol.*, 17 : 450–457.

———— (1969), Desynchronization and resynchronization of human circadian rhythms. *Aerospace Med.*, 40 : 844–849.

BAKER, J. B. E. (1960), The effects of drugs on the fetus. *Pharmacol. Rev.*, 12 : 37–90.

BALDWIN, A., KALHORN, J., & BREESE, F. (1949), The appraisal of parent behavior. *Psychol. Monogr.*, No. 299.

BARTLETT, F. C. (1932), *Remembering*. Cambridge: Cambridge Univ. Press, 1961.

BAYLEY, N. (1943), Mental growth during the first three years. In: *Child Behavior and Development*, ed. R. G. Barker, J. S. Kounin, & H. F. Wright. New York: McGraw-Hill, pp. 87–105.

———— (1949), Consistency and variability in the growth of intelligence from birth to eighteen years. *J. Genet. Psychol.*, 75 : 165–196.

———— (1955), On the growth of intelligence. *Amer. Psychol.*, 10 : 805–818.

———— (1956), Individual patterns of development. *Child Develpm.*, 27 : 45–74.

———— (1958), Value and limitations of infant testing. *Children*, 5 : 129–133.

———— (1961), *Bayley Infant Scales of Mental and Motor Development*. Berkeley: Institute of Human Development, University of California.

———— & JONES, H. E. (1937), Environmental correlates of mental and motor development. *Child Develpm.*, 8 : 329–341.

BELL, R. Q. (1959–60), Retrospective and prospective views of early personality development. *Merrill-Palmer Quart.*, 6 : 131–144.

———— (1960), Relations between behavior manifestations in the human neonate. *Child Develpm.*, 31 : 463–477.

———— (1968), A reinterpretation of the direction of effects in studies of socialization. *Psychol. Rev.*, 75 : 81–95.

WELLER, G. M., & WALDROP, M. R. (1971), Newborn and preschooler. *Monogr. Soc. Res. Child Develpm.*, 36 : 1–142.

BENDER, L. (1938), *A Visual Motor Gestalt Test and Its Clinical Use*. New York: Amer. Orthopsychiat. Res. Monogr. No. 3.

———— (1942), Childhood schizophrenia. *Nerv. Child*, 1 : 138–140.

———— (1947), Childhood schizophrenia. *Amer. J. Orthopsychiat.*, 17 : 40–56.

———— (1956a), Schizophrenia in Childhood. *Amer. J. Orthopsychiat.*, 28 : 499–506.

———— (1956b), *Psychopathology of Children with Organic Disorders*. Springfield, Ill.: Thomas.

—— (1964), A twenty-five year view of therapeutic results. In: *The Evaluation of Psychiatric Treatment,* ed. P. H. Hoch & J. Zubin. New York: Grune & Stratton, pp. 129–142.

—— & HELME, W. (1953), A quantitative test of theory and diagnostic indicators of childhood schizophrenia. *Arch. Neurol. Psychiat.,* 70 : 413–427.

BENEDEK, T. (1938), Adaptation to reality in early infancy. *Psychoanal. Quart.,* 7 : 200–214.

—— (1959), Parenthood as a developmental phase. *J. Amer. Psychoanal. Assn.,* 7 : 389–417.

BENEDETTI, P. & COCCIANTE, G. (1959), Osservazione sul comportamento della motilita reattiva a stimulazione sonore dei neonati normali prematuri e nati asfittici. *Riv. Neurol.* (Nap.), 29 : 587–593.

BENJAMIN, J. D. (1959), Prediction and psychopathologic theory. In: *Dynamic Psychopathology in Childhood,* ed. L. Jessner & E. Pavenstedt. New York: Grune & Stratton, pp. 6–77.

—— (1963), Further communication on some developmental aspects of anxiety. In: *Counterpoint: Libidinal Object and Subject,* ed. H. S. Gaskill. New York: Int. Univ. Press, pp. 121–153.

—— & TENNES, K. (1958), A case of pathological head nodding. Read at the Los Angeles Soc. Child Psychiat., and Amer. Psychoanal. Assn.

BENNETT, E. L., DIAMOND, M. C., KRECH, D., & ROSENZWEIG, M. R. (1964), Chemical and anatomical plasticity of brain. *Science,* 146 : 610–619.

BENNETT, S. L. (1968), Unpublished studies.

BEREZIN, M. A. (1964), On the constancy of style in the aging process. Read at the Amer. Psychoanal. Assn., Los Angeles.

BERGMAN, P. & ESCALONA, S. K. (1949), Unusual sensitivities in very young children. *The Psychoanalytic Study of the Child,* 3/4 : 333–352.*

BETTELHEIM, B. (1967), *The Empty Fortress.* New York: Free Press.

BEYRL, F. (1926), Über die Grössenauffassung bei Kindern. *Z. Psychol.,* 100 : 344–371.

BIBRING, G. L., DWYER, T. F., HUNTINGTON, D. S., & VALENSTEIN, A. F. (1961), A study of the psychological processes in pregnancy and of the earliest mother-child relationship. *The Psychoanalytic Study of the Child,* 16 : 9–72.

BIRCH, H. G., THOMAS, A., CHESS, S., & HERTZIG, M. E. (1962), Individuality in the development of children. *Develpm. Med. Child Neurol.,* 4 : 370–379.

BIRNS, B. (1965), Individual differences in human neonates' responses to stimulation. *Child Develpm.,* 36 : 249–256.

—— BLANK, M., BRIDGER, W., & ESCALONA, S. K. (1965), Behavioral inhibition in neonates produced by auditory stimuli. *Child Develpm.,* 36 : 639–645.

BLANK, M. (1964), Some maternal influences on infants' rates of sensorimotor development. *J. Amer. Acad. Child Psychiat.,* 3 : 668–687.

BLEULER, E. (1911), *Dementia Praecox or the Group of Schizophrenias.* New York: Int. Univ. Press, 1950.

BLOOM, B. S. (1964), *Stability and Change in Human Characteristics.* New York: Wiley.

BOSMA, J. A. (1964), Personal communication.

* *The Psychoanalytic Study of the Child.* Vols. 1–25, New York: Int. Univ. Press, 1945–1970; Vols. 26–30, New Haven: Yale Univ. Press, 1971–1975.

BOWER, T. (1972), Object perception in infants. *Perception,* 1 : 15–30.

BOWLBY, J. (1951), *Maternal Care and Mental Health.* Geneva: World Health Organization, Monogr. 2.

—— (1958a), The nature of the child's tie to his mother. *Int. J. Psycho-Anal.,* 39 : 350–373.

—— (1958b), A note on mother-child separation as a mental health hazard. *Brit. J. Med. Psychol.,* 31 : 247–248.

BRADLEY, C. (1945), Psychoses in children. In: *Modern Trends in Child Psychiatry.* New York: Int. Univ. Press, pp. 135–154.

BRAZELTON, T. B. (1962), Observations of the neonate. *J. Amer. Acad. Child Psychiat.,* 1 : 38–58.

—— (1970), Effect of prenatal drugs on the behavior of the neonate. *Amer. J. Psychiat.,* 126 : 1261–1266.

—— (1973), *Neonatal Behavioral Assessment Scale.* London: Heinemann.

—— & YOUNG, G. C. (1964), An example of imitative behavior in a nine-week-old infant. *J. Amer. Acad. Child Psychiat.,* 3 : 53–67.

BRIDGER, W. H. (1962), Sensory discrimination and autonomic function in the newborn. *J. Amer. Acad. Child Psychiat.,* 1 : 67–82.

—— & REISER, M. (1959), Psychophysiologic studies of the neonate. *Psychosom. Med.,* 21 : 265–276.

BRODY, S. (1956), *Patterns of Mothering.* New York: Int. Univ. Press.

—— (1958), Signs of disturbance in the first year of life. *Amer. J. Orthopsychiat.,* 28 : 362–367.

—— (1960), Self-rocking in infancy. *J. Amer. Psychoanal. Assn.,* 8 : 464–491.

—— (1967), Some infantile sources of childhood disturbance. *J. Amer. Acad. Child Psychiat.,* 6 : 615–643.

BUEHLER, C., HETZER, H., & BEAUMONT, H. (1935), *Testing Children's Development from Birth to School Age.* New York: Farrar & Rinehart.

BULLOWA, M., JONES, L. G., & BEVER, T. J. (1964), The development from vocal to verbal behavior in children. *Monogr. Soc. Res. Child Develpm.,* Vol. 29, No. 1.

BURLINGHAM, D. (1965), Some problems of ego development in blind children. *The Psychoanalytic Study of the Child,* 20 : 194–208.

BURNS, P., SANDER, L. W., STECHLER, G., & JULIA, H. (1972), Distress in feeding. *J. Amer. Acad. Child Psychiat.,* 11 : 427–439.

CALDWELL, B. M. (1962), The usefulness of the critical period hypothesis in the study of filiative behavior. *Merrill-Palmer Quart.,* 8 : 229–242.

CALHOUN, J. B. (1962), Population density and social pathology. *Sci. Amer.,* 206 : 139–148.

CALL, J. D. (1963), Prevention of autism in a young infant in a well-child conference. *J. Amer. Acad. Child Psychiat.,* 2 : 451–459.

—— (1964), Newborn approach behavior and early ego development. *Int. J. Psycho-Anal.,* 45 : 286–294.

—— (1968), Lap and finger play in infancy. *Int. J. Psycho-Anal.,* 49 : 375–378.

—— (1970), Games babies play. *Psychology Today,* January, pp. 34–37, 54.

—— & LIVERMAN, L. (1963), Opportunities for preventive mental health practice in a public well-child conference. *Tulane Studies in Social Welfare,* July, 1965.

CAMPBELL, R. & WEECH, A. (1941), Measures which characterize the individual during the development of behavior in early life. *Child Develpm.*, 12 : 217–236.

CAPLAN, G. (1959), *Concepts of Mental Health and Consultation.* Washington, D.C.: Children's Bureau, pp. 144, 185–187.

CAPLAN, H. (1952), Some considerations of the body image concept in child development. *Quart. J. Child Behav.*, 4 : 382–388.

—— (1956), The role of deviant maturation in the pathogenesis of anxiety. *Amer. J. Orthopsychiat.*, 26 : 94–107.

CARPENTER, G. C. & STECHLER, G. (1967), Selective attention to mother's face from week 1 through week 8. Proc., 75th Annual Convention, Amer. Psychol. Assn.

—— TECCE, J. J., STECHLER, G., & FRIEDMAN, S. (1970), Differential visual behavior to human and humanoid faces in early infancy. *Merrill-Palmer Quart.*, 16 : 91–108.

CASLER, L. (1961), Maternal deprivation. *Monogr. Soc. Res. Child Develpm.*, 26 : 1–64.

CATTELL, P. (1940), *The Measurement of Intelligence of Infants and Young Children.* New York: Psychol. Corp.

CHAMPNEY, H. (1941a), The measurement of parent behavior. *Child Develpm.*, 12 : 131–166.

—— (1941b), The variables of parent behavior. *J. Abnorm. Psychol.*, 36 : 525–541.

CHOMSKY, N. (1965), *Aspects of the Theory of Syntax.* Cambridge, Mass.: M.I.T. Press.

COBB, K., GOODWIN, R., & SAELENS, E. (1964), Spontaneous hand positions of newborn infants. Personal communication.

COLBY, K. M. (1968), Computer-aided language development in non-speaking children. *Arch. Gen. Psychiat.*, 19 : 641–651.

COLEMAN, R. W., KRIS, E., & PROVENCE, S. A. (1953), The study of variations of early parental attitudes. *The Psychoanalytic Study of the Child*, 8 : 20–47.

CONDON, W. S. & OGSTON W. D. (1967), A segmentation of behavior. *J. Psychiat. Res.*, 5 : 221–235.

—— & SANDER, L. (1974), Neonate movement is synchronized with adult speech. *Science*, 183 : 99–101.

COOPER, R. M. & ZUBEK, J. P. (1958), Effects of enriched and restricted early environments on the learning ability of bright and dull rats. *Canad. J. Psychol.*, 12 : 59–64.

CREAK, M. (1961), Schizophrenic syndrome in childhood. *Cerebral Palsy Bull.*, 3 : 501–504.

CUNNINGHAM, M. A. (1966), A five year study of the language of an autistic child. *J. Child Psychol. Psychiat.*, 7 : 143–154.

—— (1969), A comparison of the language of psychotic and non-psychotic children who are mentally retarded. *J. Child Psychol. Psychiat.*, 9 : 229–244.

—— & DIXON, C. (1961), A study of the language of an autistic child. *J. Child Psychol. Psychiat.*, 2 : 193–202.

DARWIN, C. (1873), *The Expression of the Emotions in Man and Animals.* Chicago: Univ. Chicago Press, 1963, p. 204.

—— (1877), A biographical sketch of an infant. *Mind*, 2 : 285–294.

DÉCARIE, T. GOUIN (1963), *Intelligence and Affectivity in Early Childhood.* New York: Int. Univ. Press, 1965.

DENNIS, W. (1941), Infant development conditions of restricted practice and of minimum social stimulation. *Genet. Psychol. Monogr.,* 23 : 142–189.

——— (1960), Causes of retardation among institutional children: *Iran. J. Genet. Psychol.,* 96 : 47–60.

DESMOND, M. M., WILSON, G. S., VERNIAUD, W. M., MELNICK, J. L., & RAWLS, W. E. (1969), The early growth and development of infants with congenital rubella. In: *Advances in Teratology,* ed. J. G. Mordue. London: Logos Press, 4 : 43–52.

DESPERT, J. L. (1941), Thinking and motility disorder in a schizophrenic child. *Psychiat. Quart.,* 15 : 522–536.

DONOVAN, D. E. & PAINE, R. S. (1962), Prognostic implications of neurological abnormalities in the neonatal period. *Neurology,* 12 : 910–914.

DRILLIEN, C. M. (1958), A longitudinal study of the growth and development of prematurely and maturely born children. *Arch. Dis. Child.,* 33 : 417–431.

——— (1959), A longitudinal study of the growth and development of prematurely and maturely born children: III. *Arch. Dis. Child.,* 34 : 37–45.

DUBOS, R. J. (1968), *So Human an Animal.* New York: Scribner's.

DURRELL, D. (1955), *The Durrell Analysis of Reading Difficulty.* New York: World Book Co.

EIDUSON, S., GELLER, E., YUWILER, A., & EIDUSON, B. T. (1964), *Biochemistry and Behavior.* Princeton, N.J.: Van Nostrand.

EISENBERG, L. (1966), The autistic child in adolescence. *Amer. J. Psychiat.,* 112 : 607–612.

——— & KANNER, L. (1956), Early infantile autism: 1943–1955. *Amer. J. Orthopsychiat.,* 26 : 556–566.

ELLINGSON, R. J. (1960), Cortical electrical responses to visual stimulation in the human infant. *EEG Clin. Neurophysiol.,* 12 : 663–677.

EMDE, R. N. & KOENIG, K. L. (1969a), Neonatal smiling and rapid eye movement states. *J. Amer. Acad. Child Psychiat.,* 8 : 57–67.

——— ——— (1969b), Neonatal smiling, frowning, and rapid eye movement states. *J. Amer. Acad. Child Psychiat.,* 8 : 637–656.

ENGEL, G. L. & REICHSMAN, F. (1956), Spontaneous and experimentally induced depressions in an infant with a gastric fistula. *J. Amer. Psychoanal. Assn.,* 4 : 428–452.

ENGEL, R. & BUTLER, B. V. (1963), Appraisal of conceptual age of newborn infants by electroencephalographic methods. *J. Pediat.,* 63 : 386–393.

ERIKSON, E. H. (1950a), *Childhood and Society.* New York: Norton.

——— (1950b), Growth and crisis of the healthy personality. *Psychol. Issues,* 1 : 50–100. New York: Int. Univ. Press, 1959.

——— (1956), The problem of ego identity. *J. Amer. Psychoanal. Assn.,* 4 : 56–121.

ESCALONA, S. K. (1950), The use of infant tests for predictive purposes. *Bull. Menninger Clin.,* 14 : 117–128.

——— (1952), Emotional development in the first year of life. In: *Problems of Infancy and Childhood,* ed. M. J. E. Senn. New York: Josiah Macy Jr. Foundation, 1953, pp. 11–92.

———— (1958), The impact of psychoanalysis upon psychology. *J. Nerv. Ment. Dis.*, 126 : 429–440.

———— (1965), Some determinants of individual differences. *Trans. N.Y. Acad. Sci.*, Series II, 27 : 802–816.

———— (1968), *The Roots of Individuality.* Chicago: Aldine.

———— & HEIDER, G. (1959), *Prediction and Outcome.* New York: Basic Books.

———— LEITCH, M., McFARLAND, M., BRODY, S., HEIDER, G., & HOLLINGS-WORTH, I. (1953), Early phases of personality development. *Monogr. Soc. Res. Child Develpm.*, Serial No. 54, No. 1.

EVELOFF, H. H. (1960), The autistic child. *Arch. Gen. Psychiat.*, 3 : 66–81.

FANTZ, R. L. (1967), Visual perception and experience in early infancy. In: *Early Behavior,* ed. H. W. Stevenson, E. H. Hess, & H. L. Rheingold. New York: Wiley, pp. 181–224.

———— ORDY, J. M., & UDELF, M. S. (1962), Maturation of pattern vision in infants during the first six months. *J. Comp. Physiol. Psychol.*, 55 : 907–917.

FEDER, L. (1964), Hypogalactia, syndrome of three basic traumas. Read at the West Coast Psychoanal. Soc., San Diego, Calif.

FISH, B. (1957), The detection of schizophrenia in infancy. *J. Nerv. Ment. Dis.*, 125 : 1–24.

———— (1959), Longitudinal observations of biological deviations in a schizophrenic infant. *Amer. J. Psychiat.*, 116 : 25–31.

———— (1960a), Involvement of the central nervous system in infants with schizophrenia. *Arch. Neurol.*, 2 : 115–121.

———— (1960b), Drug therapy in child psychiatry. *Compreh. Psychiat.*, 1 : 212–227.

———— (1961), The study of motor development in infancy and its relationship to psychological functioning. *Amer. J. Psychiat.*, 117 : 1113–1118.

———— (1964), Evaluation of psychiatric therapies in children. In: *The Evaluation of Psychiatric Treatment,* ed. P. H. Hoch & J. Zubin. New York: Grune & Stratton, pp. 202–220.

———— (1975), Biological antecedents of psychosis in children. In: *Biology of the Major Psychoses. Assn. Res. Nerv. Ment. Dis. Publ.*, No. 54, ed. D. X. Freedman. New York: Raven Press (in press).

———— (1976), Infants at risk for schizophrenia. *J. Amer. Acad. Child Psychiat.*, 15: 62–82.

———— & ALPERT, M. (1963), Patterns of neurological development in infants born to schizophrenic mothers. In: *Recent Advances in Biological Psychiatry,* ed. J. Wortis. New York: Plenum Press, 5 : 24–37.

———— & HAGIN, R. (1973), Visual-motor disorders in infants at risk for schizophrenia. *Arch. Gen. Psychiat.*, 28 : 900–904.

———— SHAPIRO, T., & CAMPBELL, M. (1966), Long-term prognosis and the response of schizophrenic children to drug therapy. *Amer. J. Psychiat.*, 123 : 32–39.

———— ———— ———— & WILE, R. (1968), A classification of schizophrenic children under five years. *Amer. J. Psychiat.*, 124 : 1415–1423.

———— & SHAPIRO, T. (1965), A typology of children's psychiatric disorders. *J. Amer. Acad. Child Psychiat.*, 4 : 32–52.

FOWLER, W. (1962), Cognitive learning in infancy and early childhood. *Psychol. Bull.*, 59 : 116–152.

FRAIBERG, S. (1959), *The Magic Years.* New York: Scribner's.

———— (1968), Parallel and divergent patterns in blind and sighted infants. *The Psychoanalytic Study of the Child,* 23 : 264–300.

———— (1971b), Smiling and stranger reaction in blind infants. In: *The Exceptional Infant,* ed. J. Hellmuth. New York: Brunner/Mazel, 2 : 110–127.

———— & FREEDMAN, D. A. (1964), Studies in ego development of the congenitally blind child. *The Psychoanalytic Study of the Child,* 19 : 113–169.

———— SIEGEL, B. L., & GIBSON, R. (1966), The role of sound in the search behavior of a blind infant. *The Psychoanalytic Study of the Child,* 21 : 327–357.

———— SMITH, M., & ADELSON, E. (1969), An educational program for blind infants. *J. Spec. Educ.,* 3 : 121–139.

FREEDMAN, D. G. (1961), The infant's fear of strangers and the flight response. *J. Child Psychol. Psychiat.,* 2 : 242–248.

———— (1964), Smiling in blind infants and the issue of innate vs. acquired. *J. Child Psychol. Psychiat.,* 5 : 171–184.

FREUD, A. (1936), *The Ego and the Mechanisms of Defense.* New York: Int. Univ. Press, 1966.

———— (1952), The mutual influences in the development of ego and id. *The Psychoanalytic Study of the Child,* 7 : 42–50.

———— (1965), *Normality and Pathology in Childhood.* New York: Int. Univ. Press.

———— & BURLINGHAM, D. T. (1944), *Infants Without Families.* New York: Int. Univ. Press.

FREUD, S. (1905), Three Essays on the theory of sexuality. *Standard Edition,* 7 : 125–243.*

———— (1914), On narcissism. *Standard Edition,* 14 : 73–102.

———— (1923), The ego and the id. *Standard Edition,* 19 : 12–66.

———— (1925), Negation. *Standard Edition,* 19 : 235–239.

———— (1926), Inhibitions, symptoms and anxiety. *Standard Edition,* 20 : 87–175.

———— (1937), Analysis terminable and interminable. *Standard Edition,* 23 : 209–253.

FRIES, M. E. (1937), Factors in character development, neuroses, psychoses, and delinquency. *Amer. J. Orthopsychiat.,* 7 : 142–181.

———— (1944), Psychosomatic relations between mother and infant. *Psychosom. Med.,* 6 : 159–162.

———— & WOOLF, P. J. (1953), Some hypotheses on the role of the congenital activity type in personality development. *The Psychoanalytic Study of the Child,* 8 : 48–62.

GARDNER, R., HOLZMAN, P. S., KLEIN, G. S., LINTON, H., & SPENCE, D. P. (1959), *Cognitive Controls* [*Psychol. Issues,* Monogr. 4]. New York: Int. Univ. Press.

GARMEZY, N. (1971), Vulnerability research and the issue of primary prevention. *Amer. J. Orthopsychiat.,* 41 : 101–116.

GEBER, M. & DEAN, R. F. A. (1957), Gesell tests on African children. *Pediatrics,* 20 : 1055–1065.

GESELL, A. (1925), *The Mental Growth of the Pre-School Child.* New York: Macmillan.

———— (1945), *The Embryology of Behavior.* New York: Harper.

* *The Standard Edition of the Complete Psychological Works of Sigmund Freud,* 24 Volumes. London: Hogarth Press, 1953–1974.

—— (1947), *Developmental Diagnosis,* 2nd ed. New York: Hoeber.

—— (1954), The ontogenesis of infant behavior. In: *Manual of Child Psychology,* ed. L. Carmichael. New York: Wiley, pp. 335–373.

—— & AMATRUDA, C. S. (1941), *Developmental Diagnosis.* New York: Hoeber.

GEWIRTZ, J. (1968), On designing the functional environment of the child to facilitate behavioral development. In: *Early Child Care,* ed. L. L. Dittman. New York: Atherton Press, pp. 169–213.

GITTELMAN, M. & BIRCH, H. G. (1967), Childhood schizophrenia. *Arch. Gen. Psychiat.,* 17 : 16–25.

GLOBUS, A., ROSENZWEIG, M. R., BENNET, E. L., & DIAMOND, M. C. (1973), Effects of differential experience on dendritic spine counts in rat cerebral cortex. *J. Comp. Physiol. Psychol.,* 82–83 : 175–181.

GLOVER, E. (1932), A psycho-analytical approach to the classification of mental disorders. In: *On the Early Development of Mind.* New York: Int. Univ. Press, 1956, pp. 161–186.

GOFFMAN, E. (1963), *Behavior in Public Places.* New York: Free Press.

GOLDFARB, W. (1945), Effects of psychological deprivation in infancy and subsequent stimulation. *Amer. J. Psychiat.,* 102 : 18–33.

—— (1964), An investigation of childhood schizophrenia. *Arch. Gen. Psychiat.,* 11 : 620–634.

—— BRAUNSTEIN, P., & LORGE, I. (1956), A study of speech patterns in a group of schizophrenic children. *Amer. J. Orthopsychiat.,* 26 : 544–555.

GOLDSTEIN, K. (1939), *The Organism.* New York: Amer. Book Co.

GORMAN, J. J., COGAN, D. G., & GELLIS, S. S. (1957), An apparatus for grading the visual acuity of infants on the basis of opticokinetic nystagmus. *Pediatrics,* 19 : 1088–1092.

GRAHAM, F. K. (1956), Behavioral differences between normal and traumatized newborns. *Psychol. Monogr.,* 70, Nos. 20–21 : 1–16.

—— et al. (1962), Development three years after perinatal anoxia and other potentially damaging newborn experiences. *Psychol. Monogr.,* 76, No. 3.

—— MATARAZZO, R. G., & CALDWELL, B. M. (1956), Behavioral differences between normal and traumatized newborns. *Psychol. Monogr.,* 70, Nos. 20–21 : 17–33.

GREENACRE, P. (1960), Considerations regarding the parent-infant relationship. *Int. J. Psycho-Anal.,* 41 : 571–584.

GREENMAN, G. W. (1963), Visual behavior of newborn infants. In: *Modern Perspectives in Child Development,* ed. A. J. Solnit & S. A. Provence. New York: Int. Univ. Press, pp. 71–79.

GRIFFITHS, R. (1954), *The Abilities of Babies.* London: Univ. London Press.

GROSSMAN, H. & GREENBERG, N. (1957), Psychosomatic differentiation in infancy. *Psychosom. Med.,* 19 : 293–306.

GROUP FOR THE ADVANCEMENT OF PSYCHIATRY (1957), *The Diagnostic Process in Child Psychiatry.* Report #38.

GUNTHER, M. (1961), Infant behaviour at the breast. In: *Determinants of Infant Behaviour,* ed. B. M. Foss. London: Methuen, 1 : 37–44.

HALVERSON, C. F. & WALDROP, M. (1971), Minor physical anomalies. In: *Readings in Child Development and Relationships,* ed. R. C. Smart. New York: Macmillan.

HALVERSON, H. M. (1940), Genital and sphincter behavior of the male infant. *J. Genet. Psychol.*, 56 : 95–136.

HARLOW, H. F. & HARLOW, M. K. (1962), Social deprivation in monkeys. *Sci. Amer.*, 207 : 136–146.

HARTMANN, H. (1939), *Ego Psychology and the Problem of Adaptation*. New York: Int. Univ. Press, 1958.

———— (1950a), Psychoanalysis and developmental psychology. *The Psychoanalytic Study of the Child*, 5 : 7–17.

———— (1950b), Comments on the psychoanalytic theory of the ego. *The Psychoanalytic Study of the Child*, 5 : 74–96.

———— (1952), The mutual influences in the development of ego and id. *The Psychoanalytic Study of the Child*, 7 : 9–30.

———— KRIS, E., & LOEWENSTEIN, R. M. (1946), Comments on the formation of psychic structure. *The Psychoanalytic Study of the Child*, 2 : 11–38.

———— ———— ———— (1949), Notes on the theory of aggression. *The Psychoanalytic Study of the Child*, 3/4 : 9–36.

HEBB, D. O. (1949), *The Organization of Behavior*. New York: Wiley.

HEIDER, G. M. (1966), Vulnerability in infants and young children. *Genet. Psychol. Monogr.*, 73 : 1–216.

HELLBRUGGE, T., LANGE, J. E., RUTENFRANZ, J., & STEHR, K. (1964), Circadian periodicity of physiological functions in different stages of infancy and childhood. *Ann. N.Y. Acad. Sci.*, 117 : 361–373.

HERMELIN, B. (1967), Coding and immediate recall in autistic children. *Proc. Royal Soc. Med.*, 60 : 563–564.

———— & O'CONNOR, N. (1967), Remembering of words by psychotic and subnormal children. *Brit. J. Psychol.*, 58 : 213–218.

HERNANDEZ-PEON, R., SHERRER, H., & JOUVET, M. (1956), Modification of electrical activity in cochlear nucleus during "attention" in unanesthetized cats. *Science*, 123 : 331–332.

HEWETT, R. M. (1965), Teaching speech to an autistic child through operant conditioning. *Amer. J. Orthopsychiat.*, 35 : 927–936.

HINDLEY, C. B. (1957), Symposium on the contribution of current theories to an understanding of child development. *Brit. J. Med. Psychol.*, 30 : 241–249.

HOCH, P. H. & CATTELL, J. (1959), The diagnosis of pseudoneurotic schizophrenia. *Psychiat. Quart.*, 33 : 17–43.

HOFFER, W. (1949), Mouth, hand and ego integration. *The Psychoanalytic Study of the Child*, 3/4 : 49–56.

HUMPHREY, T. & HOOKER, D. (1961), Reflexes elicited by stimulating perineal and adjacent areas of human fetuses. *Trans. Amer. Neurol. Assn.*, 86 : 147–152.

HUTT, C. & OUNSTED, C. (1966), The biological significance of gaze aversion with particular reference to the syndrome of infantile autism. *Behav. Sci.*, 11 : 346–356.

INHELDER, B. (1953), Criteria of the stages of mental development. In: *Discussions on Child Development*, ed. J. M. Tanner & B. Inhelder. New York: Int. Univ. Press, 1 : 75–107.

JACKSON, E. B., OLMSTED, R. W., FOORD, A., THOMAS, H., & HYDER, K. (1948), A hospital rooming-in unit for four newborn infants and their mothers. *Pediatrics*, 1 : 28–43.

JAMES, W. (1902), *The Varieties of Religious Experience.* New York: Modern Library.

JOINT COMMISSION ON MENTAL HEALTH OF CHILDREN, REPORT OF (1969), *Crisis in Child Mental Health: Challenge for the 1970's.* New York: Harper & Row.

JONES, E. (1953), *The Life and Work of Sigmund Freud,* Vol. I. New York: Basic Books.

JULIA, H. L. (1968), Progress Report on Adaption and Perception in Early Infancy. NICHD Project, 1965–1969.

KANNER, L. (1935), *Child Psychiatry.* Springfield, Ill.: Thomas, 3rd ed., 1957.

—— (1943), Autistic disturbances of affective contact. *Nerv. Child.,* 2 : 217–250.

—— (1944), Early infantile autism. *J. Pediat.,* 25 : 211–217.

—— (1946), Irrelevant and metaphorical language in early infantile autism. *Amer. J. Psychiat.,* 103 : 242–246.

KAPLAN, S. (1964), A clinical contribution to the study of narcissism in infancy. *The Psychoanalytic Study of the Child,* 19 : 398–415.

KARELITZ, S., KARELITZ, R., & ROSENFELD, L. S. (1960), Infants' vocalizations and their significance. In: *Mental Retardation,* ed. P. W. Bowman & H. V. Mantner. New York: Grune & Stratton, pp. 439–446.

KARLSSON, B. J. (1962), Paper read at 3rd Int. Study Group on Child Neurol., Oxford, England.

KAUFMAN, I. E. & ROSENBLUM, L. S. (1967), The waning of the mother-infant bond in two species of macaque. In: *Determinants of Infant Behaviour,* ed. B. M. Foss. London: Methuen, 4 : 41–60.

KENDON, A. (1967), Some functions of gaze-direction in social interaction. *Acta Psychol.,* 26 : 22–63.

KENT, N. & DAVIS, D. R. (1957), Discipline in the home and intellectual development. *Brit. J. Med. Psychol.,* 30 : 27–33.

KLEITMAN, N. (1939), *Sleep and Wakefulness.* Chicago: Univ. Chicago Press, 1963.

—— & ENGELMANN, T. G. (1953), Sleep characteristics of infants. *J. Appl. Physiol.,* 6 : 269–282.

KNOBLOCH, H., HARPER, P., RIDER, R., & PASAMANICK, B. (1956), The neuropsychiatric sequelae of prematurity. *J. Amer. Med. Assn.,* 161 : 581–585.

KORNER, A. F. (1964), Some hypotheses regarding the significance of individual differences at birth for later development. *The Psychoanalytic Study of the Child,* 19 : 58–72.

—— (1965), Mother-child interaction: one or two-way street? *Soc. Wk,* 10 : 47–51.

—— (1970), Visual alertness in neonates. *Percep. Mot. Skills,* 31 : 499–509.

—— (1971), Individual differences at birth: implications for early experience and later development. *Amer. J. Orthopsychiat.,* 41 : 608–619.

—— (1974), Individual differences at birth: implication for child care practices. In: *The Infant at Risk,* ed. D. Bergsma. New York & London: Intercontinental Medical Book Co., pp. 51–62.

—— & GROBSTEIN, R. (1966), Visual alertness as related to soothing in neonates. *Child Develpm.,* 37 : 867–876.

KRIS, E. (1950a), On preconscious mental processes. *Psychoanal. Quart.,* 19 : 540–560.

———— (1950b), Notes on the development and on some current problems of psychoanalytic child psychology. *The Psychoanalytic Study of the Child,* 5 : 24–46.

———— (1951), Opening remarks on psychoanalytic child psychology. *The Psychoanalytic Study of the Child,* 6 : 9–17.

———— (1962), Decline and recovery in the life of a three-year-old. *The Psychoanalytic Study of the Child,* 17 : 175–215.

KUGEL, R. B. (1970), Combatting retardation in children with Down's syndrome. *Children,* September-October, pp. 180–192.

KUGELBERG, E., EKLUND, K., & GRIMBY, L. (1960), An electromyographic study of the nocieptive reflexes of the lower limb. *Brain,* 83 : 394–410.

LACEY, J. I., BATEMAN, D. E., & VAN LEHN, R. (1953), Automatic response specificity. *Psychosom. Med.,* 15 : 8–21.

LANDRETH, C. (1958), *The Psychology of Early Childhood.* New York: Knopf.

LAURENDEAU, M. & PINARD, A. (1962), *Causal Thinking in the Child.* New York: Int. Univ. Press.

LAWICK-GOODALL, J. VAN (1971), *In the Shadow of Man.* Boston: Houghton Mifflin.

LEVINE, S. (1969), Infantile stimulation. [And] An endocrine theory of infant stimulation. In: *Stimulation in Early Infancy,* ed. A. Ambrose. New York: Academic Press, pp. 3–19, 43–71.

LEVITSKY, D. A. & BARNES, R. H. (1972), Nutritional and environmental interactions in behavioral development of the rat. *Science,* 176 : 68–71.

LEVY, D. M. (1937), Primary affect hunger. *Amer. J. Psychiat.,* 94 : 643–652.

———— (1958), *Behavioral Analysis.* Springfield, Ill.: Thomas.

LEWIN, B. D. (1950), *The Psychoanalysis of Elation.* New York: Norton.

LEWIN, K. (1936), *Principles of Topological Psychology.* New York: McGraw-Hill.

LEWIS, M., KAGAN, J., CAMPBELL, H., & KALAFAT, J. (1966), Cardiac response as a correlate of attention in infants. *Child Develpm.,* 37 : 63–71.

———— & McGURK, H. (1972), Evaluation of infant intelligence. *Science,* 178 : 1174–1177.

LEWIS, O. (1961), *The Children of Sanchez.* New York: Random House.

LINDSLEY, D. (1960), *Handbook of Physiology.* Washington, D.C.: Amer. Physiol. Soc.

LING, D. & LING, A. (1967), Speech and hearing problems in the preschool child. *Proc. Canad. Pub. Hlth Assn. (Saskatchewan) Conf.*

LIPSITT, L. P. (1967), Learning in the human infant. In: *Early Behavior,* ed. H. W. Stevenson, E. H. Hess, & H. L. Rheingold. New York: Wiley, pp. 225–247.

LIPTON, E., STEINSCHNEIDER, A., & RICHMOND, J. B. (1961), Autonomic function in the neonate. *Psychosom. Med.,* 23 : 472–484.

LIVINGSTON, R. B. (1959), Central control of receptors and sensory transmission systems. In: *The Handbook of Physiology: I. Neurology,* ed. J. Field. Baltimore: Waverly Press, pp. 741–760.

LORENZ, K. (1953), *Man Meets Dog.* Baltimore: Penguin Books, 1964.

LOURIE, R. S. (1949), Studies on bed rocking, head banging, and related rhythmic patterns. *Clin. Proc. Child. Hosp.,* 5 : 295–302.

———— (1966), Constitutional factors in the genesis of the neuroses. In: *Psychoneurosis and Schizophrenia,* ed. G. Usdin. Philadelphia: Lippincott, pp. 20–31.

LOVAAS, O. I., BERBERICH, J., PERLOFF, B., & SCHAEFFER, B. (1966), Acquisition of imitative speech by schizophrenic children. *Science,* 151 : 705–707.

LUSTMAN, S. L. (1956), Rudiments of the ego. *The Psychoanalytic Study of the Child,* 11 : 89–98.

LYNN, R. (1966), *Attention, Arousal and the Orientation Reaction.* Oxford, New York: Pergamon Press.

McCARTHY, D. (1960), Language development. *Monogr. Soc. Res. Child Develpm.,* 25, No. 3.

McGRAW, M. B. (1943), *The Neuromuscular Maturation of the Human Infant.* New York: Columbia Univ. Press.

MAHLER, M. S. (1947), Various clinical pictures of psychosis in children. Read at Schilder Soc., New York.

—————— (1952), On child psychosis and schizophrenia. *The Psychoanalytic Study of the Child,* 7 : 286–305.

—————— (1958), Autism and symbiosis, two extreme disturbances of identity. *Int. J. Psycho-Anal.,* 39 : 77–83.

—————— (1963), Thoughts about development and individuation. *The Psychoanalytic Study of the Child,* 18 : 307–324.

—————— (1968), *On Human Symbiosis and the Vicissitudes of Individuation.* New York: Int. Univ. Press.

—————— & ELKISCH, P. (1953), Some observations on disturbances of the ego in a case of infantile psychosis. *The Psychoanalytic Study of the Child,* 8 : 252–261.

—————— & FURER, M. (1960), Observations on research regarding the "symbiotic syndrome" of infantile psychosis. *Psychoanal. Quart.,* 29 : 317–327.

—————— —————— (1963), Certain aspects of the separation-individuation phase. *Psychoanal. Quart.,* 32 : 1–14.

—————— —————— & SETTLAGE, C. F. (1959), Severe emotional disturbances in childhood: psychosis. In: *American Handbook of Psychiatry,* 1 : 816–839. New York: Basic Books.

—————— & GOSLINER, B. (1955), On symbiotic child psychosis. *The Psychoanalytic Study of the Child,* 10 : 195–212.

——————, ROSS, J. R., JR., & DE FRIES, Z. (1949), Clinical studies in benign and malignant cases of childhood psychosis. *Amer. J. Orthopsychiat.,* 19 : 295–304.

MARQUIS, D. P. (1941), Learning in the neonate. *J. Exper. Psychol.,* 29 : 263–282.

MARSCHAK, M. (1960), A method of evaluating child-parent interaction under controlled conditions. *J. Genet. Psychol.,* 97 : 3–22.

—————— & CALL, J. (1965), A comparison of normal and disturbed three-year-old boys in interaction with their parents. *Amer. J. Orthopsychiat.,* 35 : 247–249.

MASON, J. W. (1968), Overall hormonal balance as a key to endocrine organization. *Psychosom. Med.,* 30 : 791–808.

MEDNICK, S. A. (1970), Breakdown in individuals at high risk for schizophrenia. *Ment. Hyg.,* 54 : 50–63.

MENSER, M. A., DODS, L., & HARLEY, J. D. (1967), A twenty-five year follow-up of congenital rubella. *Lancet,* 2 : 1347–1350.

MILLER, G. A., GALANTER, E., & PRIBRAM, K. H. (1960), *Plans and the Structure of Behavior.* New York: Holt.

MOSS, H. A. (1967), Sex, age, and state as determinants of mother-infant interaction. *Merrill-Palmer Quart.,* 13 : 19–36.

—— & ROBSON, K. S. (1967), Maternal influences in early social visual behavior. *Child Develpm.*, 39 : 401–408.

—— —— (1970), The relation between the amount of time infants spend at various states and the development of visual behavior. *Child Develpm.*, 41 : 509–517.

MUNDY, L. (1957), Environmental influence on intellectual function as measured by intelligence tests. *Brit. J. Med. Psychol.*, 30 : 194–201.

MURPHY, L. B. (1968), Assessment of infants and young children. In: *Early Child Care: The New Perspectives*, ed. L. L. Dittmann. New York: Atherton Press, pp. 107–138.

—— (1970), The problem of defense and the concept of coping. In: *The Yearbook for Child Psychiatry and Allied Disciplines*, ed. E. J. Anthony & C. Koupernik. New York: Wiley Interscience, pp. 65–86.

NORRIS, M., SPAULDING, P., & BRODIE, F. (1957), *Blindness in Children*. Chicago: Univ. Chicago Press.

O'CONNOR, N. (1956), The evidence for the permanently disturbing effects of mother-child separation. *Acta Psychol.*, 12 : 174–191.

OGDEN, K. M. & MACKIETH, R. (1955), Good nipples promote successful breast feeding. *J. Pediat.*, 46 : 210–214.

O'GORMAN, G. (1967), *The Nature of Childhood Autism*. New York: Appleton-Century-Crofts.

OMWAKE, E. B. & SOLNIT, A. J. (1961), "It isn't fair." *The Psychoanalytic Study of the Child*, 16 : 352–404.

ORLANSKY, R. (1949), Infant care and personality. *Psychol. Bull.*, 46 : 1–48.

PAINE, R. S. & OPPÉ, T. E. (1966), *Neurological Examination of Children*. London: Heinemann.

—— BRAZELTON, T., DONOVAN, D., DROBAUCH, J., HUBBELL, J., & SEARS, E. (1964), The evolution of postural reflexes in normal infants. *Neurology*, 14 : 1036–1048.

PAPOUSEK, H. (1961), Conditional head rotation reflexes in infants in the first months of life. *Acta Paediat.*, 50 : 565–576.

PARMELEE, A. H. (1961), Sleep patterns of the newborn. *J. Pediat.*, 58 : 241–250.

—— (1973), The ontogeny of sleep patterns and associated periodicities in infants. In: *Prenatal and Postnatal Development of the Human Brain*. Basel: S. Karger.

—— WENNER, W. H. & SCHULTZ, H. (1964), Infant sleep patterns. *J. Pediat.*, 65 : 576–582.

PASAMANICK, B., KNOBLOCH, H., & LILLIENFELD, A. (1956a), Socioeconomic status and some precursors of neuropsychiatric disorder. *Amer. J. Orthopsychiat.*, 26 : 594–601.

—— ROGERS, M., & LILLIENFELD, A. (1956b), Pregnancy experience and the development of behavior disorder in children. *Amer. J. Psychiat.*, 112 : 613–618.

PAVENSTEDT, E. (1961), A study of immature mothers and their children. In: *Prevention of Mental Disorders in Children*, ed. G. Caplan. New York: Basic Books, pp. 192–217.

—— (1963), Description of a research project on the influence of the maternal character structure on the development of the child's personality. Read at 4th Congr. Jap. Assn. Child. Psychiat., Ngoya Univ.

PEIPER, A. (1963), *Cerebral Function in Infancy and Childhood.* New York: Consultants Bureau.

PEIPER, D. (1956), *Die Eigenart der kindlichen Hirntätigkeit.* Leipzig: Thieme.

PIAGET, J. (1936), *The Origins of Intelligence in Children.* New York: Int. Univ. Press, 1952.

—— (1937), *The Construction of Reality in the Child.* New York: Basic Books, 1954.

—— (1945), *Play, Dreams, and Imitation in Childhood.* New York: Norton, 1951.

—— (1952), In: *History of Psychology in Autobiography,* ed. E. Boring. New York: Russell & Russell, pp. 237–256.

—— (1956), Reply to comments concerning the part played by equilibration processes in the psychobiological development of the child. In: *Discussions on Child Development,* ed. J. M. Tanner & B. Inhelder. New York: Int. Univ. Press, 1960, 4 : 77–83.

PINARD, A. & LAURENDEAU, M. (1955), Elaboration d'un examen individual de developpement mental pour les enfants de langue française age 2 à 12 ans (unpublished).

PLUTCHIK, R. & KRONOVET, E. (1959), Studies of parent-child relations. *Genet. Psychol.,* 95 : 171–176.

POTTER, H. H. (1933), Schizophrenia in children. *Amer. J. Psychiat.,* 12 : 1253–1269.

PRECHTL, H. F. R. (1958), The directed head-turning response and allied movements of the human baby. *Behavior,* 13 : 212–242.

—— (1963), The mother-child interaction in babies with minimal brain damage. In: *Determinants of Infant Behavior,* ed. B. M. Foss. New York: Wiley, 2 : 53–66.

—— (1968), Polygraphic studies of the full-term newborn infant II. In: *Studies in Infancy,* ed. M. Bax & R. C. MacKeith. London: Heinemann, pp. 22–40.

—— & BEINTEMA, O. (1964), *The Neurological Examination of the Full-Term Newborn Infant.* London: Heinemann.

—— & DIJKSTRA, J. (1959), Neurological diagnosis of cerebral injury in the newborn. In: *Prenatal Care: Symposium at Groningen and Rotterdam,* ed. B. S. ten Berge. Groningen: P. Noordhoff, 1960, pp. 222–231.

PRINGLE, M. L. K. & BOSSIO, V. (1958), A study of deprived children. *Vita Humana,* 159–170.

—— & TANNER, M. (1958), The effects of early deprivation on speech development. *Language and Speech,* 1 : 269–287.

PROVENCE, S. A. & LIPTON, R. C. (1962), *Infants in Institutions.* New York: Int. Univ. Press.

PUTNAM, M. C. (1955), Some observations on psychoses in early childhood. In: *Emotional Problems of Early Childhood,* ed. G. Caplan. New York: Basic Books, pp. 519–524.

RABIN, A. I. (1958), Infants and children under conditions of "intermittent" mothering in the kibbutz. *Amer. J. Orthopsychiat.,* 28 : 577–586.

RADEMACHER, G. G. J. (1931), *Das Stehen.* Berlin: Springer.

RANGELL, L. (1954), On the psychology of poise. *Int. J. Psycho-Anal.,* 35 : 313–332.

RANK, B. (1949), Adaption of psychoanalytic technique for the treatment of young children with atypical development. *Amer. J. Orthopsychiat.*, 19 : 130–139.

RAPAPORT, D. (1951), The autonomy of the ego. In: *Psychoanalytic Psychiatry and Psychology*, 1 : 248–258. New York: Int. Univ. Press, 1954.

—— (1960a), *The Structure of Psychoanalytic Theory* [*Psychol. Issues*, Monogr. 6]. New York: Int. Univ. Press.

—— (1960b), On the psychoanalytic theory of motivation. In: *Nebraska Symposium on Motivation*, ed. M. R. Jones. Lincoln: Univ. Nebraska Press, pp. 173–247.

RHEINGOLD, H. L. (1956), The modification of social responsiveness in institutional babies. *Monogr. Soc. Res. Child Develpm.*, 21, No. 2.

—— (1960), The measurement of maternal care. *Child Develpm.*, 31 : 565–575.

—— (1961), The effect of environmental stimulation upon social and exploratory behaviour in the human infant. In: *Determinants of Infant Behaviour*, ed. B. M. Foss. London: Methuen, 1 : 143–171.

—— & BAYLEY, N. (1959), The later effects of an experimental modification of mothering. *Child Develpm.*, 31 : 363–372.

RIBBLE, M. A. (1943), *The Rights of Infants.* New York: Columbia Univ. Press.

RICHMOND, J. B. (1962), Some direct observations of disordered behavior in infants. Abstr. in: *J. Amer. Psychoanal. Assn.*, 10 : 571–578.

—— (1965), Spasmus nutans. *J. Amer. Med. Assn.*, 192 : 1117–1120.

—— & LIPTON, E. L. (1959), Some aspects of the neurophysiology of the newborn and their implications for child development. In: *Dynamic Psychopathology of Childhood*, ed. L. Jessner & E. Pavenstedt. New York: Grune & Stratton, pp. 78–105.

—— —— & STEINSCHNEIDER, A. (1962), Observations on differences in autonomic nervous system function between and within individuals during early infancy. *J. Amer. Acad. Child Psychiat.*, 1 : 83–91.

—— & LUSTMAN, S. L. (1955), Autonomic function in the neonate. *Psychosom. Med.*, 17 : 269–275.

RICHTER, D. (1957), Biochemical aspects of schizophrenia. In: *Schizophrenia: Somatic Aspects*, ed. D. Richter. New York: Macmillan, pp. 53–75.

RIESSEN, A. H. (1950), *Arrested Vision in Frontiers of Psychological Research.* San Francisco, London: Freeman.

RIMLAND, B. (1964), *Infantile Autism.* New York: Appleton-Century-Crofts.

RITVO, S. & PROVENCE, S. A. (1953), Form perception and imitation in some autistic children. *The Psychoanalytic Study of the Child*, 8 : 155–161.

ROBSON, K. S. (1967), The role of eye-to-eye contact in maternal-infant attachment. *J. Child Psychol. Psychiat.*, 8 : 13–25.

ROFFWARG, H. P., MUZIO, J. N., & DEMENT, W. C. (1966), Ontogenetic development of the human sleep-dream cycle. *Science*, 152 : 604–619.

ROGERS, M., LILLIENFELD, A., & PASAMANICK, B. (1955), Prenatal and paranatal factors in the development of childhood behavior disorders. *Johns Hopkins Univ. School of Hyg. Pub. Hlth Bull.*

ROIPHE, H. (1968), On an early genital phase. *The Psychoanalytic Study of the Child*, 23 : 348–365.

—— & GALENSON, E. (1972), Early genital activity and the castration complex. *Psychoanal. Quart.*, 41 : 334–347.

RORKE, L. B. & SPIRO, A. J. (1967), Cerebral lesions in congenital rubella syndrome. *J. Pediat.,* 70 : 243–255.

ROSENTHAL, D. (1971), A program of research on heredity in schizophrenia. *Behav. Sci.,* 16 : 191–201.

RUDEN, J. VON (1965), The relationship between acceptance by the nurse of the method of feeding and alleviation of guilt feelings in the mother. Thesis for Master of Science in Nursing, Univ. Calif., Los Angeles.

RUESCH, H. (1956), *Nonverbal Communication.* Berkeley: Univ. California Press.

RUTTER, M. (1965), The influence of organic and emotional factors in the origins, nature and outcome of childhood psychosis. *Develpm. Med. Child Neurol.,* 7 : 518–528.

—— (1968), Concepts of autism. *J. Child Psychol. Psychiat.,* 9 : 1–25.

SAINTE-ANNE DARGASSIES, S. (1955), La maturation neurologique du prematuré. *Études Neonatales,* 4 : 2–13.

SAMEROFF, A. J. (1971), Can conditional responses be established in the newborn infant? *Develpm. Psychol.,* 5 : 1–13.

SAMLIS, H. V. (1968), Aging: the loss of temporal organization. *Perspec. Biol. Med.,* 12 : 95–102.

SAMPSON, O. C. (1945), A study of speech development in children of 18–30 months. *Brit. J. Educ. Psychol.,* 20 : 144–201.

SANDER, L. W. (1969), The longitudinal course of early mother-child interaction. In: *Determinants of Infant Behaviour,* ed. B. M. Foss. London: Methuen, 4 : 189–227.

—— (1973), Twenty-four hour distributions of sleeping and waking over the first month of life in different infant caretaking systems. Soc. Res. Child Develpm. Biennial Meeting.

—— & JULIA, H. L. (1966), Continuous interactional monitoring in the neonate. *Psychosom. Med.,* 28 : 822–835.

—— —— STECHLER, G., & BURNS, P. (1969), Regulation and organization in the early infant-caretaker system. In: *Brain and Early Behaviour,* ed. R. Robinson. London: Academic Press, pp. 311–333.

—— —— —— —— (1972), Continuous 24-hour interactional monitoring in infants reared in two caretaking environments. *Psychosom. Med.,* 34 : 270–282.

—— STECHLER, G., BURNS, P., & JULIA, H. (1970), Early mother-infant interaction and 24-hour patterns of activity and sleep. *J. Amer. Acad. Child Psychiat.,* 9 : 103–123.

SCHACHTEL, E. G. (1954), The development of focal attention and the emergence of reality. *Psychiatry,* 17 : 309–324.

SCHAEFER E. S. (1959), A circumplex model for maternal behavior. *J. Abnorm. Psychol.,* 59 : 226–235.

—— & BELL, R. Q. (1958), Development of a parental attitude research instrument. *Child Develpm.,* 29 : 339–361.

—— —— & BAYLEY, N. (1959), Development of a maternal behavior research instrument. *J. Genet. Psychol.,* 95 : 83–104.

SCHAFFER, A. J. (1960), *Diseases of the Newborn.* Philadelphia: Saunders, p. 628.

SCHAFFER, H. R. (1966), Activity level as a constitutional determinant of infantile reaction to deprivation. *Child Develpm.,* 37 : 595–602.

———— & CALLENDER, W. M. (1959), Psychologic effects of hospitalization in infancy. *Pediatrics,* 24 : 528–539.

———— & EMERSON, P. E. (1964a), Patterns of response to physical contact in early human development. *J. Child Psychol. Psychiat.,* 5 : 1–13.

———— ———— (1964b), The development of social attachments in infancy. *Monogr. Soc. Res. Child Develpm.,* 29 : 1–77, Serial #94.

SCHECHTER, M. D., SHURLEY, J. T., SEXAUER, J. D., & TOUSSIENG, P. W. (1969), Perceptual isolation therapy. *J. Amer. Acad. Child Psychiat.,* 8 : 97–139.

SCHEFLEN, A. E. (1965), Quasi-courtship behavior in psychotherapy. *Psychiatry,* 28 : 245–257.

SHAPIRO, T. & FISH, B., (1969), A method to study language deviation as an aspect of ego organization in young schizophrenic children. *J. Amer. Acad. Child Psychiat.,* 8 : 36–56.

———— ———— & GINSBERG, G. (1971), The speech of a schizophrenic child from 2–6. *Amer. J. Psychiat.,* 128 : 1408–1413.

———— ROBERTS, A., & FISH, B. (1970), Imitation and echoing in young schizophrenic children. *J. Amer. Acad. Child Psychiat.,* 9 : 548–567.

SHEIBEL, A. B. (1962), Neural correlates of psychological developments in the young organism. In: *Recent Advances in Biological Psychiatry,* ed. J. Wortis. New York: Plenum Press, 4 : 313–328.

SHIRLEY, M. M. (1933), *The First Two Years.* Minneapolis: Univ. Minnesota Press.

SIMSARIAN, F. P. & McLENDON, P. (1942), Feeding behavior of an infant during the first 12 weeks of life on a self-demand schedule. *J. Pediat.,* 20 : 93–109.

SINGER, D. B., RUDOLPH, A. J., ROSENBERG, H. S., RAWLS, W. E., & BONIUK, M. (1967), Pathology of the congenital rubella syndrome. *J. Pediat.,* 71 : 665–675.

SKEELS, H. M. (1966), Adult status of children with contrasting life experiences. *Monogr. Soc. Res. Child Develpm.,* Vol. 31, No. 3.

SKODAK, M. & SKEELS, H. M. (1949), A final follow-up study of one hundred adopted children. *J. Genet. Psychol.,* 75 : 85–125.

SLOAN, E. (1955), The Lincoln-Oseretsky scale of motor development. *Genet. Psychol. Monogr.,* 51 : 183–252.

SMITH, M. A., CHETHIK, M., & ADELSON, E. (1969), Differential assessments of "blindisms." *Amer. J. Orthopsychiat.,* 39 : 807–817.

SONTAG, L. W. (1940), Effect of fetal activity on the nutritional state of the infant at birth. *Amer. J. Dis. Child.,* 60 : 621–630.

———— (1941), Significance of fetal environmental differences. *Amer. J. Obstet. Gynecol.,* 42 : 996–1003.

———— BAKER, C. T., & NELSON, V. (1958), Mental growth and personality development. *Monogr. Soc. Res. Child Develpm.,* 23(2) : 1–143.

SPITZ, R. A. (1945a), Diacritic and coenesthetic organizations. *Psychoanal. Rev.,* 32 : 146–162.

———— (1945b), Hospitalism. *The Psychoanalytic Study of the Child,* 1 : 53–74.

———— (1946), Hospitalism: a follow-up. *The Psychoanalytic Study of the Child,* 2 : 113–117.

———— (1950), Anxiety in infancy. *Int. J. Psycho-Anal.,* 31 : 138–143.

—— (1954), Genèse des premières relations objectales. *Rev. Franç. Psychoanal.*, 38.

—— (1956), *Die Entstehung der ersten Objektbeziehungen.* Stuttgart: Klett.

—— (1957), *No and Yes.* New York: Int. Univ. Press.

—— (1959), *A Genetic Field Theory of Ego Formation.* New York: Int. Univ. Press.

—— (1963), Life and the dialogue. In: *Counterpoint: Libidinal Object and Subject,* ed. H. S. Gaskill. New York: Int. Univ. Press, pp. 154–176.

—— (1965), *The First Year of Life.* New York: Int. Univ. Press.

—— & WOLF, K. M. (1946), The smiling response. *Genet. Psychol. Monogr.*, 34 : 57–125.

STARR, P. (1954), Psychoses in children. *Psychoanal. Quart.*, 23 : 544–565.

STECHLER, G. S. (1973), Infant looking and fussing in response to visual stimulation over the first two months of life in different infant-caretaking systems. Read at Soc. Res. Child Develpm., Biennial Meeting.

—— BRADFORD, S., & LEVY, H. (1966), Attention in the newborn. *Science,* 151 : 1246–1248.

—— & CARPENTER, G. (1967), A viewpoint on early affective development. In: *The Exceptional Infant,* ed. J. Hellmuth. New York: Brunner/Mazel, 1 : 163–189.

—— & LATZ, E. (1966), Some observations on attention and arousal in the human infant. *J. Amer. Acad. Child Psychiat.*, 5 : 517–525.

STERN, D. N. (1974a), Mother and infant at play. In: *The Effect of the Infant on Its Caregiver,* ed. M. Lewis & L. Rosenblum. New York: Wiley, pp. 187–213.

—— (1974b), The goal and structure of mother-infant play. *J. Amer. Acad. Child Psychiat.*, 13 : 402–421.

—— (1975), And the beat goes on. Presented at the Loch Lomond Symposium, Scotland.

—— JAFFE, J., BEEBE, B., & BENNETT, S. (1975), Vocalizing in unison and in alternation. Trans. N.Y. Acad. Sci., Conf. on Developmental Psycholinguistics and Communication Disorders.

STERN, E., PARMELEE, A. H., & HARRIS, M. A. (1973), Sleep state periodicity in prematures and young infants. *Develpm. Psychobiol.*, 6 : 357–365.

STIRNIMANN, F. (1944), Über das Farbempfinden Neugeborener. *Ann. Pediat.*, 163 : 1–11.

STONE, A. A. & ONQUÉ, G. E. C. (1959), *Longitudinal Studies of Child Personality.* Cambridge, Mass.: Harvard Univ. Press.

STROEBEL, C. F. (1969), Biologic rhythm correlates of disturbed behavior. In: *Circadian Rhythms in Non-Human Primates,* ed. F. H. Rohles. Basel & New York: S. Karger, pp. 9–105.

THOMAS, A., CHESS, S., BIRCH, H. G., HERTZIG, M. E., KORN, S. (1963), *Behavioral Individuality in Early Childhood.* New York: New York Univ. Press.

THOMAS, ANDRÉ & SAINTE-ANNE DARGASSIES, S. (1952), *Etudes neurologiques sur le nouveau-né et le jeune nourrisson.* Paris: Masson.

THOMPSON, W. R. (1955), Early environment. In: *Psychopathology of Childhood,* ed. P. H. Hoch & J. Zubin. New York: Grune & Stratton, pp. 120–139.

—— (1960), Early environmental influences on behavioral development (unpublished research report, Wesleyan Univ.).

TINBERGEN, N. (1951), *The Study of Instinct.* Oxford: Clarendon Press.

TORS, I. (1971), The social life of the African elephant. Personal communication.

TSUMORI, M. & INAGE, N. (1958), Maternal attitude and its relationship to infant development. *Jap. J. Educ. Psychol.,* 5 : 208–218.

VICTORIA, V. (1964), Spasmus nutans. *Arch. Oftal. B. Air.,* 38 : 280–285.

WALTON, J. (1957), The limp child. *J. Neurol., Neurosurg. Psychiat.,* 20 : 144–154.

WARD, T. F. & HODDINUTT, B. A. (1968), The development of speech in an autistic child. *Acta Paedopsychiat.,* 35 : 199–215.

WEBER, M. (1921), *The Theory of Social and Economic Organization,* tr. T. Parsons. New York: Oxford Univ. Press, 1947.

WECHSLER, D. (1949), *The Wechsler Intelligence Scale for Children.* New York: Psychol. Corp.

WEECH, A. & CAMPBELL, R. (1941), The relation between the development of behavior and the pattern of physical growth. *Child Develpm.,* 12 : 237–240.

WEILAND, H. & LEGG, D. R. (1964), Formal speech characteristics as a diagnostic aid in childhood psychosis. *Amer. J. Orthopsychiat.,* 34 : 91–94.

WEISS, P. (1949), The biological basis of adaptation. In: *Adaptation,* ed. J. Romano. Ithaca, N.Y.: Cornell Univ. Press, pp. 3–22.

——— (1970), Whither life science? *Amer. Scientist,* 58 : 156–163.

WELLER, G. M. (1965), Arousal effects on the newborn infant of being first or later born. Read at Amer. Orthopsychiat. Assn., 42nd Annual Meeting, New York City.

——— & BELL, R. Q. (1965), Basal skin conductance and neonatal state. *Child Develpm.,* 36 : 647–657.

WENAR, C. (1963), The reliability of developmental histories. *Psychosom. Med.,* 25 : 505–509.

——— & WENAR, S. C. (1963), The short-term prospective model, the illusion of time and the tabula rasa child. *Child Develpm.,* 34 : 697–708.

WERNER, H. (1948), *Comparative Psychology of Mental Development.* New York: Int. Univ. Press, 1957.

——— & CRAIN, L. (1950), Marbleboard test performance in normal children. *J. Genet. Psychol.,* 77 : 217–229.

——— & WAPNER, S. (1955), Developmental study on the perception of verticality. Read at Eastern Psychol. Assn. Meetings, Philadelphia, Pa.

WEVER, R. (1970), Zur Zeitgeber-Stärke eines Licht-Dunkel-Wechsels für die circadiane Periodik des Menschen. *Pflügers Arch.,* 321 : 133–142.

WHITE, B. L. & CASTLE, P. W. (1964), Visual exploratory behavior following postnatal handling of human infants. *Percept. Mot. Skills,* 18 : 497–502.

——— ——— & HELD, R. (1964), Observations on the development of visually directed reaching. *Child Develpm.,* 35 : 349–364.

WHITE, R. W. (1960), Competence and the psychosexual stages of development. In: *Nebraska Symposium on Motivation,* ed. M. R. Jones. Lincoln: Univ. Nebraska Press, pp. 97–140.

WILLIAMS, J. R. & SCOTT, R. B. (1953), Growth and development of Negro infants. *Child Develpm.,* 24 : 103–121.

WINNICOTT, D. W. (1953), Transitional objects and transitional phenomena. *Int. J. Psycho-Anal.,* 34 : 89–97.

—— (1958), *Collected Papers.* New York: Basic Books.

—— (1960), The theory of the parent-infant relationship. *Int. J. Psycho-Anal.,* 41 : 585–595.

WOLF, K. M. (1953), Observations of individual tendencies in the first year of life. In: *Problems of Infancy and Childhood,* ed. M. J. E. Senn. New York: Josiah Macy, Jr. Foundation, pp. 97–137.

—— (1954), Observation of individual tendencies in the second year of life. In: *Problems of Infancy and Childhood,* ed. M. J. E. Senn. New York: Josiah Macy, Jr. Foundation, pp. 121–140.

WOLFF, P. H. (1959), Observations on newborn infants. *Psychosom. Med.,* 21 : 110–118.

—— (1963a), Observations on the early development of smiling. In: *Determinants of Infant Behavior,* ed. B. M. Foss. New York: Wiley, 2 : 113–138.

—— (1936b), The natural history of a family. In: *Determinants of Infant Behaviour,* ed. B. M. Foss. London: Methuen, 2 : 139–167.

—— (1965), The development of attention in young infants. *Ann. N.Y. Acad. Sci.,* 118 : 815–830.

—— (1966), *The Causes, Controls, and Organization of Behavior in the Neonate* [*Psychol. Issues,* Monogr. 17]. New York: Int. Univ. Press.

—— (1968), The role of biological rhythms in early psychological development. In: *Annual Progress in Child Psychiatry and Child Development,* ed. S. Chess & A. Thomas. New York: Brunner/Mazel, pp. 1–22.

—— (1969), What we must and must not teach our young children from what we know about early cognitive development. In: *Planning for Better Learning,* ed. P. H. Wolff & R. MacKeith. London: Heinemann, pp. 7–19.

—— & FEINBLOOM, R. I. (1969), Critical periods and cognitive development in the first 2 years. *Pediatrics,* 44 : 999–1006.

WOLFF, S. & CHESS, S. (1965), An analysis of the language of fourteen schizophrenic children. *J. Child Psychol. Psychiat.,* 6 : 29–41.

YAMAMOTO, W. S. & BROBECK, J. R., ed. (1965), *Physiological Controls and Regulations.* Philadelphia: Saunders.

YARROW, L. J. (1961), Maternal deprivation. *Psychol. Bull.,* 58 : 459–490.

—— & GOODWIN, M. A. (1965), Some conceptual issues in the study of mother-infant interaction. *Amer. J. Orthopsychiat.,* 35 : 473–481.

ZAZZO, R. (1953), Stages of psychological development of the child. In: *Discussions on Child Development,* ed. J. M. Tanner & B. Inhelder. New York: Int. Univ. Press, 1 : 161–181.

INDEX